Recent Results in Cancer Research

115

Recent Results in Cancer Research

H.-J. Senn A. Goldhirsch
R. D. Gelber B. Osterwalder (Eds.)

Adjuvant Therapy
of Primary Breast Cancer

With 65 Figures and 94 Tables

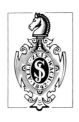

Springer-Verlag
Berlin Heidelberg New York
London Paris Tokyo

Professor Dr. Hans-Jörg Senn
Medizinische Klinik C, Kantonsspital
9007 St. Gallen, Switzerland

Priv.-Doz. Dr. Aron Goldhirsch
Servizio Oncologico Cantonale, Ospedale Civico
6900 Lugano, Switzerland

Dr. Richard D. Gelber
Division of Biostatistics and Epidemiology
Dana-Farber Cancer Institute
44 Binney Street, Boston, MA 02115, USA

Dr. Bruno Osterwalder
Abteilung für Hämatologie und Onkologie
Medizinische Klinik C, Kantonsspital
9007 St. Gallen, Switzerland

ISBN 3-540-18810-X Springer-Verlag Berlin Heidelberg New York
ISBN 0-387-18810-X Springer-Verlag New York Berlin Heidelberg

Library of Congress Cataloging-in-Publication Data
Adjuvant therapy of primary breast cancer/H.-J.Senn ... [et al.] (eds.)
p. cm. – (Recent results in cancer research; 115) Based on international conference
held in 1988. Includes index.
ISBN 0-387-18810-X (U.S.: alk. paper)
1. Breast – Cancer – Adjuvant treatment – Congresses. I. Senn, Hansjörg. II. Series.
[DNLM: 1. Adjuvants, Pharmaceutic – therapeutic use – congresses. 2. Breast Neoplasms –
drug therapy – congresses. W1 RE106P v. 115/WP 870 A2356] RC261.R35
vol. 115 [RC280.B8] 616.99'4 s-dc20 [616.99'44906] DNLM/DLC 89-11304

© Springer-Verlag Berlin Heidelberg 1989
Printed in Germany

The use of registered names, trademarks, etc. in this publication does not imply, even in the
absence of a specific statement, that such names are exempt from the relevant protective
laws and regulations and therefore free for general use.

Product Liability: The publisher can give no guarantee for information about drug dosage
and application thereof contained in the book. In every individual case the respective user
must check its accuracy by consulting other pharmaceutical literature.

Typesetting, printing, and binding: Appl, Wemding
2125/3140-543210 – Printed on acid-free paper.

Preface

The ultimate "consumer" of the data presented at conferences on the primary treatment of operable breast cancer is the patient, and when, as in this disease, the benefits of therapy are relatively modest, the availability and interpretation of the data from trials becomes an issue of primary importance. The effects of present treatment are in fact such that more patients relapse despite therapy than are estimated to benefit from it. It is, therefore, extremely difficult for the physician to recommend unequivocally one particular adjuvant treatment modality for the vast population of women with breast cancer.

The interpretation of results from clinical research-oriented programs is constantly applied, however, in the treatment of breast cancer patients *outside* of clinical trials. From presented or published data, many physicians extrapolate indications for the use of a given treatment regimen for their patients, perceiving it as the "best available therapy." It is essential that the "best available therapy" be selected individually for each patient. However, considering the modest effect of treatment upon outcome, it is imperative that those who provide the data – those who are involved in both patient care and clinical research – make it known that the best current treatment for the population of breast cancer patients is available *within the framework of clinical trials.* In this way not only present-day patients but also future ones will derive the greatest benefit.

The formats of most of the conferences on adjuvant treatment provide data and discussions which indicate specific patient care recommendations and at the same time provide new impetus for clinically oriented research. We have also attempted to highlight the fact that for this disease the "best therapy available" to the patient and her physician is to be sought in clinical research itself. Many of the issues influencing the choice of treatment remain obscure and sometimes ambiguous, and additional small but important steps toward defining more effective therapy for this disease may yet be achieved, provided that participation in clinical research meets with more widespread acceptance. The effort made at the conference to cover research- and patient-oriented issues related to adjuvant therapy in breast cancer resulted in the recognition that much remains to be understood, defined, and accomplished. The discussions of biological mechanisms and models of new approaches to adjuvant therapy in breast cancer disclosed a wide range of issues which await interpretation and results. Ongoing investigations of relative and absolute resistance to adjuvant systemic treatment and the correlation between growth factors, their receptors, and the prognosis of the patient are expected to provide further data in the near future. The results of postoperative adjuvant therapy could perhaps be substantially improved by the addition of preoperative systemic treatment. The investigation of the problems involved in controlling metastatic disease and questions about the local control of breast cancer by means of primary systemic treatment are also interesting research projects for the coming years.

The treatment of pre- and postmenopausal patients with primary breast cancer and of relapse in those who have already received adjuvant systemic therapy were the topics of most of the sessions concerned with direct patient care. The long-term advantage of adjuvant systemic chemotherapy for young women and the significant effects of endocrine systemic therapy for postmenopausal patients are representative of present achievements. Salvage therapy programs demonstrate that many patients do respond to the same treatment they received in the adjuvant setting, suggesting that the apparent resistance to adjuvant therapy may be due to a relatively resistant condition which is partially reversed at the time of proliferating metastatic disease.

More and more investigations are demonstrating that there is no qualitative difference between the responses of node-positive and node-negative cancers to adjuvant systemic therapy and that the definition of the relative magnitudes of the effect of treatment is the real problem in the choice of the treatment program for the individual patient, especially if the risk of relapse is difficult to estimate. Breast-conserving surgery has become more feasible in the treatment of women with breast cancer. Guidelines for the selection of suitable patients for breast-conserving procedures and of the appropriate sequence of the chosen treatment modalities have also to be established by future investigations. New methodologies to aid physicians and patients in the decision-making process are represented by meta-analysis and by quality-of-life-oriented research. The early detection of survival differences which can be achieved by pooling results from several trials, as well as the inclusion of additional factors such as measurements of patient well-being, suggest other stimulating possibilities for future research.

The fourth conference on the multimodal treatment of early breast cancer, scheduled for 4 years hence (February 1992), will no doubt raise still more questions and issues in this field. We hope that the data provided by the third international conference will serve to advance clinical research also among those more accustomed to making therapeutic decisions based on data rather than on actual involvement in the conduct of clinical trials.

May 1989   The Editors

Contents

List of Contributors*

Abel, U. *118, 163*
Amalric, R. *77*
Andrykowski, M. A. *272*
Assche van, C. *180*
Auclerc, G. *36*
Auclerc, M.-F. *36*
Ayme, Y. *77*
Baillet, F. *36*
Baird, R. *28*
Basco, V. *28*
Baum, M. *54, 136*
Bernhard, J. *255*
Blijham, G. *180*
Bonadonna, G. *69, 113, 175*
Boyages, J. *92*
Brambilla, C. *69, 113*
Brandone, H. *77*
Bressac, C. *77*
Brunner, K. W. *239*
Clark, G. M. *170*
Coldman, A. *28*
Connolly, J. *92*
Cuzick, J. *220*
Dittrich, D. *180*
Dunst, J. *203*
Ebbs, S. R. *136*
Frei, E. III *25*
Ganz, P. A. *244*

Gelber, R. D. *43, 153, 211, 236*
Glick, J. H. *283*
Goldhirsch, A. *43, 153, 211*
Goldie, J. H. *8, 28*
Hans, D. *77*
Harris, J. R. *92*
Heinrich, R. L. *244*
Hern, R. A. *54*
Høst, H. *186*
Houghton, J. *54*
Hryniuk, W. M. *17*
Hünig, R. *62*
Hürny, C. *255, 279*
Jacobsen, P. B. *272*
Jacquillat, C. *36*
Jakesz, R. *180*
Jonat, W. *118, 163*
Jungi, W. F. *83*
Kaufmann, M. *118, 163*
Khayat, D. *36*
Kjellgren, K. *186*
Kurtz, J. M. *62, 77*
McGuire, W. L. *170*
Mouridsen, H. T. *132, 144*
Nissen-Meyer, R. *54, 186*
Polinsky, M. *244*
Ragaz, J. *28*
Rainer, H. *180*

---

* The address of the principal author is given on the first page of each contribution.
¹ Page on which contribution begins.

Rauschecker, H. F. *203*
Rebbeck, P. *28*
Recht, A. *92*
Redd, W. H. *272*
Reiner, A. *180*
Reiner, G. *180*
Reynders, M. *180*
Riley, D. *54*
Rose, M. A. *92*
Sauer, R. *203*
Schag, C. A. C. *244*
Schauer, A. *203*
Schemper, M. *180*
Scheurlen, H. *226*
Schmid, L. *83*
Schnitt, S. *92*

Schumacher, M. *203*
Schutte, B. *180*
Senn, H.-J. *83*
Silver, B. *92*
Spitalier, J.-M. *77*
Spona, J. *180*
Stewart, H. J. *126*
Streit, A. I. *83*
Tattersall, M. H. N. *1*
Tormey, D. C. *103, 106*
Valagussa, P. *69, 113, 175*
Veronesi, U. *197*
Waldhör, T. *180*
Wallgren, A. *191*
Weil, M. *36*
Zambetti, M. *69, 113, 175*

Biological Mechanisms and Models for New Approaches to Adjuvant Therapy of Breast Cancer

Patterns of Treatment Failure – Implications for New Treatment Approaches

M. H. N. Tattersall

Department of Cancer Medicine, University of Sydney, New South Wates 2006, Australia

Introduction

A rational strategy for improving current adjuvant breast cancer treatment should be built on knowledge of the reasons for failure of the treatment currently utilised. Unfortunately, there are remarkably few data reported which identify why an adjuvant systemic treatment has failed. Most studies of adjuvant systemic treatment have found that the probability of relapse is strongly influenced by the extent of the tumour (tumour size, number of axillary lymph nodes containing metastases, etc.) before local treatment, and this has inevitably led to the assumption that treatment failure is due to the outgrowth of a tumour which is refractory to the administered adjuvant treatment. Recent evidence that relapsed tumours commonly respond to retreatment with the 'failed' adjuvant treatment (Valagussa et al. 1986; Muss et al. 1987) has led to studies of cell-kinetic modulation during adjuvant treatment (Davidson and Lippman 1987) and to reintroduction programmes. The results of these treatment programmes are not yet available.

Few studies have compared the biological or genetic characteristics of primary tumours with that of their recurrences, but this information is required before major new initiatives in adjuvant treatment can be launched. Recent reports indicate that the growth fraction of primary breast tumours may be an important prognostic factor, particularly in patients with node-negative disease (Meyer et al. 1983; Silvestrini et al. 1985; Tubiana and Koscielny 1988), and new technologies for measuring this parameter may assist in obtaining confirmatory data. While the growth fraction in a tumour at the time of relapse tends to be greater than that observed in the primary tumour (Tubiana 1982), the observation that the oestrogen- and progesterone-receptor content in a primary tumour has predictive power for endocrine response probability of metastatic disease argues for some tumour-cell homogeneity, at least in the absence of treatment, for metastatic tumours. On the other hand, with multiple systemic treatments, a number of reports indicate that the content of oestrogen or progesterone receptor in the tumour usually falls with time, an observation consistent not only with the notion of tumour dedifferentiation, but also an effect of treatment selection.

Recent Results in Cancer Research, Vol. 115
© Springer-Verlag Berlin · Heidelberg 1989

Elsewhere in this volume, molecular genetic information derived from primary and metastatic breast tumours is presented. There is a clear need for more detailed information about the prognostic importance of various genetic and phenotypic tumour characteristics in untreated patients and in those who have received adjuvant systemic treatments. These data may identify patients best treated with particular therapies.

In advanced breast cancer, there is a similar lack of detailed information about the characteristics of relapsed disease compared with the sites and biology of disease recognised prior to treatment. This information, which is potentially readily available in comparison with the adjuvant data, may provide new clues to improving adjuvant treatments.

We have analysed the patterns of disease progression in 267 patients with advanced breast cancer receiving systemic therapy (Harnett et al. 1987). Initial disease progression during therapy most commonly occurred in tissue involved by tumour at the commencement of treatment. However in 40% of patients, the first documentation of disease progression included a tissue not previously known to contain metastatic disease. This pattern of disease progression was not influenced by treatment type (i. e. endocrine or cytotoxic), tumour response to treatment, oestrogen-receptor status, prior adjuvant cytotoxic treatment or disease-free interval.

Materials and Methods

The clinical trial records of 408 patients with advanced breast cancer were examined retrospectively (Australian and New Zealand Breast Cancer Trials Group, Harnett 1987). All patients had been entered on two randomised prospective multicentre clinical trials conducted by the Australian and New Zealand Breast Cancer Trials Group of the Clinical Oncological Society of Australia. It was an eligibility requirement for these trials that patients had received no previous systemic therapy for metastatic disease and that all sites of metastatic disease were documented before commencement of treatment. These sites of disease were detected in all cases by clinical assessment and chest X-ray, and in the majority of patients, radionuclide bone scans were also performed. When additional metastatic sites were suspected, further investigations to document the extent of the disease were also performed.

The treatment regimens used in the two trials from which the patient cohorts were drawn are shown in Table 1. Individual tumour responses on therapy were categorised according to WHO criteria, and all sites of treatment failure were recorded at the time when failure was first detected. The major end points of this analysis were the identification of the tissue, e. g. bone, liver, etc., in which disease progression was first apparent and its relationship to tissues which were involved when systemic therapy had been commenced. In addition, the influence on the patterns of treatment failure of the systemic treatment type (endocrine or cytotoxic), the tumour response on systemic treatment, and the time to disease progression and prior adjuvant therapy were investigated.

Table 1. Drug regimens used

Adriamycin		50 mg/m² day 1 ⎫	repeat at 21
Cyclophosphamide		750 mg/m² day 1 ⎭	day cycles (AC)
		or	
Endocrine	Tamoxifen	20 mg daily (postmenopausal)	
	Oophorectomy (premenopausal)		
		or	
Cytotoxic + endocrine			

Results

Of the 408 entered on the two trials, 141 were not evaluable for this analysis. Of these patients, 20 were ineligible for the protocol on which they were entered, 11 have not yet relapsed, 19 died without assessment of disease status, and 89 withdrew from trial treatment because of drug intolerance or other causes before treatment failure. In two cases, trial records were incomplete. In the remaining 267 patients, it was possible to determine whether the first disease progression on randomised treatment occurred in a tissue which was known to be involved by the tumour at the commencement of therapy (i.e. an 'old' tissue), in a previously uninvolved tissue (i.e. a 'new' tissue), or both old and new tissues simultaneously. Table 2 shows that the first incident of disease progression most commonly occurred in tissues involved by tumour at the commencement of therapy. However in 40% of patients, disease progression included a tissue not previously known to contain metastatic disease and in only seven patients (i.e. 3%) was this new tissue the central nervous system. Altogether, in 15% of patients, relapse was first documented only in a new tissue, with previously known disease sites still being controlled. Table 3 presents the pattern of disease progression according to the involved tissue at the time of commencing systemic therapy. Regardless of the tissue involved before systemic therapy, new sites of metastases were identified at the time of treatment failure in one-third to one-half of patients.

Table 4 shows the tissue in which treatment failure was first documented according to the type of systemic therapy which had been given. The tissue pattern of treatment failure did not vary according to the type of treatment or its outcome, nor did oestrogen-receptor status influence the pattern of failure. The tissues' patterns of treatment failure were not detectably influenced by the prior administration of adjuvant cytotoxic therapy. The survival from the time of beginning systemic therapy for advanced disease is also shown in Table 5. Overall, the same pattern of treatment failure was observed in patients with widely differing survival duration.

Broadly similar conclusions about the patterns of treatment failure in advanced breast cancer can be drawn from the report of Fey et al. (1981). However, they observed that patients with bone, liver and brain metastases at the time of commencing systemic therapy were particularly likely to show progression in those sites.

Table 2. Patterns of disease progression in advanced breast cancer

Patient group	(n)	Tissue at first progression					
		Old		New[a]		Old and new	
		n	(%)	n	(%)	n	(%)
Total	267	160	60	39	15	68	25

[a] Seven cases relapsed within central nervous system.

Table 3. Patterns of disease progression in advanced breast cancer

Tissue involved	Total (n)	Tissue at first progression					
		Old		New		Old and new	
		(n)	(%)	(n)	(%)	(n)	(%)
Skin	57	34	60	5	9	18	31
Lymph node	104	57	55	17	16	30	29
Bone	175	117	67	17	10	41	23
Lung	86	54	63	14	16	18	21
Liver	69	43	62	7	10	19	28
Ipsilateral breast	38	20	53	4	11	14	36
Central nervous system	16	9	56	6	38	1	6

Table 4. Patterns of disease progression in advanced breast cancer

Patient group	Total (n)	Tissue at first progression					
		Old		New		Old and new	
		(n)	(%)	(n)	(%)	(n)	(%)
Treatment							
Endocrine[a]	113	74	64	15	13	26	23
Cytotoxic	80	45	56	14	18	21	26
Combined	74	43	58	10	14	21	28
Oestrogen receptor status							
RE+[b]	26	19	73	2	8	5	19
ER−	50	29	58	8	16	13	26
Response to protocol treatment							
Complete response	23	16	70	4	17	3	13
Partial response	90	46	51	13	14	31	34
Stable disease	113	72	64	18	16	23	2
Progressive disease	41	26	63	4	10	11	27

[a] Oophorectomy, 19 cases; tamoxifen, 94 cases.
[b] Oestrogen receptor (ER) positive, > 10 fmol/mg protein.

Table 5. Patterns of disease progression in advanced breast cancer

Patient group	Total (n)	Tissue at first progression					
		Old		New		Old and new	
		(n)	(%)	(n)	(%)	(n)	(%)
Disease progression							
<6 months	128	81	63	20	16	27	21
>6 months	139	79	57	19	14	41	29
Prior therapy							
None	239	143	60	37	15	59	25
L-PAM (phenylalanine mustard)	19	12	63	1	5	6	32
Disease-free interval[a]							
0[b]	46	26	57	6	13	14	30
<2 years	98	60	61	18	19	20	20
>2 years	123	74	60	15	12	34	28
Patient survival							
<1 year	66	34	52	12	18	20	30
1–2 years	84	48	57	12	14	24	29
>2 years	117	78	67	15	13	24	21

[a] Disease-free interval, interval between mastectomy and first disease recurrence.
[b] Presented with metastatic disease.

Table 6. Patterns of disease progression in advanced breast cancer

Patient group	Patients (n)	Sites of progression					
		Old		New		Old and new	
		(n)	(%)	(n)	(%)	(n)	(%)
Disease *site* at first progression							
Overall	46	19	41	18	39	9	20
Tissue at first progression							
Overall	56	33	59	13	23	10	18
Progression in old tissue by site	28	19	68	5	18	4	14

In a smaller cohort of patients with advanced breast cancer, we analysed not only whether disease progression occurred in an old or new tissue, but also whether within old tissues, disease progression was first documented in the previously involved site within that tissue or in a new site (Harnett et al. 1986). Table 6 shows that the initial site of disease progression was in a site known previously to contain metastatic disease in 41% of patients, but in 39%, progression of the disease was at a previously uninvolved site. In 20% of patients, both old and new sites of progressive disease were documented simultaneously. Thus, in over half the patients, disease progression involved the appearance of new *sites* of metastatic disease. In 18 patients, it was possible to identify an original bulk (dominant) site of disease. This was defined as measurable disease in excess of 2 cm in diameter excluding bone metastases and liver disease. In only nine of these 18 patients was the bulk site the first in which subsequent disease progression was documented.

Discussion

The main conclusion of these analyses of the sites/tissues of systemic treatment failure in patients with advanced breast cancer is that in approximately half of the patients, progressive disease was first documented in a new site and sometimes in an old metastatic site as well. This observation suggests that disease present at the time of initiating systemic treatment may often be controlled when a relapse in a new site is first detected. Under these circumstances, it may be appropriate (if possible) to *add* a new therapy to control the new site of disease rather than *substitute* for the initial treatment. The latter approach however is the one most widely adopted in clinical practice. We have initiated a randomised trial comparing substitution as opposed to addition of medroxyprogesterone acetate to patients with advanced breast cancer who have progressive disease while taking tamoxifen. The end points of this study are the pattern of disease progression, and the results will clarify which treatment strategy is optimal.

Our data make a case for adjuvant therapy using multiple drugs, and to date multi-drug endocrine adjuvants have been little studied. It should not be assumed that patients with progressive disease after receiving adjuvant treatments necessarily have a drug-resistant tumour and trials initiated by the International Breast Cancer Study Group are now investigating the effects of reintroduction of adjuvant treatment prior to a documented relapse in the hope that this strategy may prolong the disease-free interval.

The bases for the observations that at the time of relapse following adjuvant therapy, the recurrent disease is frequently sensitive are presumably either that adjuvant chemotherapy was not given for a long enough period to eliminate drug-sensitive tumour, that tumours developed *temporary* cellular resistance to therapy or that during the time that adjuvant chemotherapy was given, a significant fraction of tumour cells were either kinetically insensitive to treatment or were protected from drug access owing to local factors, e.g. fibrin clots, etc. Apart from reintroduction programmes, another approach to improving adjuvant systemic treatment which may overcome temporary resistance is to recruit out-of-cycle tumour cells into the mitotic cycle at a time when chemotherapy is being administered (Davidson and Lippman 1987). The efficacy of this sort of approach is disputed in the management of advanced breast cancer, but in the adjuvant setting, no trials have been undertaken, probably because of concern that the tumour cell recruitment strategy has the potential to worsen the outcome.

Analysing the patterns of treatment failure is an important potential means of improving treatment strategies. Goldie and Coldman (1986) have argued that a significant incidence of treatment failure in previously undetected sites is not incompatible with the somatic mutation theory of drug resistance. Improved information about changes in tumour phenotype and genotype between the primary tumour and metastatic sites is now being sought utilising modern molecular genetic techniques. Preliminary data indicate some genetic heterogeneity in a proportion of metastases compared with the primary tumour site (Harnett et al., in preparation). Additional research is required comparing parameters of primary and recurrent tumours in order to develop new rational strategies to improve the efficacy of adjuvant treatments.

References

Davidson NE, Lippman ME (1987) Stimulation of breast cancer with estrogens: how much clinical value. Eur J Cancer Clin Oncol 23: 897-900

Fey MF, Brunner KW, Sonntag RW (1981) Prognostic factors in metastatic breast cancer. Am J Clin Oncol 4: 237-247

Goldie JH, Coldman AJ (1986) Analyzing the patterns of treatment failure. J Clin Oncol 4: 825-826

Harnett PR, Kirsten F, Tattersall MHN (1986) Drug resistance in clinical practice: patterns of treatment failure in advanced breast and ovarian cancer. J Clin Oncol 4: 952-957

Harnett PR, Tattersall MHN, Coates AS, Van Couten R, Forbes J (1987) Drug resistance in clinical practice: patterns of treatment failure in patients receiving systemic therapy for advanced breast cancer. Eur J Cancer Clin Oncol 23: 1601-1605

Meyer JS, Friedman E, McCrate MM, Bauer WC (1983) Prediction of early course of breast carcinoma by thymidine labelling. Cancer 51: 1879-1886

Muss HB, Smith LR, Cooper MR (1987) Tamoxifen rechallenge: response to tamoxifen following relapse after adjuvant chemohormonal therapy for breast cancer. J Clin Oncol 5: 1556-1558

Silvestrini R, Diadone MG, Gasparia G (1985) Cell kinetics as a persistent prognostic marker in node negative breast cancer. Cancer 56: 1982-1987

Tubiana M (1982) Cell kinetics and radiation oncology. Int J Radiat Oncol Biol Phys 8: 1471-1489

Tubiana M, Koscielny S (1988) Cell kinetics, growth rate, and the natural history of breast cancer. Eur J Cancer Clin Oncol 24: 9-14

Valagussa P, Tancini G, Bonadonna G (1986) Salvage treatment of patients suffering relapse after adjuvant CMF chemotherapy. Cancer 58: 1411-1417

New Information on Drug Resistance: Implications for the Adjuvant Treatment of Breast Cancer

J. H. Goldie

Division of Medical Oncology, Cancer Control Agency of British Columbia,
University of British Columbiy, 600 West 10th Avenue, Vancouver, B.C., V5Z 4E6, Canada

Introduction

Extensive studies carried out over the past decade have abundantly confirmed the supposition that human cancer cells, both in vitro and in vivo, have an enormous capacity to develop variant phenotypes which display altered degrees of drug sensitivity. (Goldie and Coldman 1984; Von Hoff 1985). Evidence is accumulating that many of the mechanisms of specific drug resistance that have been identified in experimental systems are also likely to occur in clinical situations (Fojo et al. 1987).

Although chemotherapy is capable of curing a number of types of advanced human malignancy, it is generally agreed that breast cancer is not one of these. However, there is unambiguous evidence that systemic adjuvant chemotherapy directed at subsets of breast cancer patients with minimal tumor burdens does have the potential for significantly increasing relapse-free survival and perhaps actually eradicating residual malignancy in a proportion of patients (Buzdar et al. 1981; Bonadonna and Valagussa 1985). In this review, we will examine how certain mathematical models of the process of drug-resistance development may help to shed light on how much of the component of treatment failure in adjuvant breast cancer can be attributed to drug resistance and, by implication, how much might be related to other differing mechanisms.

A Model for the Relationship Between Tumor Mass and Curability

In previous publications our group has examined the relationships between an increasing tumor burden and the probability of cure by chemotherapy (Goldie and Coldman 1979; Coldman and Goldie 1983). The basic assumptions underlying the initial minimal model were that drug-resistant phenotypes arose randomly within a tumor cell population, but with a certain average frequency (the mutation rate). As the tumor cell population expands over time, there will be an increasing likelihood that at least one drug-resistant clone will appear within the neoplasm. If the mutant is stable, then its progeny will also be drug resistant, and moreover there will be further additions to the drug-resistant pool by other mutations from the sensitive-cell population. Over time, the proportion of drug-resistant cells will increase, and there will be an increasing probability that further mutant forms that display higher levels of drug resistance and resistance to multiple agents will develop. Given sufficient elapsed time and a sufficiently large tumor, then phenotypes resistant to all of the clinically useful antineoplastic agents may well be present at the time of clinical presentation.

Depending upon the size of the tumor and the value for the mutation rate, there will also be a probability at any given time that no resistant phenotypes will have yet emerged. This relationship is given explicitly by the function P (probability of 0 resistant cells) $= \exp(-a\{N\text{-}1\})$, where N is the number of tumor cells present and a is the mutation rate per cell generation.

If we assume that sufficient courses of treatment are given to eradicate all of the sensitive cells in the tumor, then this probability becomes equal to the probability of potential cure. This function, when plotted as probability of cure against increasing tumor burden, describes a steep sigmoid curve. The shape of the sigmoid curve is essentially that of the so-called limiting dilution Poisson distribution.

That there would be a mathematical relationship between increasing tumor burden and probability of cure is intuitively not surprising. What is perhaps counterintuitive is the steepness with which the probability of cure falls off at some critical point as the tumor burden increases. The implication for this in clinical terms is that, in any situation in which there is a reasonable probability of drug-induced cure, a delay in the initiation chemotherapy, even for short periods of time, could significantly compromise eventual treatment outcome. The corollary to this is that relatively small increases in estimates of tumor burden would likewise have a surprisingly marked impact on treatment response. This conclusion is counterintuitive because in general it is known that cancer is a chronic disease which is assumed to have a preclinical phase that may last for years and even once clinically advanced may not produce significant symptoms and morbidity for long periods of time. That such an apparently slowly evolving process can have critical transition times which will abruptly alter treatment outcome, at first examination appears surprising.

Some understanding of the mathematical basis for these sudden transition times can be developed if one bears in mind that each doubling of the tumor population adds as many cells to the tumor as were originally present at the time immediately previous. Thus, the opportunity for a rare event occurring during the last doubling of the tumor cell population is essentially equivalent to the probability of that event occurring in all the previous doublings. If treatment outcome is indeed predicated by the occurrence or nonoccurrence of certain rare random events, then the inescapable conclusion is that probability of cure will indeed fall off very steeply with elapsed time.

This theoretical approach argues very strongly for the validity of using adjuvant chemotherapy wherever feasible in the management of human malignancy. The logical question which arises is to what extent there is evidence suggesting that relatively small increases in tumor burden significantly affect treatment outcome in clinical cancer, with special reference to the adjuvant therapy of breast carcinoma.

Shortly after we published our first paper dealing with this model, Skipper of the Southern Research Institute published an extensive monograph (Skipper 1980) in which he examined large bodies of experimental data to see whether there was a correlation between predicted and observed proportions of cures in transplantable murine tumors as compared with the predictions of the mathematical model. In general, there was a surprisingly strong correlation between the predictions of the model and what was observed in a large diverse data set with a variety of antineoplastic agents in a variety of transplanted tumor cell lines. Recently, using more sophisticated mathematical and computational techniques, we have repeated this exercise on sets of experimental chemotherapy data and have confirmed that the model is capable of predicting drug treatment outcomes in transplanted tumors in mice with a high degree of precision. (Coldman and Goldie 1987). Therefore, the ability of the mathematical model to predict outcomes in experimental systems seems reasonably well established, but the issue with respect to clinical situations needs to be further clarified.

Tumor Burden and Clinical Outcome in Breast Cancer

One approach to examining this question using clinical data is to correlate treatment outcome in the adjuvant chemotherapy of breast cancer with certain measurements that are felt to be indicators of body tumor burden. In the clinical assessment of breast cancer, it has been appreciated for a number of years that the extent of axillary nodal involvement at the time of presentation carries important prognostic information. (Fisher et al. 1983; McGuire 1987). All other factors being equal (menopausal status, receptor status, histologic grade of tumor, and size of primary tumor), then the extent of nodal involvement predicts for the probability of eventual relapse and death, as well as for median duration of relapse-free survival. This strongly suggests that the extent of metastatic involvement of the axillary glands does bear a close relationship to the extent of more distant metastatic involvement, even when this is undetectable. Thus, patients with stage I breast cancer have a relatively low probability of eventual relapse, and relapse rates significantly increase with patients who fall into the stage II category.

In earlier studies in the adjuvant treatment of breast cancer, little distinction was made in the various subsets of patients in the stage II category. It was recognized in due course that patients with four or more nodes involved at the time of initial diagnosis had a worse prognosis than those with one to three nodes, but only more recently have the categories of patients with more than four nodes been further subdivided. A recent report by Jones et al. (1987) compares the survival of patients with different degrees of nodal involvement treated with chemotherapy and a matched set of controls from a natural history database. What is of particular interest in this study is that it examines the outcomes for patients groups broken down into three categories of nodal status. These are respectively one to three nodes, four to ten, and more than ten nodes.

In patients treated with the potent three-drug combination FAC (5-fluorouracil, Adriamycin, and cyclophosphamide), there was an improvement in survival and relapse-free survival for all three categories of patients as compared with the untreated patients form the natural history database. Of special interest is the fact that the groups of patients with one to three nodes and four to ten nodes responded equivalently to the FAC chemotherapy, but there was a significant decline in probability of survival above ten nodes.

One interpretation of these data is that the relationship between treatment outcome and tumor burden in stage II breast cancer follows a steep relationship perhaps similar to that predicted by the mathematical model. This is not necessarily the only explanation that can be given for these observations. It could be argued that patients who present with more than ten nodes have some as yet undefined biological property that renders them less responsive to chemotherapy than those patients who, for example, present with nine nodes. It might be easier to make this argument if one looked at the two extreme ranges, i.e., one node and for example 14 involved nodes, as being fundamentally different in their biological behavior, but it can be suggested that the fundamental difference between patients presenting with four to ten nodes and with more than ten nodes simply reflects small differences in the total metastatic burden (Skipper 1987). If these burdens are on the steep portion of the probability-of-cure curve, then the mathematical model does indeed predict that small increases in tumor extent will have a disproportionally large effect on treatment outcome.

In the absence of available techniques for accurately measuring the distant metastatic burden in these groups of patients, a definite answer to this question cannot be supplied, but we would argue that the observed data are not inconsistent with what might be expected from a drug resistance model.

Other Potential Explanations for Adjuvant Chemotherapy Failure

There are at least two other possible explanations for adjuvant chemotherapy failure in breast cancer that do not require the invoking of the emergence of drug resistance. These hypothetical explanations, however, do make different predictions as to how treatment responses could be improved utilizing chemotherapy. These will be compared with what the drug resistance model might predict.

Treatment Failure Due to Insufficient Therapy Directed at What is a Fundamentally Drug-Sensitive Tumor

Very simply put, it can be easily imagined that treatment failure could arise simply because of an inadequate course of chemotherapy either in terms of duration or the actual dose delivered. If drug resistance is not present within the tumor cell population, then it is simply necessary to kill off the tumor at a faster rate than it is regrowing until the last surviving neoplastic cell has been eliminated. If the treatment program is truncated prior to achieving this objective, then the tumor will eventually regrow. No one can be certain what the minimal or optimal duration of therapy is in a given clinical circumstance, though it is interesting to note that drug-responsive types of advanced tumors such, as non-Hodgkin's lymphoma (Klimo and Connors 1985) can be eradicated by 3–4 months of intensive treatment. If inadequate duration of therapy was a significant problem in adjuvant breast cancer, one would predict that:

1. Upon relapse, the tumor would exhibit the same degree of sensitivity and responsiveness that it initially possessed and that the institution of therapy of a longer duration would be effective in eventually eradicating the tumor
2. Programs of adjuvant chemotherapy of shorter duration would produce treatment outcomes that are progressively worse

As is well known, neither of these predictions appear to be borne out by what happens in observed instances of relapsing adjuvant chemotherapy. Although some measure of drug sensitivity may be sustained in relapsed and failed adjuvant patients, the quality and duration of responses seen are generally poor, and cures are never observed. Likewise, programs of adjuvant chemotherapy that have successively reduced the duration of treatment from 2 years to 6 months do not appear to have compromised treatment outcome. (Bonadonna and Valagussa 1987). Therefore, it seems unlikely that inadequate duration of treatment directed at what is fundamentally a drug-responsive tumor can account for many instances of treatment failure in adjuvant breast cancer.

The Persistence of Nondividing or Dormant Tumor Cells that Resist Chemotherapy

An alternative explanation that is sometimes advanced to account for treatment failure is that within the initial tumor cell population subsets of clonogenic cells exist that are not in the division cycle, but are in some form of protracted G_0 state (Hill 1982). It is postulated that in this condition the tumor cells are nearly invulnerable to chemotherpy and will therfore survive protracted programs of adjuvant treatment, to come into division at some later time and eventually cause treatment failure.

For this explanation to be credible, one has to assume that at least a proportion of these G_0 tumor cells remain dormant throughout the entire period of chemotherapeutic administration. At some later time, presumably a proportion of these randomly enter the division cycle and begin regrowing. In the simplest version of this model, if one assumes that drug resistance does not occur, then a scenario similar to what was described for inadequate courses of chemotherapy should also prevail. Namely, what is essentially a drug-sensitive tumor cell population should present itself at relapse which can then be induced into sustained remission. Even if the tumor cannot be cured, it should be possible successively to induce sustained responses and simply allow the G_0 cells to come back into cycle, regrow after a period of months or years, and then "crop" them back to a subclinical state. In theory, the patient could be treated indefinitely in this mode and live out a normal lifespan. Again, this does not conform to what is generally observed in the management of advanced or relapsed breast cancer ș̦o assuming a G_0 model in the absence of phenotypic drug resistance would appear to be an inadequate explanation. However, the possibility that G_0 cells persist within the tumor and are also a source of drug-resistant mutants could still be plausible.

The evidence supporting the presence of G_0 or dormant tumor cells in breast cancer and other neoplasms is controversial. As usually defined, G_0 is actually a physiological state that certain normal stem cells (e. g., the bone marrow) can enter into when there is diminished demand for replenishment of the differentiated pool of cells. Some of the models of the G_0 state that have been proposed for tumor cells, i.e., nutritionally deprived cells in culture, are not appropriate models for the physiological G_0 condition. However, it is conceded that the behavior of many cases of breast cancer with a prolonged disease-free interval before relapse is compatible with a dormant cell hypothesis. It should be pointed out, however, that G_0 cells, at least from the bone marrow, although less responsive to chemotherapeutic agents than rapidly dividing ones, are not totally resistant (Bruce et al. 1966). This is particularly true for drugs in the alkylating agent class.

The G_0 or dormant cell model for treatment failure would predict that protracted programs of adjuvant chemotherapy (which would include programs that have so-called reinduction regimens) should yield superior results to chemotherapy of conventional duration. The fact that worsened survival rates were not observed when chemotherapy regimens are shortened from 2 years to 6 months goes to some extent against the dormant cell hypothesis, but does not necessarily invalidate it. A more rigorous test of the dormant cell theory would be to examine the effect of adjuvant chemotherapy regimens which include prolonged duration as well as periodic cycles of more intensive reinduction therapy. These reinduction cycles would have the effect of presumably either killing less responsive dormant cells or "catching them" as they begin to enter the division cycle. Clinical trials to test this hypothesis are presently under way in a number of centers.

Predictions Related to a Drug Resistance Basis for Treatment Failure

Even if one postulates dormant cells as occurring in breast cancer, they do not seem to constitute a sufficient explanation unless drug resistance is also invoked as occurring. This takes us back to our original working hypothesis that much of the basis for treatment failure in adjuvant breast chemotherapy is attributable to drug resistance, i.e., tumor heterogeneity. What strategies therefore can be inferred by considering drug resistance to be the principle obstacle to better treatment outcome?

Improvement in treatment outcome in other, more responsive classes of neoplasm have generally involved the application of two concurrent strategies. (De Vita et al. 1987) These are *(a)* an increased degree of delivered dose intensity of chemotherapeutic agents *(b)* the introduction of additional or more potent cytotoxic drugs. Most of the adjuvant breast protocols that have been tested worldwide have been built around either the cyclophosphamide, methotrexate, 5-fluorouracil (CMF) program or the FAC protocol. While there is some evidence that both these protocols could be delivered at greater dose intensities than are commonly done (Hryniuk and Bush 1984), it is conceded that there may not be much further room for increasing the doses of these agents, given the existing protocol structure. Of the two regimens, FAC appears to be the more potent and hence may offer the most potential for further evolution and improvement. The time may be long overdue for evaluating the components of the FAC protocol to see which elements of it could be strengthened or eliminated. There seems little doubt that Adriamycin should continue to be a main component of breast cancer chemotherapy protocols. The problem with FAC may lie in the 5-fluorouracil and cyclophospha-mide components. Studies by Hryniuk et al. of the effect of 5-fluorouracil in colo-rectal cancer indicate a very steep dose-response effect (Hryniuk et al. 1987). The doses of 5-fluorouracil in most programs of FAC are at the lower end of the dose-response curve for 5-fluorouracil; therefore, this potentially potent antineoplastic agent may be being seriously underdosed in most breast cancer chemotherapy programs. The potential for enhancing the effect of 5-fluorouracil by biochemical modulation with folinic acid is another avenue for enhancing the usefulness of this agent (Petrelli et al. 1987).

Another drug which needs to be looked at critically in the chemotherapy of breast cancer is cyclophosphamide. This has been such a standard component of breast cancer (and indeed other chemotherapy protocols) that its utility never seems to be questioned. In our institution, my colleagues have recently completed a meta-analysis of the effect of cyclophosphamide in small-cell lung cancer (Mur-ray 1987). This retrospective study yielded some surprising conclusions, namely, that despite its unambiguous activity as a single agent in small-cell lung cancer, the drug appeared to have a very shallow dose-response effect when used in drug combinations and at the higher doses employed actually appeared to shorten pa-tient survival. We have therefore begun a pilot program in our center in which cy-clophosphamide has been dropped from the treatment program, allowing us to in-crease the doses of doxorubicin, etoposide, and cisplatin in the management of this tumor. Although results are still very preliminary, we have been encouraged by what has been observed to date. The possibility that cyclophosphamide may be contributing mainly hematological toxicity and reducing the ability to give more effective agents in adequate dosages needs at least to be examined in the context of the adjuvant chemotherapy of breast cancer.

Summary and Conclusions

We would suggest on the basis of our analysis that drug resistance still appears to represent a plausible explanation for drug treatment failure in adjuvant breast chemotherapy. It may not be the only factor, but, if present, clearly has to be cir-cumvented if treatment results are to be improved. Since it seems most unlikely that a new wonder drug for breast cancer will emerge in the next few years, then it is to our existing armamentarium of antineoplastic agents that we will have to turn for improved therapeutic results. Fundamental questions will need to be asked about what indeed are the most appropriate agents to be used in combination chemotherapy protocols for this disease and what are the optimal dose ratios. Our own institutional experience in a number of areas has suggested that many chemo-therapeutic protocols that are widely used represent significant underdosing and that achieving optimal results requires pushing therapeutic agents closer to the reasonable limits of tolerance. Enhanced techniques for patient support during programs of more intensive chemotherapy are now available, and it has also been our experience that patients tolerate briefer, intensive programs of chemotherapy better than they do protracted, less intensive protocols. The role of new drug com-binations that incorporate synergistic or significant biochemical modulation effects (i. e., platinum-etoposide, 5-fluorouracil-leucovorin) need to be examined in the context of the management of breast cancer. We appear to have reached something of a plateau with existing protocols and approaches, and it is time to move ahead.

References

Bonadonna G, Valagussa P (1985) Adjuvant systemic therapy for resectable breast cancer. J Clin Oncol 3: 259–275

Bonadonna G, Valagussa P (1987) Current status of adjuvant chemotherapy for breast cancer. Semin Oncol 14: 8–22

Bruce WR, Meeker BE, Veleriote FA (1966) Comparison of the sensitivity of normal hematopoietic and transplanted lymphoma colony forming cells to chemotherapeutic agents administered in vivo. J Natl Cancer Inst 37: 233–242

Buzdar A, Smith T, Blumenschein G et al. (1981) Adjuvant chemotherapy with fluorouracil, doxorubicin and cyclophosphamide (FAC) for stage II or stage III breast cancer: five year results, In: Salmon SE, Jones SE (eds) Adjuvant therapy of cancer III. Grune and Stratton Orlando, Florida pp 419–426

Coldman AJ, Goldie JH (1983) A model for the resistance of tumour cells to cancer chemotherapeutic agents. Mathematical Biosciences 65: 291–307

Coldman AJ, Goldie JH (1987) Modelling resistance to cancer chemotherapeutic agents. In: Thompson JR, Brown BW (eds) Cancer modelling. Marcel Dekker, New York, pp 315–364

De Vita VT Jr, Hubbard SM, Longo DL (1987) The chemotherapy of lymphomas: looking back, moving forward. Cancer Res 47: 5810–5824

Fisher B, Bauer M, Wickerham DL et al. (1983) Relation of number of positive axillary nodes to the prognosis of patients with primary breast cancer. An NSABP update. Cancer 52: 1551–1557

Fojo A, Cornwell M, Cardarelli C et al. (1987) Molecular biology of drug resistance. Breast Cancer Res Treat 9: 5–16

Goldie JH, Coldman AJ (1979) A mathematic model for relating the drug sensitivity of tumours to their spontaneous mutation rate. Cancer Treat Rep 63: 1727–1733

Goldie JH, Coldman AJ: (1984) The genetic origin of drug resistance in neoplasms: implications for systemic therapy. Cancer Res 44: 3643–3653

Hill BT (1982) Biochemical and cell kinetic aspects of drug resistance. In Bruchovsky N, Goldie JH (eds) Drug and hormone resistance in neoplasia, vol 1. CRC, Boca Raton, Florida, pp 21–54

Hryniuk WM, Bush H (1984) The importance of dose intensity in chemotherapy of metastatic breast cancer. J Clin Oncol 2: 1281–1288

Hryniuk WM, Figueredo A, Goodyear M (1987) Applications of dose intensity to problem in chemotherapy of breast and colorectal cancer. Semin Oncol 14 [Suppl 4]: 3–11

Jones SE, Moon TE, Bonadonna G et al. (1987) Comparison of different trials of adjuvant chemotherapy in stage II breast cancer using a natural history database. Am J Clin Oncol 10: 387–395

Klimo P, Connors JM (1985) MACOP-B for treatment of advanced diffuse large cell lymphoma. Annals Intern Med 102: 596–602

McGuire WL (1987) Prognostic factors for recurrence and survival in human breast cancer. Breast Cancer Res Treat 10: 5–9

Murray N (1987) The importance of dose intensity in lung cancer chemotherapy. Semin Oncol 14 [Suppl 4]: 20–28

Petrelli N, Herrera L, Rustum Y et al. (1987) A prospective randomized Trial of 5-FU versus 5-FU and high dose leucovorin versus 5-FU and metotrexate in previously untreated patients with advanced cerebral carcinoma. J Clin Oncol 5: 1559–1565

Skipper HE (1980) Some thoughts regarding a recent publication by Goldie and Coldman entitled "A mathematic model for relating the drug sensitivity of tumours to their spontaneous mutation rate." Booklet 9, Southern Research Institute, Birmingham, Alabama

Skipper HE (1987) Comparison of the response of MAM 16/C tumours in mice and breast cancer in women to the same three-drug combination (CAF) Using the same dose intensity units and the same normalization standards, Booklet 14, Southern Research Institute, Birmingham, Alabama

Von Hoff DD (1985) Implications of tumour cell heterogeneity for in vitro drug sensitivity testing. Semin Oncol 12: 327–331.

Correlation of Dose Intensity and Prognosis in Adjuvant Chemotherapy: An Extended Controversy

W. M. Hryniuk

Ontario Cancer Foundation; Hamilton Regional Centre, 711 Concession Street, Hamilton, Ontario L8V 1C3, Canada

Introduction

In animal model systems, the outcome of chemotherapy depends upon drug dose, tumor sensitivity, and tumor burden. In animals, optimum treatment can be determined by treating beyond lethal toxicity. This is not possible in humans, where attempts to define optimum treatment have resulted in many schedules and combinations, and attempts to avoid serious toxicity have produced many schemes to reduce doses and delay treatment. However, these schedules and schemes have obscured dose-response relationships and have led to confusion. Dose-response relationships can be rediscovered and the confusion can be cleared by expressing all treatments in terms of how much drug is given per unit time. This is dose intensity (Green and Dawson 1980). Dose intensity may be calculated from intended drug doses ("projected dose intensity") or from doses received after reductions and delays because of toxicity ("received dose intenstiy") (Hryniuk and Bush 1984).

For regimens containing only one drug, dose intensity is calculated without regard to the particular schedule specified in the protocol, and is expressed as mg/m^2/week. Dose intensity calculated in this way correlates very well with outcome for a variety of single agents in various malignant diseases (Hryniuk 1988).

For regimens containing more than one drug, dose intensity is calculated by arbitrarily choosing one regimen as the standard and expressing all other regimens relative to the arbitrarily chosen standard. For example, consider a series of cyclophosphamide, methotrexate, 5-fluorouracil (CMF) regimens. For each of the regimens, the dose intensity of C, M, and F is calculated as mg/m^2 per week (again, by disregarding the schedule), and these dose intensities are expressed as a decimal fraction of the dose intensities of C, M, and F in the arbitrarily chosen standard. The decimal fractions are then averaged for each regimen to give the "average relative dose intensity." A sample calculation is given in Table 1.

Table 1. Sample calculations: dose intensity, relative dose intensity, and average relative dose intensity

	Step 1	Step 2	Step 3
Sample Regimen (CMF Q 3 weeks)	Convert to dose intensity: mg/m²/week	Calculate relative dose intensities: decimal fraction of dose intensity in standard regimen[a]	Calculate average relative dose intensity
Cyclophosphamide 600 mg/m²/Q 3 weeks	200	200/560 = 0.36	
Methotrexate 40 mg/m²/Q 3 weeks	13.3	13.3/28 = 0.48	$\bar{x} = 0.42$
Fluorouracil 600 mg/m²/Q 3 weeks	200	200/480 = 0.42	

[a] CMF content in first 8 weeks of CMFVP regimen of Cooper et al. (1979).

Dose Intensity in Advanced Breast Cancer

When the method shown in Table 1 is used to calculate dose intensity for the various CMF regimens used against advanced breast cancer, the remission rate is clearly related to the projected dose intensity (Fig. 1 A) The remission rate is even more strongly related to received dose intensity (Fig. 1 B). Furthermore, the probability of a response for an *individual* patient receiving a particular dose intensity may be read directly from a plot of *group* response rates such as that shown by the asterisks in Fig. 1 B (Goodyear et al. 1985).

Early Breast Cancer

Dose intensity also correlates with outcome in adjuvant CMF chemotherapy of stage II breast cancer (Hryniuk and Levine 1986). For this analysis, dose intensity of various CMF regimens was also calculated as described in Table 1, using the same standard regimen. If regimens did not contain one or two drugs of CMF, a dose intensity of zero was assigned to the missing drug(s). If melphalan was used instead of cyclophosphamide, the melphalan dose was multiplied by 40 to yield the equivalent dose of cyclophosphamide. Only prospectively randomized trials were analyzed, and only those in which it was possible to identify the four subgroups according to age and nodal status. Studies were excluded if there were fewer than ten cases per subgroup, or if they contained Adriamycin (Adria) or immunotherapy or hormones other than prednisone. Projected dose intensity was thus calculated and correlated with 3-year relapse-free survival (RFS).

Figure 2 shows the results for all four subgroups: As projected dose intensity increases, 3-year RFS also increases. Figure 3 A shows that for patient under 50 years with 1–3 nodes, 3-year RFS increases rapidly, then seems to reach a pla-

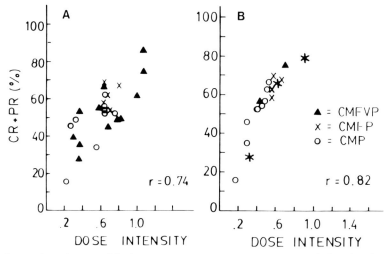

Fig. 1 A, B. Advanced carcinoma of the breast: response rate versus average relative dose intensity of various studies using CMF. Dose intensities are relative to the regimen of Cooper et al. (1979). **A** Doses projected before reductions for toxicity, **B** doses received after reductions for toxicity. The *asterisks* are responses of patients in the upper, middle, and lowest third dose intensities subdivided from the group receiving the highest dose intensity in the figure. (See Goodyear et al. 1985)

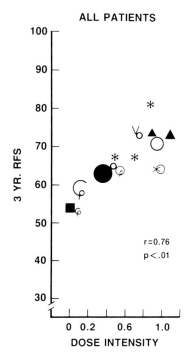

Fig. 2. Stage II carcinoma of the breast: 3-year relapse-free survival versus average relative dose intensity for adjuvant chemotherapy trials containing all four subgroups (<50 years, 1–3, and >3 positive nodes; >50 years, 1–3, and >3 positive nodes). The size of the symbols is proportional to the number of cases at each dose intensity. ■, Control; ▲, CMFVP; ♀, CMFP; ●, CpF; C, cyclophosphamide; v, CMFV; ○, CMF; ⊘, CpMF; ⚲, phenylalanine mustard; ••, trial with radiotherapy added; *, levels of CMF chemotherapy according to Bonadonna

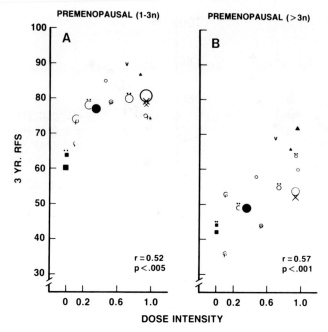

Fig. 3 A, B. Stage II carcinoma of the breast: 3-year relapse-free survival versus average relative dose intensity for adjuvant chemotherapy in women under 50. **A** 1–3 positive nodes; **B** > 3 positive nodes. *Symbols* see legend to Fig. 2

teau. In contrast, for patients under 50 years with more than three nodes, 3-year RFS increases linearly over the entire range of projected dose intensity (Fig. 3 B). In addition, the dose-response curve is shifted to the right in the patients with the heavier disease burden (compare Fig. 3 A with Fig. 3 B).

In older patients, 3-year RFS also correlates with projected dose intensity, but there is more scatter to the data. Again, there is a shift to the right for patients with heavier disease burden (compare Fig. 4 A and 4 B).

Application of Dose Intensity to Neo-Adjuvant Therapy

In the Nissen-Meyer study (Nissen-Meyer et al. 1978), cyclophosphamide was given for 5 days immediately after mastectomy and produced a 9% improvement in 3-year RFS. The dose intensity of the Nissen-Meyer regimen was only 0.02 as compared with 36 weeks of the Cooper regimen (Cooper et al. 1979) but produced an outcome equivalent to what would be expected from conventional adjuvant chemotherapy with a dose intensity of 0.24 (refer to Fig. 2). If the dose intensity of Nissen-Meyer's treatment were increased fourfold, i.e., to 0.08, this might make it equivalent in effectiveness to a more conventional CMF regimen of 0.96 dose intensity; i.e. 3-year RFS might increase to 20%. Thus, the use of the dose intensity concept might allow estimation of what postoperative chemotherapy would be required to replace much more prolonged conventional treatment. However, in ad-

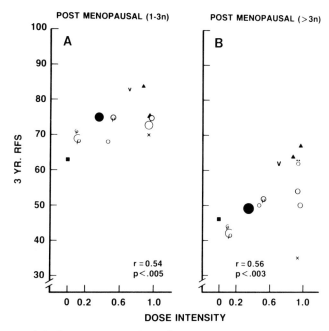

Fig. 4 A, B. Stage II carcinoma of the breast: 3-year relapse-free survival versus average relative dose intensity for adjuvant chemotherapy in women over 50. **A** 1–3 positive nodes; **B** >3 positive nodes. *Symbols* see legend to Fig. 2

dition to dose intensity, the total dose of drug may be an independent determinant of outcome (Hryniuk 1987), and the above calculations have not taken into account this possible additional factor.

Received Dose Intensity in Adjuvant Chemotherapy

Unfortunately, most reports of adjuvant treatment do not indicate what doses of chemotherapy were actually given to the patients and what the treatment delays were. Thus, it is usually not possible to calculate received dose intensity from published results of adjuvant studies. However, in one study, received levels of CMF were published (Bonadonna and Valagussa 1981), and when these levels are transformed into received dose intensities, the results fit very well with the data in Fig. 2 as shown by the superimposed asterisks. In another randomized study (Tancini et al. 1983), patients who received 6 months of adjuvant CMF had longer survival than patients receiving 12 months of adjuvant CMF. Using dose intensity analysis, it was possible to determine the probable explanation for this observed difference (Hryniuk et al. 1987a). Virtually the entire survival advantage accruing to the 6-month treatment group was concentrated in the subgroup of women over 50 years with more than three nodes. This subgroup was also the only one that, by happenstance, received more dose-intensive chemotherapy, even though the projected dose intensities were identical in the two arms of the study. This may explain why the results of adjuvant treatment appeared better in the 6-month group. We would urge that whenever trial results are published, received doses and delays should be calculated and reported. The most appropriate method would probably be the cumulative dose plot recently suggested by Coppin (1987).

Dose Intensity and Tumor Burden

Prednisone allows higher doses of CMF to be administered. This increases the received dose intensity and improves the therapeutic outcome in advanced breast cancer (Tormey et al. 1982). However, in the Ludwig trial (Ludwig Breast Cancer Study Group 1985), the addition of prednisone to CMF adjuvant therapy did not increase RFS in women under 50 with 1–3 nodes, even though the received dose intensity was increased. Reference to Fig. 3 A suggests a possible explanation why RFS was not increased: the addition of prednisone allowed an increased received dose intensity in the range of 0.94. This is on the plateau part of the dose-response curve where no benefit would be expected from relatively small increases in dose intensity. On the other hand, an increase in received dose intensity on the linear portion of the curve should improve outcome. This may explain why CMFVP was superior to CMF in patients with more than three positive nodes (Wood 1983).

The size of the tumor burden also conditions the relationship between treatment outcome and dose intensity in other situations, e. g., cisplatin therapy of testicular cancer (Samson et al. 1984) and MOPP therapy of Hodgkin's disease (Carde et al. 1983).

Dose Intensity and Adjuvant Therapy of Colorectal Cancer

Recently published analysis shows a clear relationship between the remission rate of advanced colorectal cancer and projected dose intensity of 5-FU administered by i. v. bolus. When the adjuvant colorectal cancer trials were analyzed in which 5-FU was given as a single agent, it became clear that the dose intensities used were quite low (Hryniuk et al. 1987 b). Had these dose intensities been used in advanced colorectal cancer, they would have produced responses of only 0%–17% (see Fig. 5). The only adjuvant study which did show positive effects of single agent 5-FU was also the one that used the highest dose intensity. This suggests that single agent 5-FU may have unrealized potential as an adjuvant in colorectal cancer.

Prospective Tests of the Dose Intensity Concept

Because evidence for the concept of dose intensity was generated from retrospective analyses, some skepticism has been expressed about its validity. It was suggested that patients who tolerated the most dose-intensive treatments were also in better physical condition and therefore had higher response rates or longer survival for reasons independent of dose intensity. This controversy can now be laid to

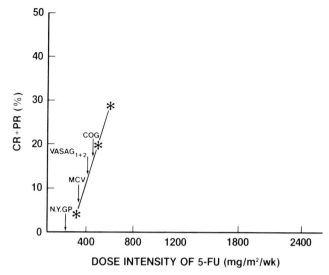

Fig. 5. Dose intensities of IV bolus 5-FU as single-agent adjuvant in colorectal cancer, superimposed on dose-response line for bolus 5-FU against advanced disease (Horton et al. 1970) *COG*, Central Oncology Group; *VASAG*, Veterans Administration Surgical Adjuvant Group; *MCV*, Medical College of Virginia; *N. Y. GP*, New York Group. For further details see Hryniuk et al. (1987b)

rest. Recent prospective randomized trials have validated the concept of dose intensity by showing that dose intensity *per se* is an important determinant of outcome independent of other factors (Beretta et al. 1986; Tannock et al. 1987; Carmo-Pereira et al. 1986a, 1986b). However, trials testing the concept should continue to be designed and implemented because the contribution of dose intensity to treatment outcome will probably depend upon the specific therapeutic situation (Pater 1987). In addition, trials must be conducted to see how dose intensity can be further increased above present levels in an attempt to approve treatment results. If these attempts are successful, we will not yet have reached the limits of what is possible to achieve with chemotherapy.

Acknowledgements. The efforts of Drs. H. Bush, L. Levin, M. Levine and M. Goodyear and the patience and skill of Mrs. Joanne McSkimming are hereby acknowledged.

References

Beretta G, Tabiadon D, Tedeschi L et al. (1986) Front line treatment with CMF variations for advanced breast carcinoma. A randomized study. Proc Am Soc Clin Oncol 5: 77
Bonadonna G, Valagussa P (1981) Dose-response effect of adjuvant chemotherapy in breast cancer. N Engl J Med 304: 10–15
Carde P, MacKintosh FP, Rosenberg SA (1983) A dose and time response analysis of the treatment of Hodgkin's disease with MOPP chemotherapy. J Clin Oncol 1: 146–153

Carmo-Pereira J, Costa FO, Henriques V et al. (1986a) A randomized trial of cyclophosphamide, methotrexate, 5-fluorouracil, and prednisone in advanced breast cancer. Cancer
Chemother Pharmacol 17: 87–90

Carmo-Pereira J, Costa FO, Henriques V et al. (1986b) Advanced breast carcinoma: a comparison of two dose levels of Adriamycin. Proc Am Soc Clin Oncol 5: 56

Cooper RG, Holland JF, Glidewell O (1979) Adjuvant chemotherapy of breast cancer. Cancer 44: 793–8

Coppin CML (1987) The description of chemotherapy delivery: options and pitfalls. Semin
Oncol 14 (4): 34–42

Goodyear M, Hryniuk W, Clark D et al. (1985) Relationship of dose intensity (DI) to outcome in chemotherapy of advanced breast carcinoma. Proc Am Soc Clin Oncol 4: 61

Green JA, Dawson AA (1980) Measurement of drug dosage intensity in MVPP therapy in
Hodgkin's disease. Br J Clin Pharmacol 9: 511–514

Hryniuk W, Bush H (1984) The importance of dose intensity in chemotherapy of metastatic
breast cancer. J Clin Oncol 2 (11): 1281–8

Hryniuk W, Levine M (1986) Analysis of dose intensity for adjuvant chemotherapy trials in
stage II breast carcinoma. J Clin Oncol 4: 1162–1170

Hryniuk W (1987) Average relative dose intensity and the impact on design of clinical trials.
Semin Oncol 14: 65–74

Hryniuk W, Bonadonna G, Valagussa P (1987a) The effect of dose intensity in adjuvant
chemotherapy. In: Jones SE, Salmon SE (eds) Adjuvant therapy of cancer, vol 5. Grune
and Stratton, Orlando, Florida, pp 13–23

Hryniuk W, Figueredo A, Goodyear M (1987b) Applications of dose intensity to problems
in chemotherapy of breast and colorectal cancer. Semin Oncol 14, (4): 3–11

Ludwig Breast Cancer Study Group (1985) A randomized trial of adjuvant combination
chemotherapy with or without prednisone in premenopausal breast cancer patients with
metastases in one to three axillary lymph nodes. Cancer Res 45: 4454–4459

Nissen-Meyer R, Kjellgren K, Malmio K et al. (1978) Surgical adjuvant chemotherapy: results with one short course with cyclophosphamide after mastectomy for breast cancer.
The Scandinavian Adjuvant Chemotherapy Study Group (SACSG) project. Cancer 41:
2088–2098

Pater JL (1987) Implications of dose intensity for cancer clinical trials. Semin Oncol 14, (4),
[Suppl 4 (December)]: 1–2

Samson JK, Rivkin SE, Jones SE et al. (1984) Dose-response and dose-survival advantage
for high versus low-dose cisplatin combined with vinblastine and bleomycin in disseminated testicular cancer. A Southwest Oncology Group (SWOG) project. Cancer 53:
1029–1035

Tancini G, Bonadonna G, Valagussa P et al. (1983) Adjuvant CMF in breast cancer: comparative 5-year results of 12 versus 6 cycles. J Clin Oncol 1: 2–10

Tannock IF, Boyd NF, Perrault DJ (1987) Randomized trial of two doses of CMF chemotherapy for metastatic breast cancer. Proc Am Soc Clin Oncol 6: 50

Tormey DC, Gelman R, Band PR (1982) Comparison of induction chemotherapies for
metastatic breast cancer. Cancer 50: 1235–1244

Wood WC (1983) Cancer and Leukemia Group B adjuvant chemotherapy trials in postmastectomy breast cancer patients. Breast Cancer Res Treat 3: 39–43

Dose Response for Adjuvant Chemotherapy of Breast Cancer: Experimental and Clinical Considerations

E. Frei III

Dana-Farber Cancer Institute, 44 Binney Street, Boston, MA 02115, USA

Preclinical experimental models of dose response in breast cancer will be presented. Dose response differs according to the agent. For example, for the alkylating agents drug resistance is generally difficult to produce experimentally, and a steep dose-response curve both in vitro and in vivo is maintained through multiple logs of cell kill (Frei et al. 1985, Frei et al., in press; Teicher et al. 1986). In contrast using nonalkylating agents, drug resistance of a high degree can be produced readily. Related to this is the fact that fractional cytoreduction is progressively compromised with increasing doses through a multilog cell kill model. In this regard, the alkylating agents more closely resemble radiotherapy. The lack of cross-resistance among the alkylating agents in both in vitro and in vivo models has important implications for clinical treatment strategies (Frei et al. 1985; Frei et al., in press; Teicher et al. 1986).

A novel in vivo model for quantifying the effect of dose on cell kill up into the high-dose transplantation range has been developed. It involves tumor excision 24 h after treatment followed by a clonal assay. This model confirms the steep dose-response curves for alkylating agents through multiple logs of cell kill. It provides an opportunity to analyze the impact of tumor volume on the dose effect. In general, the nonalkylating agents have a more curvilinear dose response, that is, a loss of fractional tumor cell kill with increasing doses (Frei et al., in press).

It has long been demonstrated experimentally that, although treatment programs have a modest effect on established tumors, they may be highly effective and even curative for microscopic disease. While tumor burden alone and first-order kinetic effects in part explain this difference, a major reason for the difference relates to microenvironmental differences. As tumors enlarge, the relative blood supply lessens, the growth fraction decreases, and other adverse micro-environmental factors such as hypoxia occur (Steele 1986).

While the adverse effect of hypoxia on X-ray response is well known, it has only recently been appreciated that experimental in vivo hypoxia may compromise the effects of a number of chemotherapeutic agents (Teicher et al. 1987). This adversity can be directed experimentally by the use of the oxygen-carrying colloid fluosol in the presence of oxygen breathing (Teicher et al. 1987). Finally, the microenvironmental situation with the limitation of certain metabolites may increase genetic plasticity, thus increasing clonal evolution, heterogeneity, and blood resistance for macroscopic tumors.

Finally, the experimental models indicate that drug resistance for alkylating agents is low level when it occurs and relative, so that it can be overcome by increasing the dosage.

Such models also attest to the fact that the opportunity for cytoeradication occurs early if it occurs at all and is best achieved when great attention is paid not only to drug selection but to dose and drug combinations. Because of the development of drug resistance, long duration of treatment is ineffective, and maximum cell kill may be achieved within 1–4 courses of treatment. This is consistent with many clinical trials of adjuvant chemotherapy indicating that we probably overtreat in terms of duration and undertreat in terms of dose.

Clinical Studies

In general, randomized comparative studies wherein dose is an independent variable have been limited, but when analyzed they show, with few exceptions, steep dose-response curves (Frei et al. 1980). This has been demonstrated conclusively in small-cell lung cancer, acute lymphocytic leukemia, and the lymphomas. In general, such studies are positive in chemosensitive tumors and less impressive in chemoresistant tumors. In short, if there is little or no response in the first place, an increase in dose is not likely to make a big difference.

In the past few years, major emphasis has been placed on retrospective dose intensity studies for a variety of chemotherapeutic regimens and a number of neoplastic diseases in both the macrometastatic and the adjuvant setting. These retrospective studies generally indicate a steep dose-response curve. This is true for patients with macrometastatic breast cancer whether analyzed across a number of studies by Hryniuk (1987), or within a given study or studies by Bonadonna. Both of these investigators have found the same to be true for adjuvant chemotherapy studies. These investigations involve a number of assumptions, and most particularly, they are retrospective and thus subject to the interpretive problems that beset such analyses. Nevertheless, they are important hypothesis-generating studies and suggest that relatively slight increments in dose (30%–50%) could make a very substantial difference in response and in the adjuvant situation in the long-term disease-free survival rate. Thus, one of the most promising and important variables which must be addressed in quantitative, prospective studies of dose response in the adjuvant situation for breast cancer is dose (Hryniuk 1987).

In the past few years, several serious studies on dose have been undertaken. It has been found that the best single agent, Adriamycin, when employed intensively, produces as much as an 80% response rate in patients with metastatic breast cancer and a 40% complete response rate (Jones et al. 1987). It has also been found that high-dose alkylating agents combined with autologous bone marrow transplantation provide very high response rates, including complete response rate in patients with advanced refractory breast cancer. The integration of these two programs, that is, high-dose Adriamycin induction therapy followed by a combination of alkylating agents and marrow autotransplantation in two early studies, produces complete response rates in the range of 75%–80%. All prior experience with adjuvant chemotherapy across a range of cancers indicates that programs which produce very high response rates and, particularly, complete response rates in patients with advanced disease have a high likelihood of improving the cure rate when applied to micrometastatic disease. Accordingly, investigators at Duke University are employing high-dose Adriamycin induction chemotherapy followed by high-dose alkylating agents and autologous bone marrow transplantation in the adjuvant breast cancer situation for high-risk patients with more than ten positive nodes (W. Peters 1988, personal communication).

Investigators in the Cancer and Leukemia Group B undertook the first randomized adjuvant breast cancer study in which dose was an independent variable. Thus, patients were randomly allocated to a twofold difference in dose level of a combination of cylophosphamide, Adriamycin, and fluorouracil. This study was constructed such that the schedule and duration of therapy were constant. The rationale, experimental design, and preliminary results of this study will be presented (CALBG Breast Adjuvant Dose Intensity Study, ongoing study).

In conclusion, experimental studies and retrospective clinical studies indicate a steep dose effect for many chemotherapeutic agents, including a steep dose effect in experimental breast cancer models and for clinical breast cancer. However, creative studies based on experimental models in quantitative clinical trials will be required to optimally exploit the dose effect – an effect which provides a major opportunity for advancing the adjuvant chemotherapy of breast cancer.

References

Frei IIIE, Canellos GP (1980) A critical factor in cancer chemotherapy. Am J Med 69: 585
Frei IIIE, Cucchi CA, Rosowsky A et al. (1985) Alkylating agent resistance: In vitro study with human cell lines. Proc Natl Acad Sci USA 82: 2158
Frei IIIE, Teicher BA, Cucchi CA et al. (in press) Resistance to alkylating agents: Basic studies in therapeutic implications. In: Bristol-Myer Cancer Symposium, vol 8
Hryniuk WM (1987) Average relative dose intensity and the impact on design of clinical trials. Semin Oncol 14: 65
Jones RB, Holland JF, Bhadardwaj S (1987) A phase I–II study of intensive dose adriamycin for advanced breast cancer. J Clin Oncol 5: 172
Steele GP (1986) The Cytokinetics of Cancer
Teicher BA, Cucchi CA, Lee JB et al. (1986) Alkylating agents: *In vitro* studies of cross resistance patterns in human cell lines. Cancer Res 46: 4379
Teicher BA, Crawford JN, Holden SA et al. (1987) Effects of various oxygenation conditions on the enhancement by fluosol of melphalan antitumor activity. Cancer Res 47: 5036

Neoadjuvant (Pre- and Perioperative) Therapy

Experimental Basis and Clinical Reality of Preoperative (Neoadjuvant) Chemotherapy in Breast Cancer

J. Ragaz, J. H. Goldie, R. Baird, P. Rebbeck, V. Basco, and A. Coldman

Cancer Control Agency of British Columbia, 600 West 10th Avenue, Vancouver, B.C. V5Z3EG, Canada

Introduction

The survival gains after conventional postoperative adjuvant chemotherapy are far from ideal. Even at best, the 25% survival improvement compared to untreated surgical controls is seldom exceeded (Bonadonna et al. 1987; Nissen-Meyer et al. 1978; Lippmann and Chabner (1986). The absence of more effective drugs for breast cancer remains consistently the main problem. At the same time, it is being increasingly recognized that the scheduling and dosing of most chemotherapeutic agents have not yet been adequately tested, as the original design of the presently utilized regimens has been largely empirical. There is a possibility that research on new scheduling of old drugs may be surprisingly fruitful. Preoperative timing of chemotherapy, along with questions on the selection and dose intensity of the chemotherapeutic drugs, emerge as one of the most exciting aspects of breast cancer clinical research. There is no question that such a development, if proven correct, will result in very significant practical alterations of the orthodox management of breast cancer. Therefore, before its full implementation, rigorous testing in clinical trials will be required.

Preoperative chemotherapy implies that the management of cancer not only necessitates the combination of at least two therapeutic approaches (the systemic and the locoregional), but also that the initial management of the newly diagnosed breast cancer will have to start with the systemic component of the therapy. Surgery, contrary to the presently established practice, will follow at a later date. Even in the absence of hard data, the neoadjuvant approach has already captured the interest of the scientific community (Jacquillat et al. 1986; Ragaz et al. 1987a; Williams et al. 1987). Such a development, no doubt is a result of the logical and scientifically appealing rationale, and is compounded by theoretical (Goldie and Coldman 1979) and animal data (Corbett et al. 1978; Fisher et al. 1968) already documenting survival advantage. However, the transfer of the well-approved theoretical approach into the realm of clinical trials and routine practice is emerging as one of the most challenging tasks in the history of cancer treatment.

Early pilot studies of preoperative and perioperative chemotherapy started several decades ago. The encouraging experimental results and common sense jus-

Recent Results in Cancer Research, Vol. 115
© Springer-Verlag Berlin · Heidelberg 1989

tified their initiation, with perioperative chemotherapy starting with breast cancer (Fisher et al. 1968; Nissen et al. 1978), followed by osteosarcoma (Sampat et al. 1987), head and neck tumors (Frei et al. 1986) and locally advanced breast cancer (Balawajder et al. 1983; Hortobagyi et al. 1987; Lippman et al. 1986b; Morris et al. 1978; Ragaz et al. 1987). More recently completed studies documenting the safety of more dose-intensive preoperative chemotherapy with anthracycline (Hortobagyi et al. 1987; Lippman et al. 1986b; Ragaz et al. 1987a) revived previous interest, resulting at present in a quest for a more organized approach towards neoadjuvant therapy (Jacquillat et al. 1986; Ragaz et al. 1986; Ragaz 1986a; Wagner et al. 1985). As larger randomized studies are planned, the rationale for the more complex approach must be clear, not only to the investigators, but also to the practitioners and their patients. Otherwise, cooperation with the accrual to the trials will not be secured.

Rationale for preoperative chemotherapy

Although each biological phenomenon will be discussed separately, they are all clearly interconnected and should be taken as equally important. The following are considered of importance:

Kinetics

The range of doubling times of systemic micrometastases, according to recent reports, may vary from as low as 17 days to as high as several months (Band and Deschamps 1983). Taking the tumors in the lower ranges of doubling time, we can recognize that in a subset of patients, a doubling or tripling of the overall tumor cell burden may be seen over 4–8 weeks. Along with the quantitative expansion of the tumor burden, transition towards aggressivity (Cifone and Fidler 1981), resistance (Goldie and Coldman 1979) or invasion of chemotherapeutic sanctuaries are all possible events. Hence, in the practice where delays of initiation of chemotherapy by 6–8 weeks are common, the system may be incurable even before the therapy is initiated.

Possible Consequences of Noncurative Surgery and Biopsy

Noncurative cytoreduction (surgery), according to the majority of animal experiments, will shift the kinetics from a flatter to a steeper portion of the growth curve, causing a measurable increase in the proliferation rate in the remaining tumor (DeWyss 1972; Fisher et al. 1983; Gorelik et al. 1978; Simpson-Herren et al. 1976). The increase of the tumor growth rate after cytoreduction may also decrease the life span of animals, as documented by elegant experiments by Simpson-Herren et al. (1976). These data have not been consistently observed in all animal systems (Van Putten 1986), and only anecdotal observations confirm their counterpart in human tumors. It may nevertheless be prudent to consider the kinetic acceleration of micrometastases after cytoreduction to be a true phenomenon, particularly at a microscopic level, and infer that in the absence of a therapeutic maneuver it may also adversely affect human malignancies. Of great interest is the phenomenon of the cell-to-cell interaction and of the overall tumor burden reacting as a whole system to a local or systemic intervention, supporting the concept of the systemic mediation of the growth control (DeWyss 1972; Dickson et al. 1986; Lippman et al. 1986a; Moses and Leof 1986; Sporn and Roberts 1985). It remains to be shown whether a sensitive interaction of mitogenic and stimulatory interplay of growth factors will have an identifiable association with kinetic alterations after cytoreduction and whether a therapeutic intervention will be possible. It is expected nevertheless that preoperative chemotherapy will reduce the tumor cell burden at surgery, and hence reduce the number of cells at risk for possible kinetic acceleration and dissemination. Also, a loss of the metastatic potential in surviving cells, (the back mutation into a more differentiated state), and the role of chemotherapeutic agents in differentiation (Bissel and Hall 1987; Jenis et al. 1987; Moses and Leof 1986; Reiss and Sartorelli 1987), represent the very promising and as yet not adequately researched aspect of the chemotherapeutic action in general.

Resistance to Chemotherapy

Recent results of DNA research indicate an association of the presence of oncogenes with several human malignancies (Bishop 1983; Lundy et al. 1986; Slamon 1987; Varmus 1984). It has yet to be shown whether DNA abnormalities, acquired or inherited, are related to the induction and maintenance of the malignancy. Taking into consideration the acquisition of genetic instability as one of the many characteristics of newly transformed cells, the loss of a previously present sensitivity to chemotherapeutic agents is yet another phenotypic feature of malignant cells. According to the interpretation of the Goldie and Coldman somatic mutation theory (1979) and of animal experiments confirming it (Skipper 1983), the appearance of the first resistant cell may be an instantaneous phenomenon, and may already occur in the early period of tumor development. Given that the presence of even one resistant cell precludes the cure by chemotherapy, and that the transitions towards resistance are ongoing, it may be essential, according to Goldie and Coldman (1979), to start chemotherapy as soon as possible after the malignancy is diagnosed. The shifting of the chemotherapy to the preoperative period is, therefore, clearly a valid approach.

Conversion of Inoperable Tumors into Operable Ones

The most visible benefit of preoperative chemotherapy is seen in locally advanced tumors, inoperable at the time of diagnosis. Preoperative chemotherapy will act simultaneously on both the systemic and the locoregional component, with the effective downstaging of the tumor enabling subsequent surgery (Frei et al. 1986). In a subset of patients in whom the systemic, but not the locoregional, component will be eradicated, such resection can be considered a curative procedure (Ragaz et al. 1987a). Recent data also indicate that as a result of debulking large tumors, surgery could not only take place, but also radical surgery may be replaced by a more conservative approach (Frei et al. 1986; Rosen et al. 1979). Over the last few years, several studies of locally advanced, inoperable breast cancer have indicated that as a result of neoadjuvant therapy, up to 70%-90% of previously inoperable tumors could be rendered operable (Balawajder et al. 1983; Hortobagyi et al. 1987; Lippman et al. 1986b; Morris et al. 1978; Ragaz et al. 1987a). It is not presently known whether surgery will be needed, after an effective initial pretreatment of the tumor, and if so, to what extent. One conclusion, however, emerges undeniably: Preoperative chemotherapy, along with the locoregional treatment modalities and hormones, has brought the entity of locally advanced tumors from the scenario of a certainty for locoregional and systemic recurrences into the arena of potentially curable human malignancies.

Practical Implications of Preoperative Chemotherapy

Role of Fine Needle Aspiration

At present, open biopsy, frequently performed as a separate surgical procedure, is the main diagnostic procedure in North America. As most breast tumors are microscopically more advanced than anticipated, the majority of open biopsies are incisional. Such an example of noncurative cytoreduction may adversely affect the system. Fine needle aspiration (FNA) can provide the initial diagnosis reliably, with the diagnostic error kept below 1% in experienced hands (Zajicek 1974). In addition to other drawbacks of open biopsy (longer waiting time, tissue trauma, use of a general anaesthetic), the less expressed kinetic alterations after the FNA make it a very appealing alternative for the initial diagnostic procedure, while a confirmatory frozen section before the definitive procedure should still be considered. FNA is receiving increasing popularity in our region (Ragaz 1986b), much as in Scandinavian countries (Zajicek 1974). Although the main official diagnostic procedure for the British Columbia Neoadjuvant Randomized Trial, FNA is still infrequently used in our study without a separate open biopsy. More experience and more publicity are needed for its uniform adoption.

Neoadjuvant Staging

In most countries, including North America, the presence of positive axillary nodes at mastectomy will determine the need for postoperative adjuvant chemotherapy. In the practice of preoperative chemotherapy, a decision to use adjuvant treatment is made soon after the tissue diagnosis is made and before the nodes have been examined. Hence, both node-positive and node-negative patients receive adjuvant chemotherapy. Although such a decision is easily made at the present time for stage III inoperable tumors, it is being questioned for stages I and II breast cancer. Several factors are of importance. Firstly, a large proportion of patients with high-risk *node-negative* cancers will recur (Silvestrini et al. 1986;

Thorpe et al. 1987; Valagussa et al. 1978, 1984). The high-risk features of node-negative breast cancer, as reviewed in the recent literature (Bonadonna et al. 1986; Huseby et al. 1988; Merkel et al. 1987; Sampat et al. 1977; Silvestrini et al. 1986; Thorpe et al. 1987; Valagussa et al. 1978, 1984), include negative hormone receptors (Merkel et al. 1987; Thorpe et al. 1987; Valagussa et al. 1984), high tumor grade (Rank et al. 1987; Silvestrini et al. 1986), vascular invasion (Sampat et al. 1977), and assessment of tumor kinetics (Meyer et al. 1983; Silvestrini et al. 1986), etc. Of particular interest are the more recent data from DNA assessment, including flow cytometry determination of S-phase percentage and ploidy (Hedley et al. 1985; Kute et al. 1985), as well as the early data emerging from the oncogenic research (Bishop 1983; Lundy et al. 1986; Slamon et al. 1987). Conceptually, it is possible that a combination of all known risk factors at diagnosis may allow a more refined risk assessment (Ragaz 1986a), determining the need for adjuvant chemotherapy while bypassing the axillary lymph nodes. With a refined selection of high-risk factors, only a subset of patients would need preoperative adjuvant chemotherapy, whereas the clearly low-risk cases would require surgical treatment only. Pending confirmation from randomized studies, such treatment could be started routinely, just after the diagnosis and after the risk assessment.

Organisational Aspects of Preoperative Chemotherapy

In the preoperative chemotherapy design, chemotherapy is given after the tissue biopsy is obtained, and before the mastectomy. Hence, the surgeon will have to initiate all the complex activity connected with the administration of adjuvant chemotherapy treatment. Surgeons will also have to take the initiative for getting the patient entered into a randomized study. In the present practice of a busy surgeon, such a complex approach to every breast cancer patient is clearly cost prohibitive, unless externally funded. The alternative is for the medical oncologist to initiate all the actions connected with the preoperative chemotherapy management. Other types of approach, practiced routinely in many European countries, would include a direct referral of newly diagnosed cancer patients to an oncological institute. In all instances, major departures from the present management of breast cancer will be required. Only very effective and clearly understood publicity aimed at general surgeons, the general population (patients), and physicians, will achieve such a major change. Indications for a clear benefit of the preoperative over the postoperative approach will be needed, however, before these alterations will be adopted uniformly.

Conclusion

Present results of postoperative adjuvant chemotherapy are far from satisfactory. Results from experimental and theoretical studies indicate that preoperative timing of systemic therapy may be a more effective treatment scheduling. Major practical alterations connected with the neoadjuvant approach will necessitate a thorough assessment of the cost benefit before it can be universally put into practice. Although preoperative chemotherapy for the management of locally advanced breast cancer can be considered already a part of the recommended management, such treatment should be practiced for stage I and II breast cancer only within the context of clinical trials.

References

Balawajder I, Antich PP, Boland J (1983) An analysis of the role of radiotherapy alone and in combination with chemotherapy and surgery in the management of advanced breast carcinoma. Cancer 51: 574–580

Band PR, Deschamps M (1983) Drug and hormone resistance in the management of breast cancer. In: Bruchovsky N, Goldie JH (eds) Drug and hormone resistance in neoplasia, CRC, Boca Raton, pp 2–27

Bishop JM (1983) Cellular oncogenes and retroviruses. Annu Rev Biochem 52: 301–54

Bissel MJ, Hall AG (1987) Form and function in the mammary gland: the role of extracellular matrix. In: Neville M, Daniel C (eds) The mammary gland development, regulation and function. Plenum, New York, pp 97–146

Bonadonna G, Valagussa P, Zambetti M (1987) Milan adjuvant trials for stage I and II breast cancer. In: Salmon SE (ed) Adjuvant therapy of cancer, vol 5. Grune and Stratton, Orlando, pp 211–21

Cifone MA, Fidler IJ (1981) Increasing metastatic potential is associated with increasing genetic instability of clones isolated from murine neoplasms. Proc Natl Acad Sci USA 78: 6949–6952

Corbett TH, Griswold DP Jr, Roberts PJ et al. (1978) Cytotoxic adjuvant therapy and the experimental model. In: Stoll BA (ed) Systemic therapy in breast cancer, vol 4. New aspects of breast cancer, Year Book Medical, Chicago

DeWyss WD (1972) Studies correlating the growth rate of a tumor and its metastases and providing evidence for tumor related systemic growth retarding factors. Cancer Res 32: 374–379

Dickson RB, Bates SE, McManaway ME et al. (1986) Characterization of estrogen responsive transforming activity in human breast cancer cell lines. Cancer Res 46: 1707–1713

Fisher B, Ravdin RG, Ausman RK et al. (1968) Surgical adjuvant chemotherapy in cancer of the breast: results of a decade of cooperative investigation. Ann Surg 168: 337–356

Fisher B, Gunduz N, Saffer EA (1983) Influence of the interval between primary tumor removal and chemotherapy on kinetics and growth of metastases. Cancer Res 43: 1488–1492

Frei E, Miller D, Krag JR et al. (1986) Clinical and scientific considerations in preoperative (neoadjuvant) chemotherapy. In: Ragaz J, Band PR, Goldie JH (eds) Preoperative (neoadjuvant) chemotherapy. Springer, Berlin Heidelberg New York Tokyo pp 1–5 (Recent results in cancer research, vol 103)

Goldie JH, Coldman AJ (1979) A mathematic model for correlating the drug sensitivity of tumors to their spontaneous mutation rate. Cancer Treat Rep 63: 1727–1733

Gorelik E, Segal S, Feldman M (1978) Growth of a local tumor exerts a specific inhibitory effect on progression of lung metastases. Int J Cancer 21: 617–625

Hedley DW, Friedlander ML, Taylor IW (1985) Application of DNA flow cytometry to paraffin embedded archival material for the study of aneuploidy and its clinical significance. Cytometry 6: 327–333

Hortobagyi G, Ames F, Buzdar A (1987) Effective multidisciplinary therapy of inoperable stage III breast cancer. Proc Am Soc Clin Oncol 6: 64

Huseby RA, Ownby HE, Frederick J et al. (1988) Node negative breast cancer treated by modified radical mastectomy without adjuvant therapies: variables associated with disease recurrence and survivalship. J Clin Oncol 6: 83–88

Jacquillat C, Weil M, Khayat D (1986) Neoadjuvant chemotherapy. John Libbey, Eurotex, Paris, pp 3–859

Jenis DM, Keyes SR, Sartorelli AC (1987) Induction of the differentiation of HL-60 promyelocytic leukemia cells by palmitoleic and myristoleic acids. Leuk Res 11: 935–939

Kute TE, Muss HB, Hopkins M et al. (1985) Relationship of flow cytometry results to clinical and steroid receptor status in human breast cancer. Breast Cancer Res Treat 6: 113–121

Lippman ME, Chabner BA (eds) Proceedings of the NIH consensus development conference on adjuvant chemotherapy and endocrine therapy for breast cancer. NCI Monogr 1: 1–159

Lippman ME, Dickson RB, Bates S et al. (1986a) Autocrine and paracrine growth regulation of human breast cancer. Breast Cancer Res Treat 7: 59–70

Lippman ME, Sorace RA, Bagley C et al. (1986b) Treatment of locally advanced breast cancer using primary induction chemotherapy with hormonal synchronization followed by radiation therapy with or without debulking surgery. NCI Monogr 1: 153–159

Lundy J, Grimson R, Mishriki Y et al. (1986) Elevated RAS Oncogene Expression Correlate with lymph node metastases in breast cancer patients. J Clin Oncol 4: 1321–1325

Merkel DE, Dressler LG, McGuire WL (1987) Flowcytometric, cellular DNA content, and prognosis in human malignancy. J Clin Oncol 5: 1690–1703

Meyer JS, Friedman E, McCrate M et al. (1983) Prediction of early course of breast cancer by thymidine labelling. Cancer 51: 1879–1886

Morris DM, Aisner J, Elias EG et al. (1978) Mastectomy as an adjunct to combination chemotherapy. Arch Surg 113: 282–284

Moses HL, Leof EB (1986) Transforming growth factor beta. In: Kahn P, Graf T (eds) Oncogenes and growth control. Springer, Berlin Heidelberg New York Tokyo, pp 51–57

NSABP Convention (1988) 31st Semiannual meeting, Palm Springs, Florida, January 1988

Nissen-Meyer R, Kjellgren K, Malmio K et al. (1978) Surgical adjuvant chemotherapy. Results with one short course with cyclophosphamide after mastectomy for breast cancer. Cancer 41: 2088–2098

Ragaz J (1986a) Emerging modalities for adjuvant therapy of breast cancer: neoadjuvant chemotherapy. NCI Monogr 7: 145–153

Ragaz J (1986b) Preoperative (neoadjuvant) chemotherapy for breast cancer: outline of the British Columbia trial. In: Ragaz J, Band PR, Goldie JH (eds) Preoperative (neoadjuvant) chemotherapy. Springer, Berlin Heidelberg New York Tokyo pp 85–94 (Recent results in cancer research, vol 103)

Ragaz J, Band PR, Goldie JH (eds) (1986) Preoperative (neoadjuvant) chemotherapy. Springer, Berlin Heidelberg New York (Recent results in cancer research, vol 103)

Ragaz J, Manji M, Olivotto I et al. (1987a) Role of mastectomy in preoperative (neoadjuvant) combined modality therapy of locally advanced breast cancer. Proc Am Soc Clin Oncol 6:55

Ragaz J, Coldman A, Salinas F, Worth A, Manji M, Goldie J (1987b) Neoadjuvant chemotherapy for breast cancer. In: Ariel F, Cleary JB (eds) Breast cancer: Diagnosis and treatment. McGraw-Hill, New York, pp 312–328

Rank F, Dombernowsy P, Jespersen NCB et al. (1987) Histologic malignancy grading of invasive ductal breast cancer. A regression analysis of prognostic factors in low risk carcinomas of 9 multicenter trial. Cancer 60: 1299–1305

Reiss M, Sartorelli AC (1987) Regulation of growth and differentiation of human keratinocytes by type beta transforming growth factor and epidermal growth factor. Cancer Res 47: 6705–6709

Rosen G, Marcove RC, Caparros B et al. (1979) Primary osteogenic sarcoma. The rationale for preoperative chemotherapy and delayed surgery. Cancer 43: 2163–2177

Sampat MB, Sirsat MV, Gangadharan P (1977) Prognostic significance of blood vessel invasion in carcinoma of the breast in women. J Surg Oncol, 9: 623–632

Second International Congress on Neoadjuvant Chemotherapy Paris, February 1988

Silvestrini R, Daidone MG, DiFronzo G et al. (1986) Prognostic implication of labelling index versus estrogen receptors and tumor size in node negative breast cancer. Breast Cancer Res Treat 7: 161–169

Simpson-Herren L, Sanford AH, Holmquist JP (1976) Effects of surgery on the cell kinetics of residual tumor. Cancer Treat Rep 60: 1749–1760

Skipper HE (1983) Some thoughts on the design and redesign of combination chemotherapy regimens for treating disseminated breast cancer. Ann Arbor, University Microfilms International 6: 3–61

Slamon DJ, Clark GM, Wong SG (1987) Human breast cancer: correlation of relapse and survival with amplification of the HER-2 NEU oncogene. Science 235: 177–182

Sporn MB, Roberts AB (1985) Autocrine growth factors in cancer. Nature 313: 745–747

Thorpe SM, Rose C, Rasmussen BB et al. (1987) Prognostic value of steroid hormone receptors: multivariate analysis of systemically untreated patients with node negative primary breast cancer. Cancer Res 47: 6126–6133

Valagussa P, Bonadonna G, Veronesi U (1978) Patterns of relapse and survival following radical mastectomy. Analysis of 716 consecutive patients. Cancer 41: 1170–1178

Valagussa P, Bignami P, Buzzoni R et al. (1984) Are estrogen receptors alone a reliable prognostic factor in node negative breast cancer? In: Jones SE, Salmon S (eds) Adjuvant therapy of cancer, vol 4. Grune and Stratton, Orlando, pp 407–415

Van Putten LM (1986) Experimental preoperative chemotherapy. In: Ragaz J, Band PR, Goldie JH (eds) preoperative (neoadjuvant) chemotherapy. Springer, Berlin Heidelberg New York Tokyo, pp 36–41 (Recent results in cancer research, vol 103)

Varmus HE (1984) The molecular kinetics of cellular oncogenes. Annu Rev Genet 18: 553–612

Wagner DJT, Blijham GH, Smeets JBE et al. (1985) Primary chemotherapy in cancer medicine. Liss, New York, pp 3–383

Williams CJ, Buchanan RB, Hall V et al. (1987) Adjuvant chemotherapy for T1–2, NO, MO estrogen receptor negative breast cancer: preliminary results of randomized trial. In: Salmon SE (ed) Adjuvant therapy of cancer, vol 5. Grune and Stratton, Orlando, pp 233–241

Zajicek J (1974) Aspiration biopsy cytology, vol 1. Cytology of supradiaphragmatic organs. Karger, New York

Neoadjuvant Chemotherapy in the Conservative Management of Breast Cancer: A Study of 252 Patients*

C. Jacquillat, M. Weil, G. Auclerc, M.-F. Auclerc, D. Khayat, and F. Baillet

Department of Medical Oncology (SOMPS), Hôpital de la Salpétrière,
47, Boulevard de l'Hôpital, 75013 Paris, France

Introduction

Concepts concerning breast cancer have been considerably modified during the last 10 years. From the concept of a local disease with secondary metastases, the thinking has changed to that of a two-component disease: local on the one hand, and generalized on the other, the latter being more critical the larger the tumor size, the faster the tumor growth rate, the greater the lymph node involvement, and the less the differentiation on histological or nuclear grading.

Although localized breast cancer patients have a 5-year survival which varies between 65% and 85%, 80% of the patients, once diagnosed as having breast cancer, will die of their cancer within 20 years (Ferguson et al. 1982). On the other hand, primary or neoadjuvant chemotherapy represents the most logical way to apply chemotherapy since it improves the effects of local treatment, whether surgery or radiotherapy. It also allows the assessment of the activity of a given combination in a given patient by measuring the amount of tumor regression, and it ensures the early management of micrometastases which will ultimately cause the death of the majority of patients.

We shall not repeat here the theoretical (Goldie and Coldman 1979), experimental (Karrer et al. 1967; Schabel et al. 1979), and clinical data (Nissen-Meyer et al. 1978; Fisher et al. 1982) in support of neoadjuvant chemotherapy.

The local treatment chosen in this study is radiotherapy. It has already been demonstrated that the 10-year survival achieved by irradiation alone is similar to that obtained by standard surgical procedures (Calle and Pilleron 1979). It has also been shown that the combination of external and endocurietherapy with irridium 192 allows a much higher rate of breast conservation for T2 and T3 patients who have had no previous tumorectomy (Otmezguine et al. 1980).

* Supported by INSERM and C.R.A.C. (Centre de Recherches Appliquées á la Chimiothérapie).

Material and Methods

Between January 1, 1980 and October 10, 1987, 252 patients entered study 03SR80, combining primary chemotherapy, locoregional radiotherapy and maintenance chemotherapy, with or without hormonotherapy. Diagnosis relied on cytology and histology obtained by aspiration and drill biopsy. Patients were stratified into four groups according to tumor size, axillary clinical lymph node status, and clinical doubling time.

The distribution of the patients according to these groups is shown in Table 1.

A total of 122 patients fulfill the criteria of locally advanced breast cancer, including all the patients in groups III and IV and six patients in group II with a tumor diameter of over 5 cm (Canellos 1984).

Distribution of age is shown in Table 2.

For all patients, a history and physical examination, complete blood count, serum chemistry, urinalysis, electrocardiogram, echocardiogram, chest roentgenograms, bone scans, liver echography, assays of carcinoembryonic antigen levels, and bilateral mammograms were performed.

The initial treatment consisted of intravenous infusion of a combination of vinblastine (6 mg/m^2), thiotepa (6 mg/m^2), methotrexate (25 mg/m^2), 5-fluorouracil (350 mg/m^2) (VTMF), delivered for 1 h, with, in groups III and IV, Adriamycin (VTMFA) (30 mg/m^2) added. VTMF was given every 14 days for three cycles in group I and every 10 days for four cycles in group II; VTMFA was administered every 7 days for four cycles in group III, and every 7 days for six cycles in group IV.

Table 1. Numbers within groups

Group	Clinical status	Patients (n)
I	T1 T2 ≤ 3 cm	48
II	T2 > 3 cm	88
	T3 ≤ 7 cm + N1b	
III	T3 > 7 cm + N1b	41
IV	T4 IBC	75
		252

Table 2. Age distribution (years) within groups

Group	20–30 (n)	31–40 (n)	41–50 (n)	51–60 (n)	> 60 (n)	Total (n)
I	1	3	11	18	15	48
II	2	4	27	28	27	88
III	0	6	7	11	17	41
IV	2	15	19	26	13	75
Total	5	28	64	83	72	252

The local treatment consisted of teleradiotherapy delivered to group I and II patients by randomization according to the classical schedule (45 Gy within 5 weeks) or delivered in two bimonthly courses of 2 consecutive days. Group III and IV patients were treated exclusively according to this hypofractionated schedule. An infusion of chemotherapy without methotrexate and Adriamycin was interspaced between these two courses. Two weeks later, after another chemotherapy dose, a booster dose at the initial tumor site, by means of endocurietherapy by iridium 192, was delivered (30 Gy).

Thereafter, maintenance chemotherapy with the same combination was given for five monthly cycles to group I, six bimonthly cycles and 12 monthly cycles to group II, six bimonthly cycles, followed by cycles every 3 weeks and then twelve-monthly cycles to groups III and IV. Adriamycin was stopped after a cumulative dose of 300 mg/m^2. In addition, tamoxifen (Nolvadex: 30 mg every day) was given to all menopausal patients. Premenopausal patients received this drug by random allocation. Preliminary results have been reported in smaller groups of patients (Jacquillat et al. 1982, 1983, 1984a, 1984b, 1985, 1988). We report here the results for 252 patients.

Results

Tumor regression of over 75% was achieved in 158 patients (63%); in all of the 252 patients, tumor regression was complete 3 months after the end of the interstitial irradiation. With a median follow-up of 48 months, actuarial disease-free survival (DFS) at 5 years is 78% in the 136 patients in groups I and II. In this group, there have been six local relapses and ten metastatic relapses as shown in Table 3, and 101 patients enjoy DFS (Fig. 1).

In the 116 patients belonging to groups III and IV, 73 enjoy relapse-free survival, 27 died from metastases, eight have active metastases, and seven have local recurrence (40 of them are free of disease). In these patients, we observe a 5-year DFS of 48%. Moreover, there is significant relationship between initial regression and long-term outcome. The incidence of relapse was 29% in 94 patients whose initial tumor regression before radiotherapy was under 75% (27 relapses) and only 20% in the 158 other patients (31 relapses). At 4 years DFS and overall survival are 61% and 74% for patients whose initial regression was less than 75%, and 74% and

Table 3. Outcome of the 252 patients

Groups	I and II (n)	III and IV (n)
Number of patients	136	116
Relapse-free survival	121 (89%)	73 (69%)
Recurrence	16	42[a]
Local recurrence[a]	6	7
Metastatic alive	4	8
Metastatic dead	6	27

[a] Three are dead and two alive with visceral metastasis.

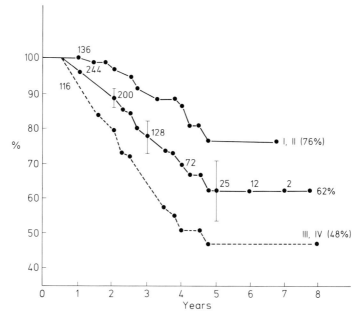

Fig. 1. DFS according to therapeutic groups

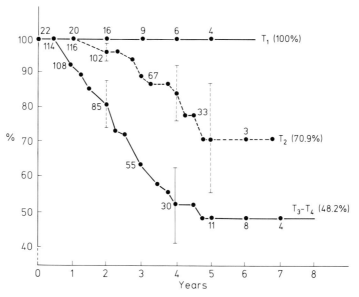

Fig. 2. DFS according to tumor size

Table 4. Influence of tamoxifen on tumor regression

Group		Regression > 75%	
		(*n*)	(%)
I, II	TAM+	66/ 93	71
	TAM−	19/ 43	44
III, IV	TAM+	54/ 79	68
	TAM−	19/ 37	51
Total		137/205	67

TAM+, tamoxifen therapy; TAM−, no tamoxifen.

88% for those whose tumor regression was over 75%. The same magnitude of difference between these two groups of patients is observed at 6 years (e.g., 54% for slow responders and 64% for good responders).

If we consider tumor size, DFS is 100% for T1, 71% for T2, and 48% for T3 and T4, as shown in Fig. 2.

As shown in Table 4, tumor regression of over 75% was more frequent in patients who received tamoxifen (Nolvadex) in addition to chemotherapy, especially in groups I and II.

Toxicity

One patient (group IV) with a family history of acute leukemia developed acute myeloblastic leukemia at 24 months and died. Clinical toxicity was dominated by nausea, fatigue, and alopecia. In most patients, hospitalization was restricted to 3 days required by endocurietherapy. In groups I and II, hematological toxicity (fewer than 1000 neutrophils/mm^3 and/or fewer than 100000 platelets/mm^3) did not require any treatment modification. In groups III and IV, one or two doses had to be delayed.

Discussion

Our study confirms the effectiveness of a combined modality approach using neoadjuvant chemotherapy and radiotherapy in the treatment of patients with breast cancer. Tumor regression of over 75% was observed in 63% of patients. Despite the large initial tumor burden observed in 122 patients with locally advanced breast cancer, the regression induced by chemotherapy allowed conservative treatment in most patients, since only 20 (8%) local relapses required secondary mastectomy: seven (5%) in groups I and II and 13 (11%) in groups III and IV.

We found a significant correlation between initial tumor regression and distant outcome: we are now testing whether treatment modifications would improve survival in relatively poor responders. The use of cytoreductive chemotherapy until maximal tumor regression occurs, prior to starting local therapy, seems appropriate. The optimal timing of radiotherapy would depend thus on the tumor burden and on the chemosensitivity since, although chemotherapy may be interspaced between radiotherapy courses, it is suboptimal chemotherapy (i.e., without methotrexate and Adriamycin).

Another unsolved problem is the optimum duration of maintenance chemotherapy. Randomized studies such as that of Tancini et al. (1983) are obviously necessary to answer this question.

In conclusion, the use of a combined treatment modality consisting of neoadjuvant chemotherapy and maintenance therapy in addition to teleradiotherapy and endocurietherapy allowed breast conservation in most patients. It may be stated already that this strategy improves DFS and survival in groups III and IV (locally advanced breast cancer) (Bonadonna et al. 1985; Chauvergne et al. 1979; Kantarjian et al. 1984; Rubens et al. 1980; Zylberberg et al. 1982). More time is necessary to confirm the same benefit for groups I and II (Papaiannou 1981). More refined knowledge of the biology of breast cancer, more complex and pharmacologically correct drug regimens, optimal timing of radiotherapy, and better schedules of hormonotherapy are now required to enhance this progress.

Acknowledgements. The authors are thankful to Amina Jindani, London, for her help with the translation.

References

Bonadonna G, Valagussa P (1985) Adjuvant systemic therapy for resectable breast cancer. Clin Oncol 3 (2): 259–275

Calle R, Pilleron JP (1979) Radiation therapy for operable breast cancer. 10 years results. Breast 5: 2–6

Canellos GP (1984) The treatment of locally advanced breast cancer. Clin Oncol 2 (3): 149–151

Chauvergne J, Durand M, Hoerni B, Cohen P, Lagarde C (1979) La chimiothérapie d'induction dans les cancers du sein à haut risque: Résultats d'une étude thérapeutique prospective. Bull Cancer (Paris) 66: 9–16

Ferguson DJ, Meier P, Karrison J, Dawson PJ, Straus FH, Lowenstein FG (1982) Staging of breast cancer and survival rates. JAMA 248: 1337–1341

Fisher B, Redmond C, Eias G, Evans J et al. (1982) Adjuvant chemotherapy of breast cancer: an overview of NSABP findings. Adv Surg Oncol 5: 65–90

Goldie JH, Coldman AJ (1979) A mathematic model for relating the drug sensitivity of tumors to their spontaneous mutation rate. Cancer Treat Rep 63: 1727–1733

Jacquillat C, Baillet F, Auclerc G et al. (1982) Initial chemotherapy and conservative radiotherapy in stage I, II and III breast cancer. Proceedings 13th International Cancer Congress, Seattle, pp 52 (abstract 3218)

Jacquillat C, Baillet F, Blondon J et al. (1983) Preliminary results of "neo-adjuvant" chemotherapy in initial management of breast cancer (BC). Proceedings ASCO, San Diego, 112 (abstract C 437)

Jacquillat C, Baillet F, Auclerc G et al. (1984a) Cancer du sein: chimiothérapie précédant le traitement loco-régional avec extension des indications du traitement conservateur. Bull Cancer (Paris) 71 (4): 354–360

Jacquillat C, Auclerc G, Baillet F et al. (1984b) Chimiothérapie première dans le cancer du sein: Résultats préliminaires. Ann Med Interne (Paris) 135 4: 1–295

Jacquillat C, Weil M, Auclerc G et al. (1985) Neoadjuvant chemotherapy in the conservative management of breast cancer. Study on 205 patients. Proc 1st Int Congress on neoadjuvant chemotherapy. Libbey, Paris

Jacquillat C, Baillet F, Weil M et al. (1988) Results of a conservative treatment combining induction (neoadjuvant) and consolidation chemotherapy, hormonotherapy, and external and interstitial irradiation. Cancer 61: 1977–1982

Kantarjian HP, Hortobagyi GN, Smith TL, Blumenschein GR, Montague E, Buzdar AU, Martin RG (1984) The management of locally advanced breast cancer, a combined modality approach. Eur J Cancer Clin Oncol 20: 1353–1361

Karrer K, Humphreys SR, Goldin A (1967) An experimental model for studying factors which influence metastases of malignant tumors. Int J Cancer 2: 213

Nissen-Meyer R, Kjellgren K, Malmio K, Mansson B, Norin T (1978) Surgical adjuvant chemotherapy: results of one short course with cyclophosphamide after mastectomy for breast cancer. Cancer 41: 2088–2098

Otmezguine Y, Martin A, Le Bourgeois JP, Maylin C, Raynal M, Sallé M, Pierquin B (1980) Etude des récidives parmi 202 cancéreuses du sein traitées conservativement par radiothérapie. J Eur Radiother 1: 115–130

Papaiannou AN (1981) Pre-operative chemotherapy for operable breast cancer. Eur J Cancer 17: 263–269

Rubens RD, Seston S, Tong D (1980) Combined chemotherapy and radiotherapy for locally advanced breast cancer. Eur J Cancer 16: 351–356

Schabel FM, Griswold DP, Corbett TH, Laster Jr, Dykes DJ, Rose WC (1979) Recent studies with adjuvant chemotherapy or immunotherapy of metastatic solid tumors of mice. In: Jones SE, Salmon SE (eds) Adjuvant therapy of cancer. Grune and Stratton, New York, pp 3–17

Tancini G, Bonadonna G, Valagussa P et al. (1983) Adjuvant CMF in breast cancer, comparative 5-year results of 12 versus 6 cycles. J Clin Oncol 1: 1–10

Zylberberg B, Salat-Baroux J, Ravina JH, Dormont D, Amiel JP, Dielbold P, Izrael V (1982) Initial chemoimmunotherapy in inflammatory carcinoma of the breast cancer 49: 1537–1543

Randomized Perioperative Therapy in Operable Breast Cancer: The Ludwig Trial V

A. Goldhirsch and R. D. Gelber*

Ludwig-Institut für Krebsforschung, Inselspital, 3010 Bern, Switzerland

Introduction

Adjuvant chemotherapy, endocrine therapy, and a combination chemo-endocrine therapy have been proven to prolong disease-free survival (DFS) and to reduce mortality in women with operable breast cancer (Bonadonna et al. 1985; Goldhirsch et al. 1986; UK-BCTSC/UICC/WHO 1984). It has been postulated that therapeutic efficacy is related to an increased tumor cell kill by higher doses of cytotoxic drugs (Bonadonna and Valagussa 1981) or by the selection of patients whose tumors are more responsive to a given treatment (e.g. patients with estrogen-receptor(ER)-positive tumors, who are receiving adjuvant endocrine therapy) (Ludwig Breast Cancer Study Group 1984). The use of sequential non-cross-resistant combinations also appears to enhance effectiveness (Perloff et al. 1986).

Adjuvant chemotherapy in the immediate postoperative period was studied during the 1960s in two randomized clinical trials and showed prolongation of survival in at least some of the treated patients as compared with the surgical controls (Fisher et al. 1975; Nissen-Meyer et al. 1978). The National Surgical Adjuvant Breast Project (NSABP) study produced a significant survival advantage in premenopausal patients with four or more metastatic nodes, using a postoperative course of thiotepa. The first Scandinavian Adjuvant Chemotherapy Group study used a 6-day course of postoperative cyclophosphamide, which yielded a survival advantage which began to appear only after 5 years, and was significant overall after 12 or more years (Nissen-Meyer et al. 1985). This benefit was almost equal for pre- and postmenopausal patients, and for those with, and without axillary node involvement. Patients (all treated in one institution) whose therapy was delayed by as little as 3 weeks showed no benefit.

These studies were based upon the hypothesis that circulating malignant cells during operation are those which will give rise to metastases, and that their elimination will result in a more effective cure. Subsequent hypotheses concerning resistance to therapy were based upon the current assumption that breast cancer is a

---

* For the Ludwig Breast Cancer Study Group (see Appendix A).

systemic disease by the time of diagnosis and operation. Experiments in animals (Schabel 1977; Fisher et al. 1983) clearly demonstrated that the time of initiation of adjuvant systemic treatment is important. Cell kinetics and drug resistance considerations (DeWyss 1972; Goldie and Coldman 1979) indicated that delayed commencement of treatment might increase the drug resistance of the tumor cells. In several randomized trials, a duration of adjuvant chemotherapy as short as 4–6 months yielded a similar outcome compared with the same treatment of longer duration (Bonadonna et al. 1981; Henderson 1987; Jungi et al. 1981).

It therefore appeared logical and important to evaluate in operable breast cancer the effects of initiating chemotherapy immediately after removal of the primary tumour, and to compare this early commencement of treatment with a "conventionally timed" start corresponding to common practice (i.e. after the removal of stitches and healing of the mastectomy wound). Since "conventionally timed" treatment involved the administration of cytotoxic drugs for 6 months, the question of the duration of adjuvant therapy was also addressed by comparing this treatment with a single course of chemotherapy given immediately after surgery.

Patients and Methods

From November 1981 to December 1985, 2628 patients with breast cancer or candidates for a surgical procedure to ascertain the presence of breast cancer were randomized to enter one of the three treatment programs described in Table 1. Because two-thirds of the patients had to start chemotherapy within 36 hrs of the completion of mastectomy, randomization prior to one-step diagnostic and definitive surgery was allowed in order to obtain consent (Gelber 1985). Owing to timing requirements, many characteristics of the disease such as nodal status, hormone receptor status and other pathological features were unknown at the time of randomization. Patients who had postoperative complications or pathological features of locally advanced disease were not excluded from the analysis.

All of the patients with breast cancer had either a total mastectomy with axillary clearance or a modified radical mastectomy. Eligibility criteria included: unilateral clinical stage [tumor node metastasis (TNM) classification] T_{1A} or $_B$, T_{2B} or $_B$, T_{3A}, N_0 or $_1$, and M_0; a peripheral white blood cell (WBC) count of $\geq 4000/mm^3$; platelet count of $\geq 100000/mm^3$; creatinine levels of ≤ 130 μmol/l; and bilirubin ≤ 60 μmol/l. The patients had to be accessible for follow-up, and they had to be informed in accordance with the practice common in their respective countries. Menopausal status had to be determined prior to randomization. Pre- and perimenopausal status was defined by at least one of the following criteria: normal menstruation, amenorrhea for less than 1 year, biochemical evidence of ovarian function, amenorrhea for 1–3 years in patients younger than 52 years of age, or hysterectomy without bilateral oophorectomy for patients younger than 56 years of age. All other patients were considered to be postmenopausal. Stratification by menopausal status and participating clinic (see Appendix A), as well as randomization, were conducted centrally by the study coordination center in Bern, Switzerland, for the European time zone (Sweden, Switzerland, Yugoslavia, Spain, Germany, Italy, South Africa) and in Sydney, Australia, for Australia and New Zea-

Table 1. Schematic design of Ludwig Breast Cancer Study V

	Operation[a]		Pathology findings	
			Node negative	Node positive
Stratify by	R			
Institution	A	– PeCT	– no further	– no further
Premenopausal v$_s$	N		treatment	treatment
Postmenopausal	D	– PeCT	– no further	– ConCT[b]
	O		treatment	
	M	– no PeCT	– no further	– ConCT[b]
			treatment	

PeCT: Perioperative therapy (begun within 36 h of mastectomy)

Cyclophosphamide	–400 mg/m^2 i.v.	
Methotrexate	– 40 mg/m^2 i.v.	} days 1 and 8
5-fluorouracil	–600 mg/m^2 i.v.	

Leucovorin[c]   15 mg i.v. 24 h after day 1 and
15 mg orally 24 h after day 8

ConCT: Conventionally timed adjuvant therapy (begun 25–32 days after mastectomy)

Cyclophosphamide (C)	–100 mg/m^2 orally	days 1–14	
Methotrexate (M)	– 40 mg/m^2 i.v.	days 1 and 8	q 28 days
5-fluorouracil (F)	–600 mg/m^2 i.v.	days 1 and 8	for 6
Prednisone (p)	– 7.5 mg/m^2 orally	daily	cycles
Tamoxifen (T)	– 20 mg orally	daily	

[a] At least total mastectomy and axillary clearance planned or performed to allow administration of first dose of perioperative chemotherapy within 36 h postsurgery (if assigned).

[b] Premenopausal women received CMFp; postmenopausal women received CMFpT.

[c] Leucovorin was added to PeCT after November 1982 on account of toxic effects attributed to interaction between methotrexate and anesthesia (nitrous oxide) (Goldhirsch et al. 1987; Ludwig Breast Cancer Study Group 1983).

land. The randomization schedule was produced using pseudo-random numbers generated by a congruence method.

Perioperative chemotherapy (PeCT) in those randomized to it was scheduled to begin immediately (within 36 hrs) after the end of the operation (Table 1). The exact time of surgery and of administration of PeCT were recorded. Patients who were subsequently classified as node-negative by routine pathological examination received no additional adjuvant therapy. This report is restricted to the patients who had metastases in axillary nodes and who were randomized to receive either PeCT alone (i.e., no additional treatment), PeCT plus conventionally timed chemotherapy (ConCT) beginning on day 29 of the perioperative course, or ConCT alone beginning between days 25 and 32 after surgery. Conventionally timed therapy consisted of six cycles of cyclophosphamide, methotrexate, 5-fluorouracil, and low-dose prednisone (CMFp) for the pre- and perimenopausal, or 6 months of CMFp and tamoxifen for postmenopausal patients (Table 1).

Of the 2628 patients who entered the study, 43 were randomized but had no cancer and did not receive the protocol treatment, seven patients had a carcinoma in situ as final local pathology diagnosis of the mastectomy specimen, and 74 pa-

Table 2. Patient characteristics by treatment assignment for women with axillary node metastases

	Total	PeCT	PeCT and ConCT	ConCT
Eligible overall	1229	413	401	415
Premenopausal	715	240	239	236
Median Age (years)	(45)	(45)	(45)	(44)
[range]	[24–60]	[24–59]	[25–60]	[25–56]
ER status				
ER+ (≥ 10 fmol)	359	113	120	126
ER– (0–9 fmol)	253	85	87	81
ER unknown	103	42	32	29
Nodal involvement				
1–3	405	132	142	131
4–9	187	70	53	64
≥ 10	123	38	44	41
Postmenopausal	514	173	162	179
Median Age (years)	(59)	(59)	(59)	(59)
[range]	[45–73]	[46–69]	[47–73]	[45–70]
ER status				
ER+ (≥ 10 fmol)	294	97	83	114
ER– (0–9 fmol)	152	51	53	48
ER unknown	68	25	26	17
Nodal involvement				
1–3	293	100	88	105
4–9	143	48	44	51
≥ 10	78	25	30	23

tients were ineligible for the following reasons: Stage $> T_{3A}$ ($n = 32$), biopsy more than 21 days prior to mastectomy ($n = 7$), previous malignancy ($n = 9$), initial laboratory results indicating ineligibility ($n = 6$), less than total mastectomy ($n = 5$), insufficient staging ($n = 4$), lactation ($n = 6$), unobtainable follow-up data ($n = 3$), medically unsuitable (arteriosclerosis) ($n = 1$), or bilateral malignancy ($n = 1$). The age limit of 65 years was introduced in 1982 because of unpredictable toxicities of the perioperative regimen (Goldhirsch et al. 1987; Ludwig Breast Cancer Study Group 1983).

Of the 2504 evaluable patients who entered the trial 1229 (49%) had nodal involvement and comprise the basis of the present report. Patient characteristics by treatment are displayed in Table 2. Hormone receptor concentrations in the primary tumors were determined by standard methods based on guidelines provided by the coordination laboratory. Estrogen receptor (ER) and progesterone receptor (PgR) results of ≥ 10 fmol/mg cytosol protein were considered positive, and lower values negative. ER results were available for 1058 patients (86.1%).

The median number of axillary nodes examined pathologically was 13, and 93% of the patients had at least eight nodes examined. The central pathology review including tumor type, grade according to a modified Bloom and Richardson's classification (Davis et al. 1986), peritumoral vessel invasion, and nodal involvement (review of all nodes found negative by routine pathological examination) is ongoing.

Clinical, hematological, and biochemical assessment of each patient was required every 3 months for 2 years, and thereafter every 6 months until death. Chest X-rays were required every 6 months. Bone scans were required every 6 months for 2 years and then once annually. All study records (on-study, treatment, toxicity and recurrence) were reviewed centrally by the medical and data management staffs.

Data available as of December 1987 (median follow-up time of 42 months, range 22–72 months) were used for this report. The time of relapse was defined as the time when recurrent disease was diagnosed or, if later confirmed, was first suspected. Disease-free survival (DFS) was the time to relapse, appearance of second primary malignancy (including contralateral breast cancer), or death, whichever occurred first. Times were measured from the date of mastectomy. Four-year DFS and overall survival (OS) percentages were estimated using the Kaplan-Meier method (Kaplan and Meier 1958). Greenwood's formula for the calculation of standard error and logrank tests for the comparison of treatment effects were also used (Gelber and Zelen 1985). Cox proportional hazard regression models (Cox 1972) were used to adjust for prognostic features (nodal and ER status). All probability values were two-sided.

Results

Patient characteristics, including ER status, tumor size, and type of mastectomy (modified radical vs. total mastectomy) were well balanced across the comparable treatment groups.

Of the 1229 patients, 509 (41.4%) relapsed or died. In both the premenopausal and postmenopausal patients, the DFS for the PeCT-treated group was significantly shorter than for those treated with ConCT alone or in combination with PeCT (Table 3 and Figs. 1, 2). Logrank and pairwise analysis of overall survival by treatment group in premenopausal and in postmenopausal patients showed only marginal differences.

Cox model analysis (Cox 1972) of pairwise comparisons between PeCT alone and treatments of longer duration within each of the menopausal subgroups provided statistically significant differences with respect to DFS. The same analyses for OS did not alter the conclusions derived from the pairwise logrank test.

Discussion

The question of duration of adjuvant chemotherapy has been clearly answered in our trial: one cycle of PeCT provides significantly less control of disease than either six or seven cycles of chemotherapy for premenopausal patients or of chemo-endocrine therapy for postmenopausal patients. A review of trials which address the question of duration (Bonadonna et al. 1981; Henderson et al. 1986; Jungi

Table 3. Four-year DFS percentages by ER status, by number of nodes (N) involved, and by treatment groups (median Follow-up 42 months)

	4-Year DFS % ± s.e.			
	PeCT	PeCT and ConCT	ConCT	P-value[a]
Premenopausal, all	40± 4	63± 4	62± 4	<0.0001
ER+	45± 6	65± 5	69± 5	0.0003
ER−	28± 6	62± 5	48± 7	0.0005
Unknown	49± 9	59±10	76±11	0.11
N+ 1–3	53± 5	77± 4	76± 4	<0.0001
N+ 4–9	26± 8	60± 8	49± 8	0.004
N+ ≧10	16± 6	19± 8	34±10	0.004
Postmenopausal, all	40± 4	55± 5	63± 4	0.0001
ER+	33± 6	63± 7	64± 5	0.0001
ER−	39± 8	35± 9	51± 8	0.27
Unknown	69±10	71±10	87± 9	0.32
N+ 1–3	51± 6	60± 7	70± 5	0.06
N+ 4–9	28± 7	69± 8	63± 7	<0.0001
N+ ≧10	24± 9	15± 9	36±11	0.42

[a] Two-sided logrank test for heterogeneity among treatment groups.

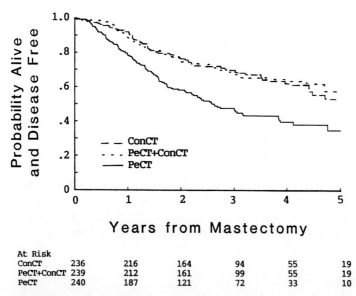

At Risk
ConCT	236	216	164	94	55	19
PeCT+ConCT	239	212	161	99	55	19
PeCT	240	187	121	72	33	10

Fig. 1. Disease-free survival by assigned treatment for 715 node-positive, pre- or perimenopausal patients at 42 months' median follow-up. Test for heterogeneity $P<0.0001$. Pairwise P values are: $P<0.0001$ PeCT vs. PeCT plus ConCT, $P<0.0001$ PeCT vs. ConCT, $P=0.86$ PeCT plus ConCT vs. ConCT

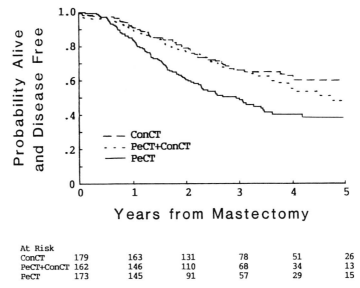

Fig. 2. Disease-free survival by assigned treatment for 514 node-positive, postmenopausal patients at 42 months' median follow-up. Test for heterogeneity $P = 0.0001$. Pairwise P-values are: $P = 0.005$ PeCT vs. PeCT + ConCT, $P = 0.0001$ PeCT vs. ConCT $P = 0.29$ PeCT + ConCT vs. ConCT

et al. 1981) leads to the conclusion that effective adjuvant chemotherapy ($\pm$ hormonal agents) might involve five or six cycles.

The question of whether continuation of endocrine therapy with tamoxifen for postmenopausal patients for a period of 2 or more years after cessation of chemotherapy remains an experimental issue. The initial use of chemo-endocrine therapy for this age group, however, represents a significant improvement over adjuvant endocrine therapy alone (Goldhirsch and Gelber 1986). Although some direct comparisons between chemo- and chemo-endocrine therapy yielded different outcomes (Ingle et al. 1986; Taylor et al. 1985) which were not significant, other trials with larger numbers of patients showed a significant improvement in results when endocrine therapy with tamoxifen was added to chemotherapy, either initially (Fisher et al. 1986; Hubay et al. 1984) or continued beyond the initial adjuvant treatment (Fisher et al. 1987).

The hypothesis that early commencement of adjuvant chemotherapy might yield better results than treatment which is delayed until after wound healing was not supported by the *preliminary findings* of this trial. Even our attempt to analyze retrospectively the outcome of patients who received PeCT alone by time from end of mastectomy (< 12 vs. $13-24$ vs. $25-36$ h) showed no trend toward improvement in results for shorter intervals between mastectomy and administration of chemotherapy. These data do not provide evidence that the mathematical model which correlates the number of resistant cells with the drug resistance mutation rate, the total burden of tumor cells, and time (DeWys 1972) has a practical implication, especially with respect to early results. It is possible, however, that the early start provides increased control of disease in those patients for whom relapses will appear later in time and in whom, therefore, a difference in outcome would be observed only later during follow-up.

Conclusions

This study is important in showing that a short course of perioperative treatment is insufficient to control relapse in early node-positive breast cancer, especially in pre- and perimenopausal patients. Six cycles of chemotherapy in premenopausal patients and 6 months of chemo-endocrine therapy in postmenopausal women provide better control of the disease.

Appendix A
Ludwig Breast Cancer Study Group: Participants and Authors

Ludwig Institute for Cancer Research, Inselspital, Bern, Switzerland

A. Goldhirsch *(Study Coordinator)*, B. Davis, R. Bettelheim, W. Hartmann, M. Neville *(Study Pathologists)*, M. Castiglione, A. Pedrazzini, D. Zava, C. Wiedmer

Harvard School of Public Health and Dana-Farber Cancer Institute, Boston, Massachusetts, U.S.A.

R. D. Gelber *(Study Statistician)*, K. Price, K. Stanley, K. Larholt, N. Snudden, M. Zelen

Frontier Science and Technical Research Foundation, Buffalo, New York, U.S.A.

M. Isley, M. Parsons, L. Szymoniak

Auckland Breast Cancer Study Group, Auckland, New Zealand (since V)

R. G. Kay, J. Probert, B. Mason, H. Wood, E. G. Gifford, J. F. Carter, J. C. Gillmann, J. Anderson, L. Yee, I. M. Holdaway, G. C. Hitchcock, M. Jagusch

Spedali Civili & Fondazione Beretta, Brescia, Italy

G. Marini, E. Simoncini, P. Marpicati, U. Sartori, A. Barni, L. Morassi, P. Grigolato, D. Di Lorenzo, A. Albertini, G. Marinone, M. Zorzi

Groote Schuur Hospital, Cape Town, Republic of South Africa

A. Hacking, D. M. Dent, J. Terblanche, A. Tiltmann, A. Gudgeon, E. Dowdle, R. Sealy, P. Palmer, P. Helman

University of Essen, West German Tumor Center, Essen, Germany

C. G. Schmidt, K. Höffken, F. Schüning, L. D. Leder, H. Ludwig, R. Callies, A. E. Schindler

University of Düsseldorf, Düsseldorf Germany

P. Faber, H. G. Schnürch, H. Bender, H. Bojar

West Swedish Breast Cancer Study Group, Göteborg, Sweden

C.-M. Rudenstam, J. Säve-Söderbergh, E. Cahlin, L. O. Haftstrom, S. Holmberg, C. Johansén, S. Nilsson, J. Fornander, H. Salander, C. Andersson, O. Ruusvik, G. Ostberg, L. Mattsson, C. G. Bäckström, S. Bergegårdh, G. Ekelund, Y. Hessman, S. Holmberg, O. Nelzén, S. Dahlin, G. Wallin, L. Ivarsson, O. Thorén, L. Lundell, U. Ljungquist

The Institute of Oncology, Ljubljana, Yugoslavia — J. Lindtner, J. Novak, D. Erzen, M. Sencar, J. Cervek, O. Cerar, B. Stabuc, R. Golouh, J. Lamovec, J. Jancar, S. Sebek

Madrid Breast Cancer Group, Madrid, Spain — H. Cortés-Funes, F. Martinez-Tello, F. Cruz Caro, M. L. Marcos, M. A. Figueras, F. Calero, A. Suarez, F. Pastrana, R. Huertas, C. Guzman

Anti-Cancer Council of Victoria, Melbourne, Australia — J. Collins, R. Snyder, R. Bennett, W. I. Burns, J. Forbes, J. Funder, T. Gale, L. Harrison, S. Hart, V. Humenuik, P. Jeal, P. Kitchen, R. Lovell, R. Mclennan, R. Reed, I. Russell, M. Schwarz, L. Sisely, P. Williams, H. Ritchie

Sir Charles Gairdner Hospital Nedlands, Western Australia — M. Byrne, P. M. Reynolds, H. J. Sheiner, S. Levitt, D. Kermode, K. B. Shilkin, R. Hähnel, G. van Hazel

SAKK (Swiss Group for Clinical Cancer Research)

Bern, Inselspital — K. Brunner, G. Locher, E. Dreher, K. Buser, H. Cottier, K. Bürki, M. Walther, R. Joss, H. Bürgi, M. Spreng, U. Herrmann, R. Kissling

St. Gallen, Kantonsspital — H. J. Senn, W. F. Jungi, R. Amgwerd, U. Schmid, Th. Hardmeier, E. Hochuli, U. Haller, O. Schildknecht

Bellinzona, Ospedale San Giovanni — F. Cavalli, H. Neuenschwander, W. Müller, C. Sessa, P. Luscieti, E. S. Passega, M. Varini, G. Losa

Basel, Kantonsspital — J. P. Obrecht, F. Harder, H. Stamm, U. Laffer, A. C. Almendral, U. Eppenberger, J. Torhorst

Geneva, Hôpital Cantonal Universitaire — P. Alberto, F. Krauer, R. Egeli, M. Aapro R. Mégevand, M. Forni, P. Schäfer, E. Jacot des Combes, A. M. Schindler, F. Misset

Lausanne, CHUV — S. Leyvraz

Neuchâtel, Hôpital des Cadolles — P. Siegenthaler, V. Barrelet, R. P. Baumann

Luzern, Kantonsspital — H. J. Schmid

Ludwig Institute for Cancer Research, and Royal Prince Alfred Hospital, Sydney, Australia — M. H. N. Tattersall, R. Fox, A. Coates, D. Hedley, D. Raghavan, F. Niesche, R. West, S. Renwick, D. Green, J. Donovan, P. Duval, A. Ng, T. Foo, D. Glenn, T. J. Nash, R. A. North, J. Beith, G. O'Connor

References

Bonadonna G, Valagussa P (1981) Dose-response effect of adjuvant chemotherapy in breast cancer. N Engl J Med 30: 10-15

Bonadonna G, Valagussa P, Rossi A, Tancini G, Brambilla C, Marchini S, Veronesi U (1981) Multimodal therapy with CMF in resectable breast cancer with positive axillary nodes. The Milan Institute experience. In: Salmon SE, Jones SE (eds) Adjuvant Therapy of Cancer III. Grune and Stratton, New York pp 435-444

Bonadonna G, Valagussa P, Rossi A, Tancini G, Brambilla C, Zambetti M, Veronesi U (1985) Ten-year experience with CMF-based adjuvant chemotherapy in resectable breast cancer. Breast Cancer Res Treat 5: 95-115

Cox DR (1972) Regression models and life tables (with discussion). J Roy Stat Soc B (Methodol) 34: 187-220

Davis BW, Gelber RD, Goldhirsch A, Hartmann WH, Zimmermann A, Locher G, Reed R, Golouh R, Säve-Söderbergh J, Hollaway L, Russell I, Rudenstam CM (1986) Prognostic significance of tumor grade in clinical trials of adjuvant therapy for breast cancer with axillary lymph node metastasis. Cancer 58: 2662-2670

DeWyss WD (1972) Studies correlating the growth rate of a tumor and its metastases and providing evidence for tumor-related systemic growth-retarding factors. Cancer Res 32: 374-379

Fisher B, Slack NH, Katrych D, Wolmark N (1975) Ten years of follow-up results of patients with carcinoma of the breast in a cooperative clinical trial evaluating surgical adjuvant chemotherapy. Surg Gynecol Obstet 140: 528-534

Fisher B, Gunduz N, Saffer EA (1983) Influence of the interval between primary tumor removal and chemotherapy on kinetics and growth of metastases. Cancer Res 43: 1488-1492

Fisher B, Redmond C, Brown A, Fischer ER, Wolmark N, Bowman D, Plotkin D, Walter J, Borstein R, Legault-Poisson S, Saffer EA (1986) Adjuvant chemotherapy with and without tamoxifen in the treatment of primary breast cancer: 5-year results from the National Surgical Adjuvant Breast and Bowel Project Trial. J Clin Oncol 4: 459-471

Fisher B, Brown A, Wolmark N (1987) Prolonging tamoxifen therapy for primary breast cancer: findings from the National Surgical Adjuvant Breast and Bowel Project clinical trial. Ann Intern Med 106: 649-654

Gelber RD (1985) Methodological and statistical aspects in perioperative chemotherapy trials. In: Metzger U, Largiader F, Senn HJ (eds) Perioperative chemotherapy. Springer, Berlin Heidelberg New York, pp 53-63 (Recent results in cancer research, vol 98)

Gelber RD, Zelen M (1985) Planning and reporting of clinical trials. In: Calabren P, Rosenberg SA, Schein P (eds) Textbook of medical oncology. MacMillan New York, pp 406-25

Goldie JH, Coldman AJ (1979) A mathematic model of relating the drug sensitivity of tumors to their spontaneous mutation rate. Cancer Treat Rep 63: 1727-1733

Goldhirsch A, Gelber RD (1986) Adjuvant treatment for early breast cancer: the Ludwig breast cancer studies. NCI Monogr 1: 55-70

Goldhirsch A, Gelber RD, Davis BW (1986) Adjuvant chemotherapy trials in breast cancer: an appraisal and lessons for patient care outside the trials. In: Forbes JF (ed) Breast disease. Clinical Surgery International. Churchill Livingston, Edinburgh, pp 123-138

Goldhirsch A, Gelber RD, Tattersall M, Rudenstam CM, Cavalli F (1987) Methotrexate/nitrous oxide toxic interaction in perioperative chemotherapy for early breast cancer. Lancet II: 151

Henderson IC (1987) Adjuvant systemic therapy of early breast cancer. In: Harris JR, Hellman S, Henderson IC, Kinne DW (eds) Breast diseases. Lippincott, Philadelphia, pp 324-353

Henderson IC, Gelman RS, Harris JR, Canellos GP (1986) Duration of therapy in adjuvant chemotherapy trials. NCI Monogr 1: 95-98

Hubay CA, Gordon NH, Crowe JP (1984) Antiestrogen-cytotoxic chemotherapy and bacillus Calmette-Guerin vaccination in stage II breast cancer: seventy-two months' follow-up. Surgery 96: 61-72

Ingle JN, Everson LK, Wieand HS, Martin JK, Wold LE, Krook JE, Ahman DL, Cullinan SA, Paulsen JK (1986) Randomized trial of adjuvant therapy with cyclophosphamide (C), 5-fluorouracil (F), prednisone (P) with or without tamoxifen (T) vs. observation following mastectomy in postmenopausal women with node-positive breast cancer. Proc Am Soc Clin Oncol 5: 70

Jungi WF, Alberto P, Brunner KW, Cavalli F, Barrelet L, Senn HJ (1981) Short- or long-term adjuvant chemotherapy for breast cancer. In: Salmon SE, Jones SE (eds) Adjuvant therapy of cancer III. Grune and Stratton, New York, pp 395-402

Kaplan EL, Meier P (1958) Nonparametric estimation from incomplete observations. J Am Stat Assoc 53: 457-481

Ludwig Breast Cancer Study Group (1983) Severe toxicity encountered in adjuvant combination chemotherapy for breast cancer administered in the immediate postmastectomy period. Lancet II: 542–544

Ludwig Breast Cancer Study Group (1984) Randomized trial of chemo-endocrine therapy, endocrine therapy, and mastectomy alone in postmenopausal patients with operable breast cancer and axillary node metastasis. Lancet I: 1256–1260

Nissen-Meyer R, Kjellgren K, Malmio K, Mansson B, Norin T (1978) Surgical adjuvant chemotherapy. Results with one short course of cyclophosphamide after mastectomy for breast cancer. Cancer 41: 2088–2098

Nissen-Meyer R, Host H, Kjellgren K, Mansson B, Norin T (1985) Short perioperative versus long-term adjuvant chemotherapy. In: Metzger U, Largiader F, Senn HJ (eds) Perioperative chemotherapy, Springer, Berlin Heidelberg New York Tokyo pp 91–98 (Recent results in cancer research, vol 98)

Perloff M, Norton L, Korzan A, Wood W, Carey R, Weinberg V, Holland JF (1986) Advantage of an adriamycin (A) combination plus halotestin (H) after initial cyclophosphamide, methotrexate, fluorouracil, vincristine and prednisone (CMFVP) for adjuvant therapy of node-positive stage II breast cancer. Proc Am Soc Clin Oncol 5: 70

Schabel Jr FM (1977) Rationale for adjuvant chemotherapy. Cancer 39: 2875–2882

Taylor SG, Kalish LA, Olson JE, Cummings F, Bennett JM, Falkson G, Tormey DC, Carbone PP (1985) Adjuvant CMFP vs. CMFP plus tamoxifen vs. observation alone in postmenopausal node-positive breast cancer patients. 3-year results of an ECOG study. J Clin Oncol 3: 144–154

UK-BCTSC/UICC/WHO (1984) Review of mortality results in randomized trials in early breast cancer. Lancet II: 1205

Is There a Role for Perioperative Adjuvant Cytotoxic Therapy in the Treatment of Early Breast Cancer?

J. Houghton[1], M. Baum[1], R. Nissen-Meyer[2], D. Riley[1], and R. A. Hern[1]

[1] CRC Clinical Trials Centre, Rayne Institue, 123 Coldharbour Lane,
London SE5 9NU, Great Britain
[2] Tyribakken 10, 0280 Oslo 2, Norway

Introduction

The use of perioperative adjuvant therapy in the treatment of breast cancer is not new; its history goes back to the mid-1960s when several groups experimented with the use of the then relatively new cytotoxic agents, giving them at about the same time as primary surgery. The conclusions drawn by the various authors show that controversy is not new to this field!

Mrazek and McDonald (1970), at a follow-up period of 8–13 years, compared patients treated by mastectomy alone with those who had mastectomy and nitrogen mustard 3 days perioperatively and three further courses, and concluded that all deaths in the chemotherapy group were unrelated to cancer. However, Finney (1971), who used cyclophosphamide for a total of 10 days beginning preoperatively, concluded that the survival rate of those treated with chemotherapy was considerably worse than those treated with surgery and radiation alone. The NSABP in a trial of over 800 patients, half of whom were randomised to receive thiotepa for 3 days perioperatively, found no significant differences in survival at 5 and 10 years, although subgroup analysis did show that premenopausal patients with four or more nodes had a significantly increased survival (Fisher et al. 1968, 1975).

The objective of this paper is to review two more recent perioperative trials, both using the same regimen, in order to determine what further information has been obtained about the role of perioperative therapy in the treatment of early breast cancer.

The Scandinavian Adjuvant Chemotherapy Study 1 (SACS-1)

The Scandinavian trial was set up in 1965 to investigate the use of a single course of cyclophosphamide (5 mg/kg/day i. v.) for 6 days perioperatively, the first dose being given immediately following the operation. Twenty-seven clinicians in 11 clinics in Finland, Norway and Sweden randomised 1026 patients between control and adjuvant treatment over a period of 11 years. The characteristics of

Table 1. Comparison of patient characteristics in the two trials (SACS-1 and CRC 2)

	SACS-1				CRC 2			
	Control		Cyclo-phosphamide		Control		Cyclo-phosphamide	
	n	(%)	n	(%)	n	(%)	n	(%)
Patients	519	(51)	507	(49)	1091	(49)	1139	(51)
Nodal status[a]								
– negative	302	(58)	310	(61)	531	(49)	560	(49)
– positive	217	(42)	197	(39)	442	(41)	462	(41)
Tumor size[a]								
– less than 2 cm	142	(27)	111	(22)	334	(31)	301	(26)
– 2 cm or more	377	(73)	396	(78)	715	(66)	703	(62)
Menopausal status[a]								
– premenopausal	222	(43)	200	(39)	398	(37)	402	(35)
– postmenopausal	285	(55)	294	(58)	563	(52)	632	(56)
Age at randomisation[a]								
– under 50 years	170	(33)	163	(32)	363	(33)	338	(30)
– 50 years and over	349	(67)	344	(68)	728	(67)	801	(70)
Patients also receiving tamoxifen					608	(56)	657	(58)

[a] In these strata, a few patients have unknown or missing data which explains why the numbers do not always add up to the totals.

patients entered into the trial are shown in Table 1. Subsequently, all these patients have been followed up and the results have been published (Nissen-Meyer et al. 1971, 1978). The relapse-free survival (RFS) (Fig. 1) shows a consistent benefit after 5 years for those patients treated with the short perioperative course ($\chi^2 = 11.03$, $P = 0.0009$). The overall survival (OS) (Fig. 2) does not reach conventional statistical significance ($\chi^2 = 3.17$, $P = 0.075$), but the advanced age of the patients, and therefore the high proportion of non-breast cancer deaths in the latter years of follow-up, probably accounts for this (Nissen-Meyer 1986).

Cancer Research Campaign Adjuvant Breast Trial (CRC2)

In 1980, the Cancer Research Campaign initiated a new study to repeat two previous trials; the SACS-1 and the Nolvadex Adjuvant Trial (NATO). The design used therefore was a 2×2 factorial one (Fig. 3), in which "main effects analysis" enables the use of all patients for either the cyclophosphamide or the tamoxifen comparisons. For example, to determine the effects of cyclophosphamide, patients in the cyclophosphamide-alone arm are compared with those in the control (no adjuvant therapy) arm, and this result is added to that obtained from the comparison between patients treated with cyclophosphamide and tamoxifen and those treated with tamoxifen alone.

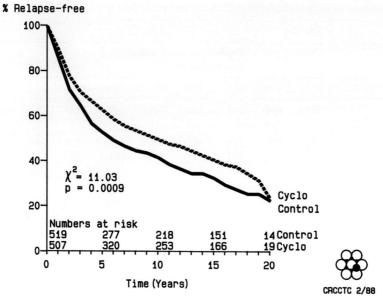

Fig. 1. SACS-1 Trial of perioperative cyclophosphamide: relapse-free survival. The number at risk represents the number of patients alive and event-free in each group at the beginning of each 5-year interval

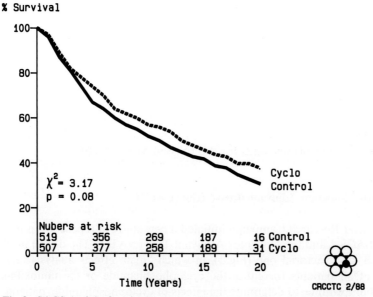

Fig. 2. SACS-1 trial of perioperative cyclophosphamide: overall survival

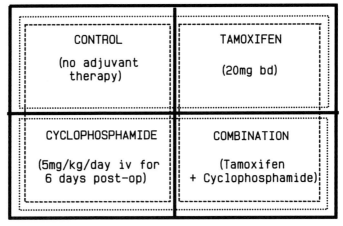

Fig. 3. 2×2 factorial design used in CRC Adjuvant Breast Trial (CRC 2). The *dashed line* represents main effects analysis for cyclophosphamide and the *dotted line,* for tamoxifen

The treatment regimens in the trial were designed to repeat exactly those in the previous study; cyclophosphamide was given at 5 mg/kg/day i.v. for 6 days immediately following primary surgery, the first injection being administered within 24 h of operation. Tamoxifen was given at 20 mg per day for 2 years, as in the NATO trial. All patients with clinical stage I or II disease and under the age of 75 years were eligible for randomisation. Initially, primary therapy was total mastectomy and axillary sampling, with radiotherapy for node-positive patients, or total mastectomy with full axillary clearance and no radiotherapy. However, owing to the increase in the number of clinicians performing lumpectomy as the primary surgical procedure, surgeons were allowed to randomise such patients from June 1983. Seventy-nine surgeons from 61 centres, mainly within the UK but also some from Eire, Greece and Australia, randomised 2230 patients in an approximately 5-year period. Patient characteristics are given in Table 1.

The main effects analysis for cyclophosphamide for first event (recurrence, new tumour or death) is shown in Fig. 4. Although a significant result has been reported previously, the present analysis does not reach conventional statistical significance ($\chi^2 = 3.09$). However, the trend still remains for benefit in the cyclophosphamide group. When stratified according to nodal and menstrual status or age, the relative risk is in favour of the cyclophosphamide group in each stratum (Table 2). Currently, there is no effect on survival ($\chi^2 = 0.25$, $P = 0.62$).

Toxicity

The toxicity of the regimen was mild compared with that reported from patients treated with multiple drug chemotherapy. The most commonly reported side effects in the CRC trial were alopecia (43% patients), with 20% requiring wigs, and nausea (20% patients). Severe leucopenia at 14 days was reported in only 6.8% patients. That the therapy was well tolerated is indicated by the fact that, of the patients allocated to cyclophosphamide, over 90% completed the 6-day course.

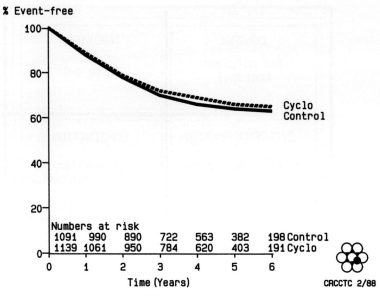

% Event-free

Fig. 4. CRC Adjuvant Breast Trial: cyclophosphamide main effect analysis for first event

Table 2. Logrank analysis of the effect of cyclophosphamide on first event stratified by nodal and menstrual status

	Control		Cyclophosphamide		
	n	O/E	n	O/E	χ^2
Node-negative	531	1.09	560	0.92	1.77
Node-positive	442	1.03	462	0.97	0.36
Overall stratified[a]	973	1.05	1022	0.95	1.64
Premenopausal[b]	398	1.02	402	0.98	0.08
Postmenopausal	563	1.10	632	0.91	3.34
Overall stratified[a]	961	1.06	1034	0.94	2.47
Under 50 years	363	1.02	338	0.98	0.06
50 years and over	728	1.07	801	0.94	2.34
Overall stratified[a]	1091	1.05	1139	0.95	1.99

O/E is the ratio of the observed events to the expected events calculated from a lifetable.
[a] Histological node and menstrual status was not known in all cases.
[b] The premenopausal group is defined as patients having had their last period within 2 years.

Overview of SACS-1 and CRC 2

The data from the two trials can be combined in a similar way in which the breast cancer trials overview has been performed (Anonymous 1984). The results of this analysis for first event are shown in Table 3 for the main strata (node-negative and -positive, pre- and postmenopausal). Since the CRC trial has a median follow-up

Table 3. Overview analysis of first even in nodal and menstrual strata of SACS-1 and CRC 2 trials

	n	O-E	Relative risk[a]	χ^2	P
Node-negative					
SACS-1	612	− 14.09			
CRC 2	1091	− 10.02			
	1703	− 24.11	0.78 (0.64–0.95)	5.85	0.016
Node-positive					
SACS-1	414	− 17.81			
CRC 2	904	− 5.94			
	1318	− 23.75	0.86 (0.74–1.00)	3.45	0.06
Overall	3021	− 47.86	0.83 (0.74–0.94)	8.71	0.003
Premenopausal					
SACS-1	422	− 18.26			
CRC2	800	− 2.26			
	1222	− 20.52	0.83 (0.68–0.99)	3.90	0.048
Postmenopausal					
SACS-1	579	− 12.50			
CRC 2	1195	− 17.33			
	1774	− 29.83	0.82 (0.70–0.96)	5.82	0.016
Overall	2996	− 50.35	0.82 (0.73–0.93)	9.73	0.002

[a] 95% confidence interval given in parentheses.

Table 4. Summary overview analysis of survival in nodal and menstrual states of SACS-1 and CRC 2

	Relative risk	95% confidence interval	χ^2	P
Node-negative	0.81	0.61–1.08	2.08	0.15
Node-positive	0.99	0.81–1.20	0.01	0.91
Premenopausal	0.79	0.63–1.02	3.36	0.07
Postmenopausal	1.00	0.80–1.25	0.00	0.97

of only approximately 4 years, the data from the SACS-1 have also been limited to the first 5 years. Doubling the observed minus expected value gives the approximate number of patients who would have been saved from having an event (or death) had all the patients received treatment. A negative value indicates that the treated group is doing better than the control group. For each stratum, patients treated with cyclophosphamide show some benefit, and only in the node-positive patients does this fail to reach conventional statistical significance. There is no evidence that any particular subgroup achieves a greater response rate than the others.

Discussion

As already discussed, the role of perioperative adjuvant therapy has long been under investigation, and the results from the SACS-1 trial were first published many years ago. However, apart from some Scandinavian groups, perioperative therapy has been little used in the routine management of early breast cancer, although other groups are now carrying out further investigations in the context of clinical trials. The overview presented in this paper suggests that one short perioperative course of cyclophosphamide increases RFS in all subgroups, unlike prolonged chemotherapy, which seems to be effective primarily in the younger age group (Anonymous 1984). Therefore, the question of whether perioperative therapy produces its effect through the same mechanism of action is raised. Nissen-Meyer (1979) has suggested that the short course of cyclophosphamide kills cells shed at about the time of operation, and it is this cell-killing effect which produces the prolonged difference in RFS.

In fact, the whole question of the timing of adjuvant chemotherapy in breast cancer has received little attention. The second Scandinavian trial (SACS-2) has compared the administration of a single perioperative cyclophosphamide, methotrexate, 5-fluorouracil (CMF) course with perioperative plus six cycles of CMF, and demonstrated an increased RFS for the prolonged therapy group but at a cost of increased toxicity (Nissen-Meyer 1986). The Ludwig group has run a similar study, and their preliminary results are to be presented at this meeting (Goldhirsch and Gelber, this volume). Therefore, trials are still needed to further elucidate the best timing and the duration of adjuvant chemotherapy.

Is there, then, a role for a single course of cyclophosphamide in the management of early breast cancer? The consistent increase in RFS and the tendency towards increased OS for a regimen which is well tolerated and easy to administer would suggest that there is. In many centres, conventionally timed chemotherapy is only given once the nodal status has been determined, but perioperative cyclophosphamide could be given routinely to all women undergoing surgery for early breast cancer, since it seems to have a similar effect in all prognostic subgroups. Patients who are later found to have a poor prognosis could then be started on longer-term adjuvant therapy, while node-negative patients could well have benefited from the single course.

Acknowledgements. The authors wish to thank the Cancer Research Campaign for their continued financial support, the SACSG for allowing meta-analysis of their data and all the participating clinicians in both trials for their extra unrewarded work.

References

Anonymous (1984) Review of mortality results in randomised trials in early breast cancer. Lancet II: 1035–1036

Finney R (1971) Adjuvant chemotherapy in the radical treatment of carcinoma of the breast – a clinical trial. Am J Roentgenol III: 137–141

Fisher B, Ravdin RG, Ausman RK, Slack NH, Moore GET; Noor RJ (1968) Surgical adjuvant chemotherapy in cancer of the breast; results of a decade of cooperative investigation. Ann Surg 168: 337–356

Fisher B, Slack N, Katryu D, Wolmark N (1975) Ten year follow-up of breast cancer patients in a cooperative clinical trial evaluating surgical adjuvant chemotherapy. Surg Gynecol Obstet 140: 528–534

Goldhirsch A (1988) Early results of randomised perioperative therapy in operable breast cancer: the Ludwig Breast Cancer Study V, presented at 3rd international conference on adjuvant therapy of primary breast cancer.

Mrazek RG, McDonald GO (1970) Surgery and adjuvant chemotherapy in treatment for breast carcinoma. Oncology – Proceedings of the tenth international cancer congress, Houston, Texas, p. 501

Nissen-Meyer R (1979) Adjuvant cytostatic and endocrine therapy: increased cure rate or delayed manifest disease. In: Commentaries on research in breast disease 1. Liss, New York.

Nissen-Meyer R, Kjellgren K, Mansson B (1971) Preliminary report from the Scandinavian adjuvant chemotherapy study group. Cancer Chemotherapy Reports 55: 561–566

Nissen-Meyer R, Kjellgren K, Malmio K, Mansson B, Norin T (1978) Surgical adjuvant chemotherapy. Results with one short course with cyclophosphamide after mastectomy for breast cancer. Cancer 41: 2088–2098

Nissen-Meyer R, Host M, Kjellgren K, Mansson B, Norin T (1986) Treatment of node-negative breast cancer patients with short course of chemotherapy immediately after surgery. NCI Monogr 1: 125–134

Problems of Rational Follow-up and Salvage Therapy

Radiation Therapy in Prevention and Salvage of Local Relapse: Its Prognostic Implication

R. Hünig und J. M. Kurtz

Department of Radiation Oncology, University Hospital, 4031 Basel, Switzerland

Introduction

"Adjuvant" radiotherapy has the same meaning as "elective" radiotherapy, an expression introduced considerably earlier by radiation oncologists. This refers to the irradiation of potentially involved areas, which have been judged operatively or clinically to be free of cancer. As is the case with adjuvant systemic therapy, the indication for elective radiotherapy depends upon the probability with which a recurrence in the given area is to be expected. How great the likelihood of recurrence need be in order to justify an adjuvant therapy is a value judgement, influenced, at least in part, by the expected therapeutic efficiency as well as the potential side effects and risks of such treatment. In addition, it must be taken into consideration in what ways the adjuvant therapy might interfere or interact with other treatments which might be required either simultaneously or at a later time.

The local effectiveness, as well as the local and the general side effects of radiotherapy, are influenced by the following four physical factors: target volume, the maximum and minimum dose within this volume, the fractionation (dose/time), and the dose distribution in adjacent normal tissues (dependent, as is the dose distribution within the target volume, upon the therapy technique).

Based on the analysis of retrospective data, Fletcher et al. (1968) were first to postulate that subclinical tumor manifestations could be sterilized in most cases by the application of 45-50 Gy in 4.5-5 weeks. This observation has since been confirmed by numerous studies. It is also worth mentioning in this regard that adjuvant radiotherapy with modern equipment and techniques is generally well tolerated.

Potential Benefits of Adjuvant Radiotherapy

If adjuvant radiotherapy following mastectomy is to have an influence on prognosis, this can be achieved only when the treatment reduces the frequency of local-regional recurrences, and when this leads as a result to a reduction in the frequency of distant metastases. This is possible only in a subgroup of patients who have

Recent Results in Cancer Research, Vol. 115
© Springer-Verlag Berlin·Heidelberg 1989

Table 1. Randomized trials concerning adjuvant radiotherapy after radical, modified radical or simple mastectomy

Number	Trial	Year of onset	References
1. A	Manchester Q	1949	Paterson 1962; Easson 1968
B	Manchester P	1952	Palmer and Ribeiro 1985
2. A	Oslo I	1964	Host et al. 1986
B	Oslo II	1968	
3.	Stockholm	1971	Wallgren et al. 1986
4.	Manchester Regional	1970	Lythgoe and Palmer 1982
5.	CRC	1970	Cancer Research Campaign Working Party 1980
6.	NSABP-BO4	1971	Fisher et al. 1985
7.	Edinburgh I	1974	Duncan et al. 1975

local-regional subclinical disease present and, at the same time, have no other occult tumor manifestations in distant sites. This subgroup which might benefit from adjuvant radiotherapy is likely to be rather small in patients with breast cancer. Whether or not such a subgroup exists or has clinical relevance could be demonstrated only by properly designed and conducted randomized clinical trials. Up to the present time, nine trials of this sort have been reported (Table 1).

The methodology and results of trials 1, 2 A, 4–5, and 7 have been critically reviewed on numerous occasions (Bedwinek 1984; Cuzick et al. 1987; Levitt and Potish 1980; Levitt 1986). Based on accepted rules for the conduct of clinical trials and/or contemporary standards of radiotherapy practice, these five studies need no longer be accepted as authoritative. At the very least, these studies do not rule out the possibility that adjuvant radiotherapy conducted under optimal conditions might have a beneficial effect on prognosis.

The following comments are based exclusively on the Second Oslo Trial (Host et al. 1986), the Stockholm Trial (Wallgren et al. 1986), and the NSABP Trial B-04 (Fisher et al. 1985), in which megavoltage therapy was employed according to uniform guidelines. First, regarding local-regional recurrences, the following can be accepted as established: (a) Adjuvant radiotherapy leads to a marked diminution in local-regional recurrences in both node-negative and node-positive tumors, (b) Adjuvant radiotherapy not only delays recurrences, it prevents their appearance. This is demonstrated by the local-regional disease-free survival curves, which show no tendency to come together with time.

As indicated by the title of this paper, the possible influence of adjuvant radiotherapy on overall survival is the principal concern of this analysis. In the Oslo Trial, adjuvant radiotherapy led to a small, non-significant ($P = 0.15$) improvement in overall survival, but only in patients with node-positive tumors. Similarly, in the Stockholm Trial there was also a statistically insignificant survival benefit for the patients with irradiated node-positive tumors ($P = 0.09$), which was 54% after 8 years in comparison with 47% in the controls treated by surgery alone.

In the NSABP B-04 Trial, clinically node-negative patients were randomized to three arms (radical mastectomy versus simple mastectomy with or without radiotherapy) and clinically node-positive patients to two arms (radical mastectomy versus simple mastectomy with radiotherapy). After 10 years, there was no advantage in any of the arms for either risk group, suggesting that adjuvant radiotherapy had no significant effect on overall and distant disease-free survival.

Several additional interesting observations can be made from these trials: in the Oslo Trial, node-positive patients with central or medial tumors had a 20% better overall survival after 10 years in the irradiated group. Because of the small number of patients in these subgroups, the difference did not reach statistical significance ($P=0.08$), or perhaps the difference is not real. This tendency could not, however, be confirmed by the B-04 study.

In addition, in the Oslo Trial, irradiated node-negative patients suffered a significantly higher mortality from myocardial infarctions than their nonirradiated counterparts. This presumably reflected the direct irradiation of the mediastinum with cobalt-60, employing rather large daily doses.

In the Stockholm Trial, the following conclusions could be drawn regarding node-positive patients:

1. Radiation therapy led to significant reduction in the cumulative rate of distant metastases (from 60% to 47% after 11 years, $P=0.01$).
2. The survival benefit associated with radiation therapy was of the same magnitude as that observed in the Milan Adjuvant cyclophosphamide, methotrexate, 5-fluorouracil (CMF) Trial after 8 years (Bonadonna et al. 1983; Wallgren et al. 1986).

As a result of their experience, Wallgren et al. voiced the opinion that, with the proper techniques, adjuvant radiotherapy has fewer side effects than chemotherapy. They concluded that for many high-risk patients adjuvant radiotherapy might be considered as a worthy alternative to adjuvant chemotherapy.

Combined Adjuvant Radio- and Chemotherapy

Since the above studies demonstrate that elective radiotherapy results in a marked reduction in local-regional recurrences and possibly a small reduction in distant metastases, it would be of great interest to investigate the use of radiotherapy in combination with adjuvant chemotherapy. Of the prospective studies addressing this question, three are particularly worthy of mention. The first, from the Southeastern Cancer Study Group (Velez-Garcia et al. 1987), randomized mastectomized patients with four or more positive nodes to three arms: 6 or 12 months CMF chemotherapy or radiotherapy followed by 6 months CMF. After a median follow-up of 5 years, there was no significant difference between the three arms with respect to overall and disease-free survival, local-regional recurrences, or distant metastases, although there was a trend in favor of the combined modality arm (Table 2).

In the second study, which was performed in Boston (Griem et al. 1987), mastectomized stage II and selected stage III patients were divided into a moderate and a high-risk group, according to tumor size and the extent of lymph node involvement. Moderate-risk patients were randomized between two different chemotherapy regimens, CMF and methotrexate, 5-fluorouracil (MF). High risk patients

Table 2. Sites and frequency of relapse in patients with four or more positive nodes (Velez-Garcia et al. 1987)[a]

Treatment arm	(n)	Local-regional		Local-regional and distant		Distant only	
		(n')	(%)	(n')	(%)	(n')	(%)
6 months CMF	122	14	11	7	6	49	40
12 months CMF	55	4	7	5	9	24	44
RT + 6 months CMF	119	6	9	3	3	41	34

RT, radiation therapy; CMF, cyclophosphamide + methotrexate + 5-fluorouracil.
[a] Median follow-up, 60 months.

were randomized between five or ten cycles of a more aggressive chemotherapy program (cyclophosphamide adriamycin, (A)). In addition, both risk groups were randomized to receive or not receive adjuvant radiotherapy upon completion of chemotherapy. With a median follow-up of 53 months for the CMF/MF patients, the local failure rate was 0% and 5% with and without radiotherapy (statistically not significant). For the CA patients after a median follow-up 45 months, local failure was observed in 2.3% of the patients receiving radiotherapy, compared with 20% receiving chemotherapy alone ($P = 0.007$). In each group, one patient developed local recurrence during chemotherapy.

With respect to overall survival and disease-free survival, there was no advantage for patients randomized to radiotherapy in either risk group. It should be mentioned, however, that 34 patients randomized to receive radiotherapy were not irradiated, and one patient who had been randomized to observation received radiotherapy. The cardiotoxicity of the CA arm was studied and was identical for patients receiving or not receiving radiotherapy.

The third study (Kleefström et al. 1987) comes from Helsinki, where 119 patients with operable clinical stage III cancers (T3 N0–2) were randomized to three treatment arms: adjuvant radiotherapy, adjuvant radiotherapy followed by adjuvant chemotherapy, and adjuvant chemotherapy. All patients were randomized in addition to receive or not to receive levamisole. Chemotherapy consisted of six cycles of vincristine, Adriamycin and cyclophosphamide (VAC). The minumum follow-up was 5 years. Both disease-free and overall survival were significantly better in the combined therapy arm than in either of the single-modality arms. Levamisole produced an additional overall improvement.

The following conclusions may be drawn from these studies:

1. Adjuvant chemotherapy alone does not solve the local recurrence problem for high-risk patients (four or more involved nodes, large tumors).
2. Although the addition of radiotherapy to the adjuvant program reduces local recurrence rates, significant survival benefit from this combination has yet to be demonstrated.
3. The use of the both modalities together need not be associated with unacceptable toxicity.

Salvage of Local Relapse

As mentioned previously, control of recurrence by means of local therapies can favorably influence prognosis only if this represents the only remaining disease manifestation, under the assumption that the recurrence can act as a source of later metastases. If recurrence is simply the expression of pre-existing dissemination, then "curative" local treatment of the recurrence will hardly have any significant effect on prognosis. In the first situation, an aggressive treatment of recurrence is certainly justified. In the latter case, its principal value lies in the prevention of the unpleasant physical and psychological consequences of uncontrolled local-regional disease.

Unfortunately, there are so far no results from prospective studies allowing definitive conclusions to be drawn regarding the following important questions:

1. What influence do initial tumor stage and initial therapy have on the disease course and prognosis following recurrence?
2. Which patient-related and/or biological factors influence the disease course and prognosis following initial therapy as well as after recurrence?
3. What is the prognostic significance of the disease-free interval between primary therapy and the clinical manifestation of recurrence?
4. What combination of surgery, radiotherapy, and systemic therapy is under given conditions the most effective for the control of local recurrence and associated subclinical metastases?

The results of retrospective studies suggest that the course of the disease after recurrence can be extremely variable. Survival after recurrence correlates with a variety of factors, which are at least in part mutually interdependent. These include initial tumor extent, disease-free interval, the macroscopic aspect of the recurrence (single nodule, multiple nodules, diffuse), and possibly hormone receptor status. In addition, most studies suggest that prognosis after recurrence depends upon whether or not local control could be permanently achieved. It is impossible to state whether this represents a direct effect of treatment or simply an expression of the various patient and tumor-related factors mentioned previously. The available literature does not allow a more precise analysis of the complex inter-relationships between these parameters.

It should be emphasized that, even under optimal conditions, local control or recurrent disease can only be achieved in 50%–70% of recurrences. Although resectable recurrences have a more favorable prognosis and excision probably contributes to local disease control, only a minority of recurrences are amenable to surgical treatment. The effectiveness of therapy therefore appears to depend most strongly upon the quality of the radiation treatment. Several retrospective analyses have attempted to demonstrate the direct influence of radiotherapy on prognosis. Given the multiplicity of techniques and doses, local control rates were quite variable. Bedwinek et al. (1981) were able to show that "adequate" radiotherapy was associated with a local control rate of 72%, in contrast to 28% for "inadequate" radiotherapy (Table 3). The control rate was the same whether or not surgical excision had been performed and overall survival was unaffected by local control. Similar conclusions regarding local control rates were made by Patanaphan et al.

Table 3. Local-regionally recurrent breast cancer: effect of RT on subsequent local control

Author	Therapy	Local-regional control (%)
Bedwinek et al. (1981)	"adequate" RT	72
	"inadequate" RT	28
Patanaphan et al. (1984)	"adequate" RT	72
	"inadequate" RT	48
Magno et al. (1987)	"adequate" RT	50
	"inadequate" RT	32

Table 4. 5-Year survival following isolated chest wall recurrence: influence of response to treatment on survival

Author	Local disease status	5-year survival (%)
Chen et al. (1985)	controlled	63
	uncontrolled	34
Stadler et al. (1987)	controlled	40–45
	uncontrolled	20
Magno et al. (1987)	controlled	42
	uncontrolled	5

(1984) and by Magno et al. (1987). Chen et al. (1985), Stadler and Kogelnik (1987), and Magno et al. (1987) also analyzed survival as a function of local control and found marked differences at 5 years, ranging from a factor of 2 to 5 (Table 4).

As mentioned previously, it is possible that the positive correlation between local control and survival is not directly related to the beneficial effect of therapy, but rather to differing distribution of relevant prognostic factors between the treatment groups.

Can radiotherapy alone or as an adjuvant in the treatment of recurrence have a significant influence on prognosis? A clear answer to this question must await completion of properly designed and carefully executed randomized clinical trials.

References

Bedwinek JM (1984) Adjuvant irradiation for early breast cancer. An on-going controversy. Cancer 53: 729–739
Bedwinek JM, Fineberg B, Lee J, Ocwieza M (1981) Analysis of failures following local treatment of isolated local-regional recurrence of breast cancer. Int J Radiat Oncol Biol Phys 7: 581–585
Bonadonna G, Rossi A, Tancini G, Valagussa P (1983) Adjuvant chemotherapy in breast cancer. Lancer I: 1157

Cancer Research Campaign Working Party (1980) Cancer Research Campaign (King's/ Cambridge) trial for early breast cancer. Lancet II: 55-60

Chen KK-Y, Montague ED, Oswald JM (1985) Results of irradiation in the treatment of locoregional breast cancer recurrence. Cancer 56: 1269-1273

Cuzick J, Stewart H, Peto R, Baum M, Fisher B, Host H, Lythgoe JP, Ribeiro GG, Scheurlen H, Wallgren A (1987) Overview of randomized trials of postoperative adjuvant radiotherapy in breast cancer. Cancer Treat Rep 71: 15-29

Duncan W, Forrest APM, Gray N, Hamilton T, Langlands AO, Prescott RJ, Shivas AA, Stewart HJ (1975) New Edinburgh primary breast cancer trials. Br J Cancer 32: 628-630

Easson EC (1968) Post-operative radiotherapy in breast cancer. In: Forrest APM, Kunkler PB (eds) Prognostic factors in breast cancer. Churchill Livingstone, Edinburgh, pp 118-127

Fisher B, Redmond C, Fisher ER, Bauer M, Wolmark N, Wickerham L, Deutsch M, Montague E. Margolese R, Forster R (1985) Ten-year results of a randomized clinical trial comparing radical mastectomy and total mastectomy with or without radiation. N Engl J Med 312: 674-681

Fletcher GH, Montague ED, White EC (1968) Evaluation of irradiation of peripheral lymphatics in conjunction with radical mastectomy for cancer of the breast. Cancer 21: 791-797

Griem KL, Henderson IC, Gelman R, Ascoli D, Silver B, Recht A, Goodman RL, Hellman S, Harris JR (1987) The 5-year results of a randomized trial of adjuvant radiation therapy after chemotherapy in breast cancer patients treated with mastectomy. J Clin Oncol 5: 1546-1555

Host H, Brennhovd IO, Loeb M (1986) Postoperative radiotherapy in breast cancer - Long-term results from the Oslo study. Int J Radiat Oncol Biol Phys 12: 727-732

Kleefström P, Gröhn P, Heinonen E, Holsti L, Holsti P (1987) Adjuvant postoperative radiotherapy, chemotherapy, and immunotherapy in stage III breast cancer. II. 5 year-results and influence of Levamisole. Cancer 60: 936-942

Levitt SH (1986) The role of radiation therapy as an adjuvant in the treatment of breast cancer. Int J Radiat Oncol Biol Phys 12: 843-844

Levitt SH, Potish RA (1980) The role of radiation therapy in the treatment of breast cancer: The use and abuse of clinical trials, statistics and unproven hypotheses. Int J Radiat Oncol Biol Phys 6: 791-798

Lythgoe JP, Palmer MK (1982) Manchester regional breast study - 5 and 10 year results. Br J Surg 69: 693-696

Magno L, Bignardi M, Micheletti E, Bardelli D, Plebani F (1987) Analysis of prognostic factors in patients with isolated chest wall recurrence of breast cancer. Cancer 60: 240-244

Palmer MK, Ribeiro GG (1985) Thirty-four-year follow up of patients with breast cancer in a clinical trial of postoperative radiotherapy. Br Med J 291: 1088-1091

Patanaphan V, Salazar OM, Poussin-Rosillo H (1984) Prognosticators in recurrent breast cancer. Cancer 54: 228-234

Paterson R (1962) Breast cancer: A report of two clinical trials. J R Coll Surg Edinb 7: 243-254

Stadler B, Kogelnik HD (1987) Local control and outcome of patients irradiated for isolated chest wall recurrences of breast cancer. Radiother Oncol 8: 105-111

Velez-Garcia E, Carpenter JT, Moore M, Vogel CL, Marcial V, Ketcham A, Raney M, Smalley R (1987) Postsurgical adjuvant chemotherapy with or without radiotherapy in women with breast cancer and positive nodes: Progress report of a Southeastern Cancer Study Group (SEG) trial. In: Salmon SE (ed) Adjuvant therapy of cancer V. Grune and Stratton, Orlando, pp 347-355

Wallgren A, Arner O, Bergström J, Blomstedt B, Granberg P-O, Rät L, Siltverswärd C, Einhorn J (1986) Radiation therapy in operable breast cancer: Results from the Stockholm trial on adjuvant radiotherapy. Int J Radiat Oncol Biol Phys 12: 533-537

Salvage Treatments in Relapsing Resectable Breast Cancer*

P. Valagussa, C. Brambilla, M. Zambetti, and G. Bonadonna

Istituto Nazionale Tumori, Via Venezian, 1, 20133 Milano, Italy

Introduction

There is convincing evidence that the natural history of resectable breast cancer can be perturbed by adjuvant medical intervention. In fact, a highly significant reduction in the recurrence rate has been documented, which was reflected in a highly significant reduction in the odds of death following adjuvant chemotherapy, especially in premenopausal women (Bonadonna and Valagussa 1988; Consensus Conference 1985; Henderson 1987). Nonetheless, despite improvements in primary treatments, a considerable proportion of women who receive adjuvant therapy subsequently develop recurrent disease. The proper management of these patients, can present a therapeutic problem. In fact, the prognostic variables at the time of first treatment failure can be considerably different as far as disease-free interval, the anatomical extent of recurrence, patient performance status, menopausal and steroid-receptor status are concerned. Limited case series have been reported so far in medical literature (Bitran et al. 1983; Buzdar et al. 1981; Chlebowsky et al. 1981; Morris et al. 1985; Wendt et al. 1980), and all concerned women who relapsed after adjuvant chemotherapy. The conclusions about the efficacy of salvage therapy have been somewhat contradictory; controversies also exist about whether previous adjuvant therapy, especially chemotherapy, could adversely affect survival after recurrence (Brincker et al. 1987).

In this report, we update our previous publication (Valagussa et al. 1986) on first salvage treatments in patients who failed after surgery alone (control) compared with cyclophosphamide, methotrexate, and fluorouracil (CMF)-treated patients.

* Supported in part by Contract NO1-CM-07338 with the Division of Cancer Treatment, National Cancer Institute, National Institutes of Health.

Patients and Methods

Starting in June 1973, we enrolled 1065 women with resectable breast cancer and histologically-positive axillary nodes into two successive randomized trials and into a non-randomized study. A total of 179 patients were subjected to radical or modified radical mastectomy alone, whereas in the remaining 886 women the adjuvant treatment consisted of CMF chemotherapy administered for 12 or 6 monthly cycles (Bonadonna et al. 1985). The treatment outcome was recently reported within the context of the experience achieved by our Institute on postoperative adjuvant chemotherapy (Bonadonna et al. 1987).

The records of 578 primary treatment failures were reviewed. The details regarding eligibility criteria for entry into adjuvant programs, drug administrations, timing, and methods of follow-up have previously been reported in detail (Bonadonna et al. 1985; Valagussa et al. 1981).

A total of 127 failures were documented among the 179 patients of the control group, and 451 relapses were observed among 886 women scheduled to receive either 6 or 12 cycles of adjuvant CMF. The type of first salvage treatment was not systematically planned in the original study protocols. The treatment choice varied according to whether adjuvant CMF had already been administered, disease presentation, age and clinical situation, length of disease-free interval, and estrogen-receptor (ER) assay availability. For the purpose of the present analysis, a total of 137 failures (23%) were not considered evaluable (controls: 23 women or 18%; CMF: 114 or 25%) for the following reasons. Contralateral breast cancer as the first and only site of new disease manifestation was documented in 40 of 137 patients; 17 patients refused to take any form of treatment at the time of relapse; 29 women, two of whom were in the control group, died of rapidly progressive disease before anticancer treatment could be instituted. Finally, 44 patients received their first salvage therapy outside the Institute, and details on the types of treatment were not available, whereas seven women presented new disease manifestations less than 3 month prior to the date of present analysis.

A total of 441 patients (control: 104; CMF: 337) were therefore available for the analysis of response to various salvage treatments. The main salvage modalities are reported in Table 1. As can be seen, systemic therapy was given to 90% of the patients in the control group and to 95% of women in the CMF group.

Despite efforts always to administer systemic treatment, a total of 26 patients were treated with local-regional therapy alone, i.e., radiotherapy and/or surgery.

Table 1. Main salvage treatments in relapsing operable breast cancer

	Control		Adjuvant CMF	
	(n)	(%)	(n)	(%)
Local therapy	10	10	16	5
Castration	12	12	55	16
Endocrine therapy	17	16	139	41
Combined chemoendocrine therapy	10	10	29	9
Chemotherapy	55	52	98	29

Fourteen patients presented with local-regional recurrence alone and five other patients with a single bone lesion. Two patients presenting with metastasis to the choroid, in one case associated with a single bone lesion, and four women with brain involvement underwent local irradiation. Finally, one patient presented with a single pulmonary nodule, and lobectomy was performed for diagnostic as well as for therapeutic purposes. It is worth mentioning that the majority of these 26 patients were treated and followed up outside the Outpatient Medical Oncology Clinic.

The details on types and schedules of systemic treatments have previously been reported (Valagussa et al. 1986). It is worth noting that about half of the patients in the control group were given salvage chemotherapy, whereas 57% of women in the adjuvant CMF group received salvage endocrine therapy (Table 1).

Evaluation of Treatment Response

Complete remission (CR) was defined as the complete disappearance of all symptoms and signs of disease with recalcification of osteolytic bone metastases. In this category, we also entered a total of 28 patients, whose first new disease manifestation was surgically removed and whose disease-free status lasted for a minimum of 6 months. There were 26 women who presented with soft tissue involvement (mainly local-regional recurrences), one patient with metastases to the ovary, and one patient with a single pulmonary nodule. Partial remission (PR) was classified as a 50% or greater reduction in the product of the two largest diameters of the indicator lesions without appearance of new sites of disease manifestation and with partial recalcification of osteolytic lesions. Patients who did not achieve either CR or PR were categorized as treatment failures. This category also includes patients with osseous involvement, whose disease remained stable for longer than 6 months.

Statistical Analysis

The duration of remission and survival were estimated by the Kaplan-Meier product-limit method (1958) and were computed from the starting date of salvage treatment. In the subset of patients taking part in the first adjuvant program, overall survival was also computed from the date of surgery.

Results

Following salvage local-regional treatment, the response rate was 40% in the control group and 44% in the CMF group and, apart from the two patients presenting with metastasis to the choroid and with a single pulmonary nodule, treatment response was observed primarily in soft tissue lesions. Despite this fact, response duration was short, lasting a median of 14 months in the control group and 13 months in the CMF-treated group.

Table 2. Therapeutic castration

	Control		CMF	
	(n)	(%)	(n)	(%)
NED prior to castration	3/12	25	4/55	7
With ovarian metastases only	1/12	8	0	
CR plus PR	1/8	12	10/51	20
With amenorrhea				21
No amenorrhea				19
Response duration,	12		20	
median in months				
(range)	(8–133$^+$)		(4–54$^+$)	

NED, no evidence of disease (local-regional recurrence surgically removed).

Combined chemoendocrine treatments were administered to a total of 39 patients (control: 10; CMF: 29). Eight patients in the control group achieved CR plus PR, whereas a response was documented in 52% of women in the CMF group. The median response duration was 15 and 18 months, respectively.

A total of 223 patients (control: 29; CMF: 194) were subjected to various endocrine manipulations. Table 2 details the results achieved with therapeutic castration in 67 premenopausal women. Three patients in the control group and four women in the CMF group underwent castration following surgical removal of soft tissue involvement, while one additional patient had disease limited to the ovary. It is worth emphasizing that the frequency of remission was unrelated to CMF-induced amenorrhea. In fact, in patients with measurable disease, the CR plus PR rate was 21% in women with drug-induced amenorrhea and 19% in patients in whom CMF did not induce cessation of menses. ER assay was available only in a minority of patients, and the objective response related to ER-positive tumors was as follows: control group, 0 of 2; CMF group, 8 of 30 cases.

Additive endocrine therapy was administered to 17 failures in the control group and to 139 CMF-treated women. In the control group, about half of patients given salvage endocrine treatment presented with soft tissue lesions as compared with approximately one-third of women failing in the adjuvant therapy group. The treatment results somewhat reflect this different pattern of presentation with a higher response rate (59% vs. 37%) and a longer remission duration (32 vs. 25 months) favoring control patients. Tamoxifen was administered to 14 patients in the control group and to 122 women in the CMF group, with a response rate of 62% and 40%, respectively. Estrogen-receptor assays, performed either at the time of mastectomy or upon relapse were available in 70 patients in the CMF series and the response rate in ER-positive tumors was 42%.

Salvage chemotherapy was administered to a total of 153 women (control: 55; CMF: 98). Table 3 presents the essential findings. In the control group, 45 women received therapeutic CMF, whereas in the CMF series, 35 patients were retreated with CMF, and 58 were given adriamycin (ADM) or regimens containing ADM. The remaining 10 control and 15 CMF patients mainly received single alkylating agents. Overall, more than 40% of women given chemotherapy as first salvage treatment presented with visceral involvement. In the control group, therapeutic

Table 3. Chemotherapy as first salvage treatment

	CTR	CMF	
	CMF ($n=45$)	CMF ($n=35$)	ADM Regimens ($n=58$)
Dominant disease in viscera (%)	42	43	48
CR + PR (%)	38	37	38
RFS ≤ 12 months[a]		0	31
RFS > 12 months[a]		48	45
Response duration, median in months	20	22	17
(range)	($11-81^+$)	($8-100^+$)	($7-91$)

[a] From end of adjuvant CMF.

CMF was able to induce CR plus PR in 38% of women for a median response duration of 20 months from the start of therapy.

In the adjuvant CMF failures, salvage chemotherapy was able to induce remission in 38% of women, but treatment response was influenced by the relapse-free interval (RFS) from the end of adjuvant therapy. In fact, when RFS was less than 12 months, none of the eight patients retreated with CMF could achieve remission, which was attained in nine of 29 women treated with salvage ADM regimens. By contrast, when RFS lasted longer than 12 months, the treatment response was similar following CMF retreatment (13 of 27, or 48%) and ADM regimens (13 of 29, or 45%). It is important to stress that patterns of disease presentation were unrelated to the length of RFS. It is worth mentioning that four women given CMF in the control group and five women retreated with CMF refused to continue treatment after six cycles while the disease was in remission, and tamoxifen was then administered. Similarly, seven responders in the ADM regimens were given tamoxifen or medroxyprogesterone acetate once the cumulative dose of adriamycin was approaching 450 mg/m^2. While sequential endocrine treatment was unable to improve the extent of remission in partial responders, the median response duration in these patients was 38, 30, and 54 months, respectively.

The median duration of overall survival was calculated for the entire series of patients (control: 104; CMF: 337) as well as for patients taking part in the first CMF program (control: 104; CMF: 90) to allow a proper comparison in women with a similar length of follow-up. The results are presented in Table 4, and their

Table 4. Median survival in months

	Control	CMF
Total series		
From relapse	35	31
First CMF program		
From relapse	35	34
From mastectomy	60	60

similarity is quite impressive. In fact, regardless of whether adjuvant CMF was administered, the median overall survival from relapse is less than 3 years, while the median survival from mastectomy is 60 months.

Discussion

The results of our retrospective analysis on first salvage treatment in relapsing resectable breast cancer can be summarized as follows:

1. Survival from first relapse was no different in patients whose primary treatment consisted in local-regional therapy alone and in those started on adjuvant CMF.
2. Regardless of salvage treatment(s) applied, survival from mastectomy was also similar in relapsing women started on adjuvant CMF (20% alive at 12 years) compared with relapsing women in the control group (16%).
3. Regardless of primary therapy and despite relatively high remission rates, all forms of salvage treatment failed to provide, in unselected cases, long-term control of relapsed breast cancer.

A few points deserve some additional comments. Secondary treatment upon relapse could not be instituted or effectively administered in about 5% of our patients because of rapidly progressive disease. Furthermore, a few patients (approximately 3% in the present series) refuse any form of treatment primarily because of negative psychological reactions toward the eventual treatment outcome.

In contrast to other investigators (Brincker et al. 1987; Clark et al. 1987; Chlebowsky et al. 1981; Morris et al. 1985), our data do not support evidence that survival after recurrence was significantly poorer in patients with previous adjuvant chemotherapy than in control patients. When survival was analyzed for all 578 primary failures, no difference was detected between control and CMF-treated patients.

Our series of patients has some unique features which render our conclusions more plausible. First of all, it is a large series, and despite the fact that in about 8% of patients details on salvage treatments were not available, the majority of our patients are being treated and followed up in one single institution. The type of first salvage therapy was not systematically planned in the original study protocols, but the same treatment strategy was almost always applied, both in women failing after primary local-regional modality as well as in patients relapsing after adjuvant CMF. This would help dispel the impression that superior results can possibly be achieved in patients without prior exposure to adjuvant chemotherapy.

The somewhat low response rate reported in our series is mainly due to the fact that this represents an *unselected* case series. This is especially true in women subjected to salvage chemotherapy. In this subgroup, patients presenting with massive abdominal involvement or disease in the central nervous system were also entered and evaluated. Nevertheless, a 38% response rate could be documented.

The observation that retreatment with CMF in women relapsing less than 12 months from the end of adjuvant therapy is unable to achieve disease remission is clinically relevant. It is conceivable that these patients were indeed resistant to the drugs utilized. This observation is further emphasized by the fact that in a similar patient population ADM regimens were able to attain a 31% response rate. By contrast, retreatment with CMF in patients failing more than 12 months from the end of adjuvant therapy is able to achieve a 48% response rate, a figure which is similar to that documented following ADM regimens (45%). Similar results on re-treatment with the same chemotherapy regimen were also reported by Buzdar et al. (1981).

In our series, in both treatment groups, endocrine therapy yielded objective tumor remission as well as a duration of response which were in the range of published findings when women were not selected through the results of an ER assay. It is interesting to point out that the response rate after castration was comparable between the subsets with and without CMF-induced amenorrhea. The findings confirmed once more that amenorrhea following treatment with anticancer drugs is not tantamount to ovarian failure and that the main therapeutic effect of CMF (or comparable drug combinations) is not mediated through chemical castration.

In conclusion, following relapse after mastectomy, first salvage therapy has failed to show superior results in women subjected to the local-regional modality alone compared with those treated with primary adjuvant therapy. Thus, the reported increased relapse-free and survival rates favoring combined modality treatment (Bonadonna and Valagussa 1988) can be ascribed to the early administration of CMF. Despite the fact that any form of salvage treatment seems unable to achieve a lasting remission duration in the vast majority of patients, physicians should be encouraged always to administer adequate systemic treatments at the time of first relapse, regardless of prior exposure to cytotoxic agents.

References

Bitran JD, Desser RK, Shapiro CM, Michel A, Kozloff MF, Billings AA, Recent W (1983) Response to secondary therapy in patients with adenocarcinoma of the breast previously treated with adjuvant chemotherapy. Cancer 51: 381–384

Bonadonna G, Valagussa P (1988) The contribution of medicine to the primary treatment of breast cancer. Cancer Res 48: 2314–2324

Bonadonna G, Valagussa P, Rossi A, Tancini G, Brambilla C, Zambetti M, Veronesi U (1985) Ten-year experience with CMF-based adjuvant chemotherapy in resectable breast cancer. Breast Cancer Res Treat 5: 95–115

Bonadonna G, Valagussa P, Zambetti M, Buzzoni R, Moliterni A (1987) Milan adjuvant trials for stage I–II breast cancer. In: Salmon SE (ed) Adjuvant therapy of cancer. V. Grune and Stratton, Orlando, pp 211–221

Brincker H, Rose C, Rank F, Mouridsen HT, Jakobsen A, Dombernowsky P, Panduro J, Andersen KW on behalf of the Danish Breast Cancer Cooperative Group (1987) Evidence of a castration-mediated effect of adjuvant cytotoxic chemotherapy in premenopausal breast cancer. J Clin Oncol 5: 1771–1778

Buzdar AU, Legha SS, Hortobagyi GN, Yap H, Wiseman CL, DiStefano A, Schell FC, Barnes BC, Campos LT, Blumenschein GR (1981) Management of breast cancer patients failing adjuvant chemotherapy with adriamycin-containing regimens. Cancer 47: 2798–2802

Clark GM, Sledge GW Jr, Osborne CK, McGuire WL (1987) Survival from first recurrence: relative importance of prognostic factors in 1015 breast cancer patients. J Clin Oncol 5: 55–61

Chlebowsky RT, Weiner JM, Luce J, Hestorff R, Lang JE, Reynolds R, Godfrey T, Ryden VMJ, Bateman JR (1981) Significance of relapse after adjuvant treatment with combination chemotherapy or 5-fluorouracil alone in high risk breast cancer. Cancer Res 41: 4399–4403

Consensus Conference (1985) Adjuvant chemotherapy for breast cancer. JAMA 254: 3461–3463

Henderson IC (1987) Adjuvant systemic therapy for early breast cancer. Curr Probl Cancer 11: 125–207

Kaplan EL, Meier P (1958) Non-parametric estimation from incomplete observations. J Am Stat Assoc 53: 457–481

Morris DM, Elias EG, Didolkar MS, Brown SD (1985) The response to further chemotherapy in patients with carcinoma of the breast who progressed while receiving adjuvant therapy. J Surg Oncol 29: 154–157

Valagussa P, Tesoro-Tess JD, Rossi A, Tancini G, Banfi A, Bonadonna G (1981) Adjuvant CMF effect on site of first recurrence, and appropriate follow-up intervals, in operable breast cancer with positive axillary nodes. Breast Cancer Res Treat 1: 349–356

Valagussa P, Tancini G, Bonadonna G (1986) Salvage treatment of patients suffering relapse after adjuvant CMF chemotherapy. Cancer 58: 1411–1417

Wendt AG, Jones SE, Salmon SE (1980) Salvage treatment of patients relapsing after breast cancer adjuvant chemotherapy. Cancer Treat Rep 64: 269–273

Time Course and Prognosis of Mammary Failure Following Breast-Conserving Therapy

J. M. Kurtz[1], J.-M. Spitalier[2], R. Amalric[2], H. Brandone[2], Y. Ayme[2], C. Bressac[2], and D. Hans[2]

[1] Department of Radiation Oncology, University Hospital, 4031 Basel, Switzerland
[2] Académie Mediterranéenne d'Oncologie Clinique, Marseille, France

Introduction

Since the combination of conservative surgery and radiation therapy is being implemented with increasing frequency both in Europe and in North America, it is of considerable interest that the problem of recurrent cancer in the treated breast be studied in depth. As breast recurrence following adequate treatment is an uncommon event and many years of follow-up must be accrued in order to evaluate subsequent prognosis, few treatment centers are in a position to carry out such an analysis. As the combination of primary limited surgery and megavoltage radiotherapy has been practiced at the Marseille Cancer Institute since the early 1960s (Spitalier et al. 1986), we have had the opportunity of treating many local recurrences and observing their subsequent course (Kurtz et al. 1988a). The purpose of this paper is to analyze the development of breast recurrence as a function of time, as well as to study the prognosis following treatment of local failure.

Materials and Methods

The study population consists of 1593 patients with clinical stage I and II breast cancers (American Joint Committee 1983) treated between November 1963 and December 1982 at the Cancer Institute and associated clinics in Marseille, employing primary limited surgery followed by megavoltage radiotherapy. Patient selection criteria, a description of treatment techniques, and the results of therapy have appeared in previous publications (Amalric et al. 1982; Amalric et al. 1983; Spitalier et al. 1986).

Briefly, the surgical treatment for all patients involved a macroscopically complete tumor removal by simple tumorectomy or wide excision. In addition, 681 more recent patients were subjected to an axillary dissection, which was usually limited to the lower two levels. Radiotherapy involved treatment of the entire breast, as well as of the draining lymph node areas, generally with administration of 50-60 Gy (5000-6000 rad) in 5-6 weeks employing a telecesium or telecobalt machine (Amalric and Spitalier 1982). Additional "boost" radiation was given to

Recent Results in Cancer Research, Vol. 115
© Springer-Verlag Berlin · Heidelberg 1989

the tumor bed, most commonly with electron-beam therapy (mean total prescribed dose, 78 Gy).

Although 580 selected pre- and perimenopausal patients were surgically castrated, adjuvant medical therapy was not commonly employed prior to 1980. A total of 218 patients received some form of hormone therapy, and 145 patients adjuvant chemotherapy, most commonly as a single alkylating agent in the peri-operative period.

The follow-up from time of primary therapy ranged from 5 to 24 years, with a median of 11 years. Actuarial calculations were performed by the life table method, as recommended by the American Joint Committee (American Joint Committee 1983). Actuarial freedom from mammary recurrence was calculated using the effective number of breasts at risk during the interval in question, with documented failure in the parenchyma or skin or the treated breast as the end point. Patients who developed distant metastases, died, or were lost to follow-up were treated as censored observations. In the calculation of actuarial overall survival rates, all causes of death were included, with patients lost to follow-up censored at time of the last consultation. Patients dying of unknown causes were considered to have died of cancer. Differences between survival curves were tested for significance using the logrank test.

Results

Time Course of Recurrence

As of December 1987, recurrent cancer in the ipsilateral breast, without prior distant metastases, had been documented in 178 of the 1593 patients (11%). The actuarial freedom from mammary recurrence was 93% at 5 years, 86% at 10 years, 82% at 15, and 80% at 20 years. Isolated axillary recurrences were recorded in an additional 32 patients; these are not considered further in this report.

The annual actuarial risk of breast recurrence, as calculated from life tables, averaged 1.5% per year during the first two 5-year periods. For 442 breasts at risk at the beginning of the 11th year, the residual risk averaged 1.1% per year between 10 and 15 years. For 120 breasts at risk at the beginning of the 16th year, three additional recurrences were observed (at 198, 252, and 259 months).

Location of Recurrences within the Breast

An effort was made retrospectively to distinguish between regrowth of cancer within the vicinity of the original primary tumor and "new tumor" formation elsewhere within the breast. Recurrent tumors were considered true recurrences if they occurred within the tumor bed or in its vicinity, not more than a few centimeters form the edge of the electron boost field. In contrast, a recurrence was classified as clearly distant when it could be judged to be at least 5 cm away from the original primary tumor. In case of doubt, recurrences were preferentially placed in the true recurrence category, as were seven cases for which the available descriptions were inadequate.

Only 38 of the recurrences (21%) clearly arose at a distance from the original tumor bed. These "new" tumors tended to occur later, with a mean time to diagnosis of 88.5 months, compared with 54.5 months for localized true recurrences. Only four of 40 (10%) recurrences diagnosed during the first 2 years were clearly new tumors, in contrast to nine of 14 failures (64%) occurring after 10 years, including all three recurrences after 15 years. The great majority of operable recurrences occurring during the first decade appeared to be localized within the vicinity of the primary tumor (135 of 164, or 82%).

Prognosis of Mammary Failure

Of 178 patients with breast recurrences, only seven were diagnosed concomitantly as having distant metastases, and an additional three patients developed local failure following the appearance of distant disease. These ten patients had a median survival after recurrence of 21 months. Twelve patients had recurrences which were so advanced as to preclude surgical treatment, usually with extensive skin involvement ("inflammatory recurrence"). All but one of these patients has died of breast cancer, with a median survival of 9 months.

All but three of the patients whose recurrences were operable (159 of 178, or 89%) were treated by salvage surgery, with or without adjuvant chemotherapy and/or hormonal manipulation. Secondary surgery consisted of some form of total mastectomy in 79 patients and a wide excision of the recurrent tumor in 77 selected cases. Adjuvant hormone therapy was liberally employed, but combination chemotherapy was reserved for recurrences which were thought to have an unfavorable prognosis, especially in premenopausal patients.

For all 159 patients with operable recurrences, overall survival following salvage therapy was 69% at 5 years and 57% at 10 years. Of the various parameters investigated as potential prognostic factors for overall survival after recurrence, the most important appeared to be the disease-free interval between primary therapy and the diagnosis of recurrence. Patients relapsing after 5 years had a very favorable prognosis, with an overall survival rate of 84% 5 years after recurrence. For patients relapsing before 5 years with operable recurrence, the 5-year overall survival was 61% ($P<0.057$). In addition, all inoperable recurrences were observed prior to 5 years.

Since the prognosis of late recurrences appeared to be uniformly favorable, the remainder of the analysis was restricted to the 89 patients developing operable mammary recurrence before 5 years. The following factors were found to have no significant influence on survival after recurrence: age at time of initial therapy (younger than 50 versus 50 or older), initial clinical tumor stage (T1 versus T2), pathologic nodal status (N-negative vs. N-positive), estrogen receptor (ER) status (ER-positive vs. ER-negative), location of recurrent tumor (near tumor bed vs. elsewhere), and type of salvage operation (mastectomy vs. breast conserving).

Table 1 presents factors correlating with overall survival following operable early recurrence. Even within the time frame of 5 years, the disease-free interval played a significant role, with recurrences diagnosed prior to 2 years having an unfavorable prognosis. Histologic grade, using a modified Bloom-Richardson grad-

Table 1. Factors correlating with overall survival following operable mammary recurrence diagnosed within 5 years of primary treatment ($n = 89$)

Factor	(n)	5-Year survival (%)	P-value
Disease-free intervall			
2–5 years	58	68	
≤2 years	31	48	0.027
Histologic grade			
G 1–2	24	72	
G 3	18	40	0.003
Unknown	47	61	
Extent of recurrence[a]			
Limited	37	74	
Extensive	36	42	0.018
Adjuvant therapy			
None	44	59	0.313
Hormonal	28	74	
Chemotherapy	17	47	0.03

[a] See text for definition of limited and extensive recurrence.

ing system (Contesso et al. 1987), was also significantly correlated with prognosis. Recurrences of limited extent (2 cm or smaller, without axillary recurrence) had a favorable prognosis compared with more extensive recurrences. The effects of adjuvant therapy at time of recurrence were difficult to evaluate. Neither hormone therapy nor chemotherapy was associated with a statistically superior survival rate compared with no adjuvant therapy, but patients treated with hormone treatment (including oophorectomy) fared better than patients receiving chemotherapy. The latter patients, however, generally had less favorable recurrences.

Local Control Following Salvage Treatment

With a median follow-up of 53 months after mammary failure, 31 of the 159 patients developed further recurrence in the preserved breast, on the chest wall, or in the regional nodal areas. The actuarial freedom from second local-regional recurrence for patients treated by salvage mastectomy was 88% at 5 years. For patients treated with breast-conserving salvage surgery, the corresponding figure was 64%. Many of the recurrences in the latter patients could be treated by additional surgery.

Discussion

The two most commonly employed methods for treatment of the breast in early mammary carcinoma are total (or modified radical) mastectomy alone and tumor excision in conjunction with breast irradiation. Although it is well established that

5-year local failure rates are similar (Sarrazin et al. 1984; Fisher et al. 1985; Veronesi et al. 1986), our experience serves to highlight some important differences between the local recurrences associated with the two treatment approaches.

A unique feature of breast-conserving therapy is the continued risk of tumor formation in the treated breast. Although chest wall recurrence after 5 years is not rare in early-stage disease (Montague 1984), late recurrences are decidedly more common with breast preservation (Recht et al. 1988). In our experience, the yearly recurrence risk continues to approximate 1% per year through the first half of the second decade; after 15 years, the risk appears to be quite small. Most recurrences occurring after 10 years were at some distance from the primary tumor and could be viewed as new tumors.

The intimate association between chest wall recurrence and distant metastases has been well documented. Distant metastases are clinically manifest in one-fourth to one-half of cases by the time local recurrence is diagnosed, and 5-year survival after the treatment of "isolated" chest wall recurrence in unselected surgical series ranges from 18% to 32% (Donegan et al. 1966; Fentiman et al. 1985; Gilliland et al. 1983; Heitanen et al. 1986). In contrast, mammary recurrence is almost always an isolated event, with only ten of 181 patients in this series having the prior or concomitant diagnosis of metastatic disease. In addition 85%–95% of isolated breast recurrences are operable, and patients can be rendered disease-free by potentially curative salvage surgery.

In contrast to recurrence in the chest wall after mastectomy, prognosis following mammary failure is comparatively favorable, especially for late failures. For operable recurrences occurring prior to 5 years, the subsequent outlook appears to be determined both by the biologic aggressiveness of the disease (as expressed by histologic grade and disease-free interval) and by the extent of the local-regional disease process at time of recurrence. Patients with small recurrences confined to the breast have a favorable prognosis, especially if the recurrence is diagnosed after 2 years. The further definition of prognostic factors and their interrelationships will require additional study.

Local-regional control following the treatment of recurrence has been satisfactory, with a 12% probability of subsequent recurrence in the chest wall or nodal areas 5 years after salvage mastectomy. Since many patients continue to desire breast preservation even in the face of local recurrence, we have turned increasingly to wide excision as surgical therapy of small, well-localized recurrences (Kurtz et al. 1988). Most patients suffering subsequent local recurrence can then be treated by additional surgery. The actuarial risk of subsequent recurrence in the breast after conservative salvage surgery (36% at 5 years) is similar to local recurrence rates reported after segmental mastectomy alone as primary treatment (Fisher et al. 1985).

In summary, mammary failure differs from chest wall recurrence both in its more protracted time course and in its more favorable prognosis. Painstaking lifelong follow-up by experienced physicians is clearly an important element in the breast conserving treatment strategy. Salvage mastectomy represents effective local therapy for recurrences in the breast, and wide excision appears to be an adequate alternative for selected, limited recurrences in patients continuing to desire breast preservation. The indications for adjuvant hormonal of chemotherapy in this setting remain to be defined. The use of such therapies for unfavorable recurrences appears justified. It is unclear, however, whether patients with late recurrence or patients with small recurrences limited to the breast would benefit from adjuvant medical treatment. Such questions require study within the framework of a prospective clinical trial.

References

Amalric R, Santamaria F, Robert F et al. (1982) Radiation therapy with or without primary limited surgery for operable breast cancer. Cancer 49: 30-34

Amalric R, Santamaria F, Robert F, et al. (1983) Conservation therapy of operable breast cancer: results at five, ten and fifteen years in 2216 consecutive cases. In: Harris JR, Hellman S, Silen W (eds) Conservative management of breast cancer. Lippincott, Philadelphia, pp 15-21

Amalric R, Spitalier JM (1982) Radiation as the sole mode of treatment in carcinoma of the breast. In: Zuppinger A, Hellriegel W (eds) Handbuch der medizinischen Radiologie, vol 19, Part 2, Springer, Berlin Heidelberg New York Tokyo, pp 301-346

American Joint Committee on Cancer (1983) Manual for staging of cancer. Lippincott, Philadelphia, pp 127-133

Contesso G, Mouriesse H, Friedman S et al. (1987) The importance of histologic grade in long-term prognosis of breast cancer: a study of 1010 patients, uniformly treated at the Institute Gustave-Roussy. J Clin Oncol 9: 1378-1386

Donegan WL, Perez-Mesa CM, Watson FR (1966) A biostatistical study of locally recurrent breast carcinoma. Surg Gynecol Obstet 122: 529-540

Fentiman IS, Matthews PN, Davison OW et al. (1985) Survival following local skin recurrence after mastectomy. Br J Surg 72: 14-16

Fisher B, Bauer M, Margolese R et al. (1985) Five year results of a randomized clinical trial comparing total mastectomy and segmental mastectomy with or without radiation in the treatment of breast cancer. N Engl J Med 312: 665-673

Gilliland MD, Barton RM, Copeland EM (1983) The implications of local recurrence of breast cancer as the first site of therapeutic failure. Ann Surg 197: 284-287

Heitanen P, Meittinen M, Mäkinen J (1986) Survival after first recurrence in breast cancer. Eur J Cancer Clin Oncol 22: 913-919

Kurtz JM, Amalric R, Brandone H et al. (1988) Results of salvage surgery for mammary recurrence following breast-conserving therapy. Ann Surg 207: 347-351

Kurtz JM, Amalric R, Brandone H et al. (1988) Results of wide excision for local recurrence after breast-conserving therapy. Cancer 61: 1969-1972

Montague ED (1984) Conservation surgery and radiation therapy in the treatment of operable breast cancer. Cancer 53: 700-704

Recht A, Silen W, Schnitt SJ et al. (1988) Time-course of local recurrence following conservative surgery and radiotherapy for early stage breast cancer. Int J Radiat Oncol Biol Phys 15: 255-261

Sarrazin D, Lé M, Rouëssé J et al. (1984) Conservative treatment versus mastectomy in breast cancer tumors with macroscopic diameter of 20 millimeters or less. Cancer 53: 1209-1213

Spitalier JM, Gambarelli J, Brandone H et al. (1986) Breast-conserving surgery with radiation therapy for operable mammary carcinoma: a 25-year experience. World J Surg 10: 1014-1020

Veronesi U, Banfi A, Del Vecchio M et al. (1986) Comparison of Halsted mastectomy with quadrantectomy, axillary dissection, and radiotherapy in early breast cancer: long-term results. Eur J Cancer Clin Oncol 22: 1085-1089

Detection of Recurrence:
A Critical Assessment of Existing Methods and Programs

W. F. Jungi, A. I. Streit, L. Schmid, and H.-J. Senn

Medizinische Klinik C, Kantonsspital, 9007 St. Gallen, Switzerland

Introduction

Recurrence is the most dreadful event for the woman who has undergone surgery for breast cancer. Every effort possible should be made therefore to prevent a recurrence or – at least – to detect it as early as possible with a high degree of reliability in the hope of prolonging survival. This is and has been the goal of all the various follow-up programs. While the physical methods employed are mostly the same, the laboratory tests vary considerably. The respective contribution of each method to the detection of specific metastatic sites has been analyzed several times with conflicting results. Earlier reports were mostly positive and reassuring, whereas more recent analyses question the value of single tests or combinations of tests.

All follow-up programs have been developed under the hypothesis that the earlier the recurrence is found, the better the chance of response to subsequent treatment should be. Even if the relapse indicates incurability, survival of the patient should be improved and prolonged.

Have these goals really been achieved? Are these assumptions valid? This has been contested recently by several authors (Dewar and Kerr 1985; Ormiston et al. 1985; Paulick and Caffier 1985; Tomin and Donegan 1987). They claim that most recurrences are not detected earlier in patients followed regularly than in those who are not and – more important – that survival is not prolonged by early detection and treatment of recurrence. They explain this by three biases (Tomin and Donegan 1987):

1. *Detection methods:* Routine methods find lesions at biologically favorable sites, like skin, soft tissue, nodes, but not in the prognostically decisive visceral organs.
2. *Length bias:* Tumors detected asymptomatically grow more slowly and less aggressively.
3. *Lead time:* The time gained by earlier detection of a recurrence – in fact 6–12 months – is no real gain in survival. Only the time with known recurrence is prolonged.

Recent Results in Cancer Research, Vol. 115
© Springer-Verlag Berlin·Heidelberg 1989

The purpose of this paper is to analyze critically the methods most commonly used in the follow-up of breast cancer patients, in the following order:

1. Medical history and physical examination
2. Radiologic tests and those making use of nuclear medicine
3. Laboratory tests

We would like to answer four questions:

1. Which is the best method for detecting a specific metastatic site?
2. What is the optimal follow-up schedule?
3. Should low- and high-risk patients be differentiated?
4. Are there true tumor markers for breast cancer?

We present data from our own OSAKO analysis (Streit et al. 1987), as well as those of other groups.

Medical History and Physical Examination

All authors agree that medical history and clinical examinations are the most important, simplest, and most effective means of detecting breast cancer recurrences. Horton calls it "the dominant feature of any follow-up examination" (Horton 1984). This has been extensively documented, for example by Cantwell et al. (1982), Horton (1984), Pandya et al. (1985) (for the Eastern Cooperative Oncology Group [ECOG]). Scanlon et al. (1980), Schnitt et al. (1985), Tomin and Donegan (1987), Winchester et al. (1979), and ourselves. Among our patients, the medical history and physical examination were positive for 96% of our relapsing patients (Table 1).

By definition, the patient's history reveals symptomatic recurrences. Up to three-quarters of all relapsing patients have some complaints, which are elicited sometimes only through systematic questioning by an experienced person. The symptom most often reported is pain, followed by coughing, anorexia, general fatigue, and weakness, whereas dyspnea, weight loss, and nausea occur less frequently (Eisemann et al. 1982; Tomin and Donegan 1987). Bony and visceral metastases cause symptoms more often than soft tissue lesions. An additional 20% of mostly soft tissue recurrences are detected by a thorough clinical examination, half of these being without accompanying symptoms (Dewar and Kerr 1985). Loco-regional recurrences and secondary cancers in the other breast can be detected at a

Table 1. Detection of recurrence by medical history and physical examination

	Cases (%)
Pandya et al. 1985	73
Tomin and Donegan 1987	74
Valagussa et al. 1982	78
Winchester et al. 1979	90
Streit et al. 1987	96

stage where a curative approach is still possible. Initial relapses within the treated areas or in the contralateral breast were found significantly more often at routine visits than were initial distant metastases. This also resulted in a significantly better survival rate than for those whose local recurrence was detected at an interval visit (Dewar and Kerr 1985). Would the patient herself not best suited to find any locoregional recurrence? Every patient should be instructed to examine herself and to report any new finding to her doctor.

We must question the value of a regular follow-up, if most recurrences are not detected at routine visits, as documented by Dewar and Kerr (1985), Ormiston et al. (1985), and Tomin and Donegan (1987). Dewar and Kerr (1985) calculate that a curable relapse was detected at only 1% and a successfully treated relapse at only 0.4% of all routine visits. He argues – as Ormiston et al. (1985) do – in favor of "reduc[ing] the intensity of the follow-up without any adverse effect on prognosis but with appreciable financial and other benefits." How many recurrences are missed or found too late if we adhere to a strict follow-up schedule? Zwaveling et al. (1987) gives a figure of 73%, in contrast to only 27% diagnosed as a result of a routine examination. Other authors (Ormiston et al. 1985; Tomin and Donegan 1987) confirm that there is no difference in survival between patients presenting an account of symptoms and those with relapses detected at regular follow-up.

Radiologic and Ultrasonic Investigations

Chest X-Rays

A radiologic chest examination is the only way of detecting asymptomatic recurrences in the lungs, pleura, and intrathoracic lymph nodes. It has high diagnostic accuracy, 75% for the lungs, 85% for adenopathy, 89% for pleura, as reported for the Milano group by Valagussa et al. (1982). Of the patients who subsequently developed metastases within a 5-year period, 47% had metastases detected by chest radiography. However, only 5%–20% of asymptomatic isolated lesions are found this way (Chaudary et al. 1983; Ciatto and Herd-Smith 1983; Pandya et al. 1985). Also in our analysis (Streit et al. 1987), the contribution is small (Fig. 1). There is

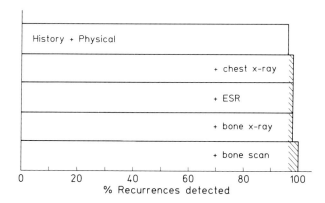

Fig. 1. Percentage of recurrences detected by various methods

no gain in survival owing to early diagnosis of lung metastases (Ciatto and Herd-Smith 1983), in spite of a lead time of 1–24 months. All patients became symptomatic within a year, and the diagnosis of lung metastases is associated with an incurable state (Horton 1984).

Mammography

There is little data on the value of routine mammographic screening of the contralateral breast after mastectomy for breast cancer, in sharp contrast to the abundant literature on primary screening. Mammography detected 20% of other soft tissue recurrences in the ECOG analysis (Pandya et al. 1985), in a quarter of the cases of Schnitt et al. (1985), and 35 of 81 impalpable tumors in McSweeney and Egans patients (1985). Mammography was more effective than clinical examination (McSweeney and Egan 1985). In the Royal Marsden Series (reported by Bailey 1981), a second primary tumor is detected at an earlier stage in patients examined regularly than it is in patients not on a regular basis screened (McSweeney and Egan 1985; Nielsen et al. 1985). The prognosis is not impaired by a second cancer. Bailey's patients with a metachronous second primary – likely to be a selected group – had a significantly better prognosis than patients with unilateral cancer (Coombes et al. 1981). In contrast to other investigators, including our own experience (Schenker 1983), Chaudary et al. (1984) calculate a constant rate of 7.6 per 1000 secondary cancers per year in the follow-up. If the first cancer arises before the age of 40, the risk is three times higher. The detection rate of nonsynchronous bilateral tumors may have been increased owing to more general use of mammography. There seems to be good reason for regular, lifelong routine mammography. Its postoperative starting point and optimal interval have still to be determined prospectively.

Skeletal Survey

Routine bone X-rays have been abandoned on account of their low sensitivity, high radiation exposure, and cost. Valagussa et al. (1982) gives an excellent analysis of bone X-rays, which are more often positive in symptomatic than in asymptomatic and in lytic than in mixed lesions.

Bone Scan

The use of bone scans has replaced the skeletal survey and was first praised as an ideal screening method for bone metastases (Burkett et al. 1979; Front et al. 1979; Gerber et al. 1977; Roberts et al. 1976). Owing to its high diagnostic accuracy – 73.8% in Valagussa et al.'s (1982) series 100% in our series – it is one of the most sensitive indicators of evolving metastatic disease. However, it is not specific enough and has a high false-positive rate (12%–34%). Its place in most follow-up programs has been questioned recently as a consequence of analyses of large cooperative trials. Burkett et al. (1979) found only 1.3% occult bone recurrences,

Wickerham 0.6% (1984), and Winchester (1979) none, but Schuster et al. (1984) 12%. In one-third of Thomsen's (1984) patients, the last bone scan was reported to be negative, and therefore not predictive. In other analyses, the predictive value, i.e., the percentage of times that a positive test indicates a diseased individual, was 11.8% (Burkett 1979) 18% (Pandya et al. 1985), and 23.5% (Pedrazzini et al. 1986). But of the 87% patients with a normal scan in the Ludwig Series, 6.9% developed bone metastases within 4 years – which is not statistically significantly different from the 11.2% among the 11% doubtful scans in the series reported by Pedrazzini et al. (1986). These authors calculate that early detection by scan would have been possible in 2.4% of cases, but that 80 scans would have been done for each initial relapse in bone. Our personal experience is too limited to allow a conclusion. We agree with most others that, after a baseline examination, bone scans should not be routinely repeated, but should be performed only as dictated by the clinical situation. It is however mandatory in the staging of patients at first recurrence.

Ultrasonic Liver Scans

Ultrasonic examination has replaced liver scintigraphy in the search for liver metastases. Its place and value in routine follow-ups have not been determined so far. Its results depend on the skill of the examiner and are hardly quantifiable. To our knowledge, there has been no critical analysis of this method in the postoperative follow-up of breast cancer patients.

Despite this fact, it is included in many follow-up programs, especially in German-speaking countries (Sauer et al. 1987). There is good reason to question the accuracy of ultrasound in this indication considering its low specificity with a high rate of false-positive results.

Laboratory Tests

The situation gets even more complicated and diffuse when we try to discern which laboratory test or which combination of tests allows us to detect recurrence in general or more specially, liver or bone metastases at an asymptomatic stage.

Erythrocyte Sedimentation Rate

In our own analysis of 113 breast cancer patients, the erythrocyte sedimentation rate (ESR) was elevated in almost half the recurrences. This has been confirmed by Cantwell et al. (1982) and others. Coombes et al. (1980, 1981) criticizes the low specificity of this test, as well as the lack of lead time.

Enzymes

Most investigators attribute some value to alkaline phosphatase (AP) and gamma-glutamyl transpeptidase (γGT), especially for the early diagnosis of *liver* metastases. They all point to the high rate of false-positive results (low specificity).

Pedrazzini et al. (1986) cannot see any clinical use for *bone* metastases at all. Coombes et al. (1981) document a lead time of up to 8 months with these two enzymes. None of the many other enzymes has ever gained wide acceptance as an indicator. Tests involving multicombinations of enzymes ("Enzymstatus") are quite popular in many countries, but do not provide more information.

Carcinoembryonal Antigen

Carcinoembryonal antigen (CEA) levels are frequently elevated in breast cancer in proportion to the tumor mass present. Unfortunately this indicator is not at all specific, and its sensitivity is also questionable. It may be helpful to some extent in the follow-up of breast cancer patients, as shown by Cantwell et al. (1982), Coombes et al. (1980, 1981), Lüthgens, Schlegel (1981) and Paulick and Caffier (1985). CEA levels are sometimes elevated more than 8 months before a recurrence becomes symptomatic (Coombes et al. 1981). Other oncofetal antigens are less widely accepted as indicators. Only tissue polypeptide antigen (TPA) has been investigated and promoted by Caffier and Brandau (1983).

Combinations

Excellent analyses are given by Coombes et al. (1980/81) and Kamby et al. (1987a, b). In the Royal Marsden Series of 47 patients with recurring tumors, AP, CEA, and γGT were the most sensitive tests, resulting in a lead time of over 3 months and making all other laboratory tests superfluous. Kamby et al. (1987a, 1987b) compare bilirubin + AST (aspartate aminotransferase) with AP + LDH (lactic dehydrogenase). If all four tests are negative, a relapse can be excluded with 99% certainty; if more than two are positive, metastatic disease is proven with 99% certainty. Cantwell et al. (1982) has seen elevated CEA, AP, and ESR levels in 14 of 18 relapsing patients, though with 38.8% false-positive tests. In our series, at least one laboratory parameter was abnormal in two-thirds of cases. Hemoglobin and white blood count were of no diagnostic value, nor were serum calcium, AP, and transaminases (Streit et al. 1987). In the ECOG study, blood chemistry was helpful in detecting 12.1% of bone and 31.8% of liver metastases (Pandya et al. 1985).

Conclusions

Three conclusions may be drawn from our review:

1. There is nothing new at all.
2. Nothing is clear.
3. There is no truly reliable test and no real tumor marker to detect breast cancer.

These conclusions may be logically correct – but in this case, the logical consequence would be to discard all follow-up examinations after surgery for breast cancer as long as no better, more sensitive, and specific methods are available. Some authors, e.g., Dewar and Kerr (1985), Ormiston et al. (1985), Scanlon et al. (1980), Tomin and Donegan (1987), and Zwaveling et al. (1987), point in this direction.

But what would the average breast cancer patient do in this situation? Would she really examine herself correctly, and should she be able to distinguish between harmless changes or normal findings and the first signs of relapse – which are mostly also the first signs of incurable disease? Would this not increase her anxiety and lead her to the many people outside of established medicine, who claim convincingly to know how to detect and even to prevent recurrent disease for sure? We personally recommend not completely abandoning regular follow-up, but reducing it to a reasonable extent. It should be offered to the great majority of patients who desire it, but should be forced upon nobody.

The optimal follow-up schedule has still to be defined. It should be tailored to the risk of the patient and to the recurrence time pattern of the specific risk group. We have to concentrate our efforts on the first 3 years, when more than 80% of all recurrences arise. Thereafter, further visits could depend on the needs of the patient, who should be well informed. Useful recommendations are given by Hughes (1985) and Joss et al. (1985). Medical history and physical examination are definitely the most effective methods, assuming the cooperation of the patient. Laboratory investigations could be safely reduced to a very few tests, e.g., assays of ESR, AP, and CEA, as proposed by Coombes et al. (1980). Chest X-rays and bone scans should only be performed during the initial work-up, but not repeated routinely later on, even in clinical trials. The role of routine contralateral mammography has to be investigated further.

References

Burkett FE, Scanlon EF, Garces RM, Khandekar JD (1979) The value of bone scan in the management of patients with carcinoma of the breast. Surg Gynecol Obstet 149: 523–525

Caffier H, Brandau H (1983) Serum tumor markers in metastatic breast cancer and course of disease. Cancer Detect Prevent 6: 451–457

Cantwell B, Fennelly JJ, Jones M (1982) Evaluation of follow-up methods to detect relapse after mastectomy in breast cancer patients. Ir J Med Sci 157

Chaudary MA, Maisey MN, Shaw PJ, Rubens RD, Hayward JL (1983) Sequential bone scans and chest radiographs in the postoperative management of early breast cancer. Br J Surg 70: 517–518

Chaudary MA, Millis RR, Hoskins EOL, Halder M, Bulbrook RD, Cuzick J, Hayward JL (1984) Bilateral primary breast cancer: a prospective study of disease incidence. Br J Surg 71: 711–714

Ciatto S, Herd-Smith A (1983) The role of chest x-ray in the follow-up of primary breast cancer. Tumori 69: 151–154

Coombes RC, Powles TJ, Gazet JC, Nash AG, Ford HT, McKinna A (1980) Assessment of biochemical tests to screen for metastases in patients with breast cancer. Lancet I: 296–298

Coombes RC, Powles TJ, Ford HT, Gazet JC (1981) Breast cancer management. Grune and Stratton, New York

Dewar JA, Kerr GR (1985) Value of routine follow-up of women treated for early carcinoma of the breast. Br Med J 291: 1464–1467

Doyle MA (1987) Practices of breast self examination in women with a known breast neoplasm. Breast Cancer Res Treat 10: 115

Eisemann B., Robinson WA, Steele G (1982) Follow-up of the cancer patient. Thieme-Stratton, New York

Front D, Schneck SO, Frankel A, Robinson E (1979) Bone metastases and bone pain in breast cancer, JAMA 242: 1747-1748

Gerber FH, Goodreau JJ, Kirchner PT, Fouty WJ (1977) Efficacy of preoperative and postoperative bone scanning in the management of breast carcinoma. N Engl J Med 297: 300-303

Horton J (1984) Follow-up breast cancer patients. Cancer 53: 790-797

Hughes LE, Courtney SP (1985) Follow-up of patients with breast cancer. Br Med J [Clin Res] 290: 1229-1230

Joss R, Metzger U, Brunner KW (1985) Nachkontrollen beim kurativ behandelten Krebspatienten. Zweck, Durchführung, Dauer? Schweiz Med Wochenschr 115: 714-721

Kamby C, Dirksen H, Vejborg I, Daugaard S, Guldhammer B, Rossing N, Mouridsen HT (1987a) Incidence and methodologic aspects of the occurrence of liver metastases in recurrent breast cancer. Cancer 59: 1524-1529

Kamby C, Vejborg I, Daugaard S, Guldhammer B, Dirksen H, Rossing N, Mouridsen HT (1987b) Clinical and radiologic characteristics of bone metastases in breast cancer. Cancer 60: 2524-2531

Lüthgens M, Schlegel G (1981) Verlaufskontrolle mit Tissue Polypeptide Antigen und Carcinoembryonalem Antigen in der radioonkologischen Nachsorge und Therapie. Tumor Diagnostik 2: 179-188

McSweeney MB, Egan RL (1985) Bilateral breast carcinoma. In: Brünner S, Langfeldt B (eds) Early detection of breast cancer. Springer, Berlin Heidelberg New York Tokyo (Recent results in cancer research, vol 105)

Nielsen M, Christensen L, Dyreborg U, Andersen JA (1987) Contributions to the diagnosis of contralateral malignancies in women with invasive breast cancer. In: Brünner S, Langfeldt B (eds) Breast cancer. Springer, Berlin Heidelberg New York Tokyo (Recent results in cancer research, vol 105)

Ormiston MC, Timoney AG, Qureshi AR (1985) Is follow-up of patients after surgery for breast cancer worthwhile? J R Soc Med 78: 920

Pandya KJ, McFadden ET, Kalish LA, Tormey DC, Taylor SG, Falkson G (1985) A retrospective study of earliest indicators of recurrence in patients on eastern Cooperative Oncology Group Adjuvant Chemotherapy Trials for breast cancer. Cancer 55: 202-205

Paulick R, Caffier H (1985) Klinische Bedeutung erhöhter CEA-Werte in der Nachsorge von Patientinnen mit Mammakarzinom. Geburtshilfe Frauenheilkd 45: 774-779

Pedrazzini, A, Gelber R, Isley M, Castiglione M, Goldhirsch A (1986) First repeated bone scan in the observation of patients with operable breast cancer. J Clin Oncol 4: 389-394

Roberts JG, Bligh AS, Gravelle IH, Leach KG, Baum M, Hughes LE (1976) Evaluation of radiography and isotopic scintigraphy for detecting skeletal metastases in breast cancer. Lancet I 237

Sauer H, Eiermann, W, Possinger K et al. (1987) Empfehlungen zur Diagnostik, Therapie und Nachsorge bei Brustkrebs. Onkologie 10 [Suppl 1]: 5-44

Scanlon EF, Oriedo MA, Cunningham HP et al. (1980) Preoperative and follow-up procedures on patients with breast cancer. Cancer 46: 977-979

Schenker C (1983) Verlaufsmammographie der kontralateralen Brust bei kurativ reseziertem Mammakarzinom. Dissertation, Basel

Schnitt SJ, Connolly JL, Recht A, Silver B, Harris JR (1985) Breast relapse following primary radiation therapy for early breast cancer. II. Detection, pathologic features and prognostic significance. J Rad Oncol Biol Phys 11: 1277-1284

Schuster R, Lenzhofer R, Pirich K, Dudzak R, Gabl F (1984) Ist die routinemäßige Skelettszintigraphie in der Nachsorge des Mammakarzinoms gerechtfertigt?, Dtsch Med Wochenschr 109: 1639-1642

Streit A, Schmid L, Jungi WF, Senn HJ (1987) Welche Untersuchungen sind zur Diagnose von Rezidiven beim operablen Mammakarzinom geeignet? Schweiz Med Wschr 117: 1615–1619

Thomsen HS, Lund JO, Munck O, Andersen KW, Støckel M, Rossing N (1984) Bone metastases in primary operable breast cancer. The role of serial scintigraphy. Eur J Cancer Clin Oncol 20: 1019–1023

Tomin R, Donegan WL (1987) Screening for recurrent breast cancer its effectiveness and prognostic value. J Clin Oncol 5: 62–67

Valagussa P, Tesoro Tess JD, Rossi A, Tancini G, Banfi A, Bonadonna G (1982) Adjuvant CMF effect on site of first recurrence, and appropiate follow-up intervals, in operable breast cancer with positive axillary nodes. Breast Cancer Res Treat 1: 349–356

Wickerham L, Fisher B, Cronin W and NASBP (1984) The efficacy of bone scanning in the follow-up of patients with operable breast cancer. Breast Cancer Res Treat 4: 303–307

Winchester DP, Sener SF, Khandekar JD, Oviedo MA, Cunningham MP, Caprini JA, Burkett FE, Scanlon EF (1979) Symptomatology as an indicator of recurrent or metastatic breast cancer. Cancer 43: 956–960

Zwaveling A, Albers GHR, Felthuis W, Hermans J (1987) An evaluation of routine follow-up for detection of breast cancer recurrences. J Surg Oncol 34: 194–197

Factors Associated with Local Recurrence as a First Site of Failure Following the Conservative Treatment of Early Breast Cancer

J. Boyages, A. Recht, J. Connolly, S. Schnitt, M. A. Rose, B. Silver, and J. R. Harris

Department of Radiation Therapy, Joint Center of Radiation Therapy, Harvard Medical School, 50 Binney Street, Boston, MA 02115, USA

Introduction

Conservative surgery and radiation therapy (CS + RT) has been shown to be an effective method of local treatment of early breast cancer, with survival rates equivalent to those following mastectomy. In view of this, more attention is now being focused on risk factors of local recurrence following CS + RT in an attempt to refine selection criteria and treatment techniques.

Risk factors for local recurrence following mastectomy have been well established. Multiple studies have consistently indicated that the risk of local recurrence following mastectomy, principally radical mastectomy, is primarily related to the presence and extent of axillary lymph node involvement (Fisher et al. 1981; Valagussa et al. 1978). The consistency of this observation is largely due to the strict definition of the surgical procedure and the absence of adjuvant therapies.

Risk factors for local recurrence following CS + RT are less well established. The use of this form of local treatment is more recent, and fewer long-term studies are available. More importantly, perhaps, there is a large amount of variation in the implementation of the treatment. The extent of surgery, for example, has ranged form needle biopsy (Bataini et al. 1978) to simple gross excision with a minimal margin of surrounding breast tissue (Harris et al. 1981), excision with tumor-free margins (Fisher et al. 1985), and resection of the involved quadrant, or "quadrantectomy" (Veronesi et al. 1986). There are also differences in the doses and volumes of tissue irradiated, as well as differences in the use of adjuvant systemic therapy. It is not surprising, therefore, that different centers have found different risk factors for local recurrence following CS + RT. In this paper, we review the available data for risk factors for local recurrence after CS + RT, stressing the results obtained at the Joint Center for Radiation Therapy in Boston.

Materials and Methods

Between July 1968 and December 1981, 733 female patients with UICC-AJC clinical stage I or II invasive breast cancer were treated by primary radiation therapy. Of these, 14 underwent treatment for contralateral breast carcinoma during that

Recent Results in Cancer Research, Vol. 115
© Springer-Verlag Berlin · Heidelberg 1989

period, making total of 747 evaluable breasts. To minimize the possible confounding effects of potentially inadequate treatment, 30 patients who had only a needle or incision biopsy (i.e., gross residual disease was left by the surgeon) and 110 patients whose breast received a total dose of less than 60 Gy to the region of the primary tumor site have been excluded from the following analysis. Thus, the study population consisted of 597 patients with 607 breast cancers.

Follow-up was obtained as of January 1988, with a median follow-up time of 86 months for surviving patients (range, 37–200 months). The majority of live patients (99%) had follow-up of at least 5 years, and 34 (7%) had been followed for more than 10 years. The median age at diagnosis was 51 years, with a range of 25–87 years.

The details of treatment have been described previously (Svensson et al. 1980; Harris et al. 1981; Recht et al. 1985). In that time period, an excisional biopsy was defined as a gross macroscopic resection of the primary tumor, without regard as to whether the margins were later found to be microscopically involved. An axillary dissection, usually limited to level I and II nodes, was performed in 441 patients. A "boost" dose of radiation was delivered by an iridium 192 implant in 556 treated breasts (two or more planes in 65%) and by photons or electrons in 41 breasts. The total dose to the region of the primary tumor ranged from 60 to 84 Gy (median, 68 Gy).

Adjuvant chemotherapy [usually cyclophosphamide, methotrexate, and 5-fluorouracil (CMF)] was given to 135 patients, including 120 of the 148 patients with histologically positive axillary lymph nodes.

Pathologic analysis was limited to 445 of the 607 breasts (73%) in which the predominant type of invasive tumor was infiltrating ductal carcinoma and sufficient breast tissue was present adjacent to the primary tumor for pathologic evaluation. Details of the evaluation have been previously described (Schnitt et al. 1984). It is note worthy that, during these years, it was not routine practice to remove the breast mass in a single specimen, nor was it routine to ink the margins of resection. As a result, the microscopic margins of resection could not be evaluated in most specimens.

Our prior experience has shown the most important predictor of breast cancer recurrence to be what we have defined as an "extensive intraductal component" (EIC) in the primary excision specimen (Schnitt et al. 1984). This is defined as the presence of both intraductal carcinoma within the primary tumor, comprising at least 25% of the tumor mass, *and* the presence of intraductal carcinoma clearly extending beyond the infiltrating margin of the tumor or present in grossly normal adjacent breast tissue.

Local recurrence is defined as the detection of cancer in the parenchyma and/or skin of the treated breast occurring before or simultaneously with the discovery of distant metastases. The pattern of local recurrence was classified as either: true recurrence (TR), marginal miss (MM), recurrence elsewhere in the breast (E), or a skin recurrence (S). A local recurrence which could not be categorized because of insufficient clinical or pathologic information was termed unclassified (U) (see Recht et al. 1985 for definitions).

The risk of local recurrence was evaluated by the use of actuarial calculations and by crude incidence. Actuarial curves were calculated by the Kaplan-Meier

(1958) method and comparisons between curves were made using the two-tailed "naive" log-rank test. The Kaplan-Meier estimates, however, can be shown to be unbiased and maximum likelihood estimates only if time to distant and time to local failure are statistically independent. This assumption can be questioned in this data set. Such nonindependent censoring could cause the log-rank test to be biased in either direction (too significant or not significant enough). Breasts were censored from the calculation of local recurrence at the time of last follow-up, the detection of metastatic disease, the discovery of regional disease without local recurrence or death from intercurrent illness. "Freedom from distant disease" calculations were done by censoring patients at the time of death from intercurrent illness or at last follow-up, scoring failure at the time of first discovery of disease outside the treatment field. All intervals were calculated from the date of commencement of radiation therapy. Differences between proportions were tested by the chi-squared test, with P-values of 0.05 or less considered statistically significant.

Results and Review of Literature

The 5- and 10-year actuarial local recurrence rates for the 747 treated breasts were 11% and 18%, respectively. With follow-up times ranging from 37 to 209 months (median, 87 months), 94 of the 747 treated breasts developed a local recurrence (13%). The 5- and 10-year actuarial rates were more than doubled in the 30 patients in whom a less than excisional biopsy was performed (34% and 40%). The importance of at least an excisional biopsy in maximizing local control has also been reported by others (Almaric et al. 1983; Bedwinek et al. 1980; van Limbergen et al. 1987). In order to minimize bias due to the inclusion of patients treated in a nonuniform manner, we have restricted further analysis to 597 patients with 607 breast cancers treated with an excisional biopsy *and* given a total dose of at least 60 Gy to the region of the primary site (that is, patients treated by our current practice). In this group of patients, the 5- and 10-year actuarial local recurrence rates were 10% and 16% (corresponding to a crude recurrence rate of 71 of 607 breasts or 12%). We have examined the effect of various clinical, pathologic, and treatment characteristics as potential risk factors for local recurrence and have compared our findings with those reported by other institutions.

Clinical Characteristics

Patient Factors

We examined the risk of local recurrence related to patient age. Young patients (aged 34 or less) were more likely to develop a local recurrence than older patients. In younger patients, 12 of 47 (26%) developed a recurrence in their treated breast, compared with 59 of 560 (11%) of the older patients ($P=0.005$). The corresponding 5-year actuarial local recurrence rates were 27% and 9% ($P=0.0001$). The patients in the two age groups were similar in their distribution of T stage,

N stage, and median number of positive nodes. They differed in their frequency of extensive intraductal carcinoma, which will be discussed below. The incidence of other histologic features, including blood or lymphatic vessel invasion, high nuclear grade, high histologic grade, and tumor necrosis, was not significantly different in these patients. We also examined the incidence of distant relapse for the two age groups. We found no difference in the 5-year actuarial freedom from distant relapse, being 82% for the older patients and 78% for patients aged 34 or less [P=not significant (NS)].

Young age as a significant adverse prognostic factor for breast cancer relapse has also been reported by other centers, particularly when a cut-off age of between 32 and 40 was used (Calle et al. 1986; Delouche et al. 1987; Kurtz et al. 1987; Muscolino et al. 1987; Nobler et al. 1985; Vilcoq et al. 1981; van Limbergen et al. 1987), but this finding has not been universal (Solin et al. 1987).

Tumor Factors

Table 1 shows the relationship between the risk of local recurrence and tumor stage, tumor location, clinical nodal status, and UICC-AJC clinical stage. None of these tumor factors were associated with an increased risk of local recurrence. The lack of influence of tumor size as a risk factor for local recurrence was also reported by Fisher et al. (1985) in the NSABP B-06 trial. In that study, local recurrence for T1 tumors (6.5%) did not significantly differ from that occurring for T2 lesions (9.6%). Similarly, the Milan group (Luini et al. 1987) reported a nearly identical rate of local recurrence in a cohort of 83 patients with T2 tumors (treated on an

Table 1. Five-year actuarial breast recurrence as affected by tumor factors (JCRT)[a]

Factors	Total (*n*)	% 5-Year LR (*n*)	*P*-value
Tumor location			
Lateral	351	11	NS
Central	38	9	NS
Medial	217	9	NS
T stage			
T1	329	10	NS
T2	278	10	
N stage			
N0/1A	531	11	NS
N1B	76	7	
Stage (UICC)			
I	305	10	NS
II	302	10	

LR, Local breast recurrence; NS, not significant.
[a] All patients treated by excisional biopsy and given at least 60 Gy to the region of the primary tumor

off-trial basis) to that of patients with T1 tumors who were included in their randomized trial (Veronesi et al. 1986). In the experience of the Institut Gustave-Roussy (Clarke et al. 1985), 20 of 345 pathologic stage T1 tumors recurred (6%) compared with one of 35 T2 tumors (3%). Similarly at that institution, tumor location or UICC clinical stage were not predictors of breast recurrence.

In a previous study from our institution (Connolly et al. 1987), patients with multiple synchronous ipsilateral cancers of the breast were found to have a higher rate of local recurrence following primary radiation therapy compared with patients with only one cancer. Four of ten such patients developed a recurrence in the treated breast, despite the gross resection of all identified tumors, compared with 77 of 707 patients (11%) with single lesions ($P=0.02$).

Pathological Characteristics

Histologic Nodal Status

An analysis of histologic nodal status as an independent risk factor was not possible in our series, as the majority of node-positive patients also received adjuvant chemotherapy. Bearing this in mind, the 5-year actuarial local recurrence rate for patients found to have histologically negative nodes (13%) did not differ significantly from that of patients with one to three, or four or more positive nodes involved (10% and 8% respectively). At the Institute Gustave-Roussy, local recurrence was observed in 4% of patients with negative nodes and in 7% in patients with positive nodes ($P=NS$), both groups not having received chemotherapy (Clarke et al. 1985).

Intraductal Component of Tumor

We examined the risk of local recurrence in relation to the histopathologic factors of the primary tumor. The only feature which was shown to have a significant effect on local tumor control was the presence of an EIC. Figure 1 shows the probability of local recurrence based on the intraductal component. Patients with significant intraductal carcinoma at both sites [i.e., within +, adjacent + (W+A+) or EIC] had a 25% actuarial risk of local recurrence at 5-years, compared with 6% for patients with intraductal carcinoma only in the adjacent tissue (W−A+), 5% for those patients with significant intraductal carcinoma in the primary tumor alone (W+A−), and 3% for patients with neither feature (W−A−). Overall, 36 of 143 patients (25%) with EIC developed a local recurrence compared with 17 of 302 patients (6%) without EIC ($P<0.0001$). The 5-year actuarial freedom from distant relapse was similar in the two groups. It was 84% for patients with EIC compared with 78% for those without EIC ($P=NS$).

We related the pattern of local failure in the treated breast to the presence or absence of EIC. Of the 36 patients with an EIC who relapsed, 32 patients (89%) developed a TR or MM, two patients (6%) had a recurrence outside the primary tumor site, one patient had a recurrence in the skin of the breast and one patient

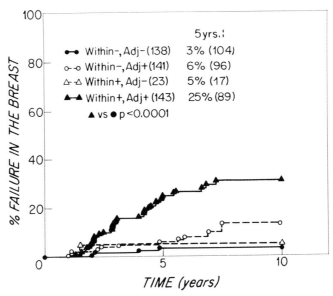

Fig. 1. Effect of intraductal component on local tumor control. *Numbers in parentheses* represent the number of patients in each pathologic subgroup and the number of patients at risk at 5 years. *Within +* indicates the presence of prominent intraductal carcinoma within the primary tumor; *Adj +* indicates the presence of intraductal carcinoma outside the infiltrating margin of the tumor

Table 2. Pattern of local failure as affected by the degreee of intraductal component (JCRT)[a]

Intraductal Component	Breasts (*n*)	LF	Pattern of local failure				
			TR *n* (%)	MM *n* (%)	E *n* (%)	S *n* (%)	U *n* (%)
Within − ADJ −	138	5	3 (60)	1 (20)	1 (20)	0	0
Within − ADJ +	141	11	4 (36)	0	3 (28)	4 (36)	0
Within + ADJ −	23	1	1 (100)	0	0	0	0
Within + ADJ +	143	36	18 (50)	14 (39)	2 (5)	1 (3)	1 (3)

TR, true recurrence; MM, marginal miss; E, elsewhere; S, skin failure; U, unclassified; Adj, adjacent; LF, local failure.
[a] All patients treated by excisional biopsy and dose to the primary site $\geq$ Gy, infiltrating ductal histology, with evaluable specimen.

had a recurrence which could not be classified. Of the 17 patients without EIC who relapsed, nine (53%) developed a TR or MM, four (23.5%) had a recurrence elsewhere in the breast, and four (23.5%) patients had a recurrence in the skin (Table 2).

We also examined the relationship between the presence of an EIC in the tumor specimen and the patient's age at diagnosis in order to assess whether the two factors may be confounded. We found that, although the incidence of an EIC was somewhat higher in younger patients (44% vs. 31%; $P=0.13$), this did not appear to account totally for the difference in breast recurrence rates. Among patients with EIC, both young and older patients had a high 5-year actuarial rate of local recurrence (38% and 23% respectively, $P=$ NS). Among patients without EIC, the 5-year risk of local recurrence was 25% for young patients compared with only 3% in older patients ($P<0.0001$). Of note, however, is that there were only 23 patients aged 34 or less without an EIC. As a result, firm conclusion on this point cannot be made.

Other Histologic Prognostic Factors

Other reported risk factors for local recurrence have included a high Bloom grade. Clark et al. (1985) reported that 12 of 297 (4%) patients with tumors of Bloom grade I and II suffered a recurrence, compared with 8 of 66 (12%) patients with grade III tumors ($P=0.001$).

The effect of involved margins of resection as an adverse risk faktor is not clear, particularly as there is variation in the definition of histologic involvement. A positive margin may be defined as the presence of cancer at an inked surface or the presence of cancer that lies within some arbitrary distance from an inked margin. Despite this, the available studies which have addressed this issue (Alpert et al. 1978; Clarke et al. 1985; Hüning et al. 1983; Solin et al. 1986) have not reported a higher risk of local recurrence for patients with involved margins over that in other patients.

Treatment Characteristics

Radiation Factors

We examined the risk of local recurrence in relation to the interval between excision of the primary tumor and the initiation of radiation therapy. We did not find a significantly higher 5-year actuarial relapse rate for the patients in whom the interval between excision of the primary tumor and the commencement of radiation was less than 7 weeks, compared with those patients in whom the delay was 7 weeks or greater (11% vs 10% respectively, $P=$ NS). On the contrary, Clarke et al. (1985) found a local recurrence rate of 14% compared with 5% for the same time intervals ($P=0.01$).

We also examined whether the total dose prescribed to the primary tumor site or the volume of implant had an impact on tumor recurrence. No association was found between either the total dose to the primary site or the volume of the boost and the risk of local recurrence. Local recurrence occurred in 11% of the 143 treated breasts which received a total dose to the primary tumor site of 70 Gy or more, compared with 10% for the 464 breasts which received a lower dose ($P=$ NS). Similarly, in 546 patients in whom the volume of implant (as determined by the total number of seeds) was known, the breast recurrence rate was 12% for patients whose implant contained up to 50 seeds, 9% for those implanted with 51–74 seeds, and 10% for those who received 75 or more seeds ($P=$ NS). Of note, however, is that since the choice of doses and volumes were at the discretion of the attending clinician, it is likely that significant selection biases were present.

In view of the high risk of relapse in patients with an EIC in their tumor, we also examined whether differences in radiation dose and volume had any effect on the incidence or pattern of local recurrence in this subset of patients. Here, too, variations in total dose and boost volume were not associated with differences in the total risk of local recurrence. It should be noted, however, that the risk of local relapse was high even in the 18 patients with EIC who received the highest radiation dose and largest volume of implant (that is, ≥ 70 Gy and ≥ 75 seeds). In this select subgroup, the 5-year actuarial breast recurrence rate was 33%, compared with 23% for other patients with EIC ($P = 0.41$).

The reason for the association of EIC with a high risk of local recurrence is not entirely clear. In a recent study performed at our institution (Schnitt et al. 1987), we found that patients who underwent an initial gross excision of the tumor and were found to have an EIC in the initial specimen were more likely to have residual cancer in a re-excision specimen than other patients without EIC (88% vs 44%, $P = 0.002$). More importantly, patients with EIC were more likely to have extensive residual carcinoma on re-excision compared with non-EIC patients, and that residual carcinoma was principally intraductal in nature. Among patients with EIC, 44% had extensive residual intraductal carcinoma on re-excision compared with only 2% for patients without EIC ($P < 0.0001$). These results indicate that tumors exhibiting an EIC have a greater residual tumor burden after tumor excision than patients without EIC. This larger tumor burden may be too great and too extensive to be eradicated by the conventional doses and technique of radiation used.

The impact of time-dose factors of radiotherapy on the risk of developing a local recurrence has been addressed in a number of studies. Kurtz et al. (1983) found that local recurrence was greater when a dose of 8 Gy or less was administered per week compared with less protracted treatment times. This finding has also been reported by the Institut Gustave-Roussy (Clark et al. 1985) and by investigators at the Royal Marsden Hospital (Osborne et al. 1984).

There is not universal agreement on the usefulness of a boost dose of radiation to the region of the primary tumor site in reducing the incidence of local recurrence. The major study in which a boost was not used was the NSABP B-06 trial. In that study, the 5-year actuarial rate of breast failure was 8% (Fisher et al. 1985). Given the protracted course of local recurrence, however, longer follow-up will be required to assess the results of treatment without a boost. It is likely that the necessity of performing a boost needs to be considered in relation to the extent of breast surgery. A boost may be more important after an excisional biopsy than after very wide excision or quadrantectomy.

Effect of Adjuvant Chemotherapy

We have attempted to examine the influence of adjuvant chemotherapy on local tumor control by comparing 120 node-positive patients who received adjuvant chemotherapy in addition to radiation therapy, with 28 node-positive patients who only received radiation therapy. The respective local recurrence rates were not significantly different (9% vs 15%). This comparison was limited by the confounding of the use of adjuvant chemotherapy and patient age. Younger patients were more likely to receive adjuvant chemotherapy. Further analysis of the effect of chemotherapy on local tumor control in relation to patient age was hampered by the fact that there were only seven premenopausal patients (defined here as age at diagnosis of 50 years or less) who were node-positive and who did not receive chemotherapy. It was of some interest, however, that of these seven patients, three (43%) had developed a local recurrence, compared with 9 (11%) of the 81 premenopausal patients who also received chemotherapy ($P=0.07$). The corresponding 5-year actuarial rates of local recurrence were 58% and 11% respectively ($P=0.003$). In the Milan and NSABP B-06 study (Veronesi et al. 1986; Fisher et al. 1985), the local recurrence rate was also found to be low in patients treated by combined radiation therapy and chemotherapy. In the NSABP B-06 trial, the local recurrence rate was lower in node-positive patients who received adjuvant chemotherapy in addition to radiation therapy, than in node-negative patients who only received radiation therapy. These results suggest that radiation therapy and chemotherapy may be interactive in influencing local tumor control after breast-conserving surgery.

Discussion

In this report, we have examined possible prognostic factors for local recurrence as a first site of failure in a cohort of patients treated in a consistent manner. Our analysis was restricted to patients who underwent an excisional biopsy, without regard to microscopic margins of resection, and who received a total dose to the primary tumor site of at least 60 Gy. In this analysis, we found that the most important factors associated with local recurrence as a first site of failure were patient age and the presence of an extensive intraductal component. Clinical tumor characteristics, including tumor size, tumor site, and stage, were not found to be associated with the risk of local recurrence.

The most important factor associated with a local recurrence in our experience was the presence of a significant intraductal component in the primary tumor specimen *and* the presence of an intraductal component in the adjacent normal tissue (EIC). We found that those patients whose tumors had this factor had a 5-year local recurrence rate of 25% compared with only 5% for patients not having this feature ($P<0.0001$). We also found that variations in radiation dose and volume were not associated with differences in the risk of local recurrence. Even those patients with EIC who received the highest dose and largest implant volume ($\geqslant 70$ Gy and $\geqslant 75$ seeds) had a substantial risk of recurrence.

The presence of EIC has not been noted to be an important risk factor for local recurrence in studies reported by other centers (Calle et al. 1986; Clarke et al. 1985; Delouche et al. 1987; van Limbergen et al. 1987). In our view, the most likely explanation for this are differences in the definition of EIC and variations in treatment technique. In this regard, the extent of the initial tumor resection may be a major factor. We have found in our re-excision study (Schnitt et al. 1987) that patients with EIC have a larger residual tumor burden than patients whose tumors

do not have an EIC. A simple gross excision is not as likely to be effective in reducing this larger residual tumor burden as compared with a wider local excision
or resection of the involved quadrant. This may be the reason for the lack of EIC
as a risk factor in the Milan study (Veronesi 1988, personal communication). However, in order to test the validity of this hypothesis, we are currently performing an
outcome study on patients with EIC treated at our institution during a later time
period who underwent a re-excision of the primary tumor site prior to radiation
therapy.

The findings presented in this paper have altered the practice of CS + RT at our
institution. Patients now initially undergo a limited resection of the primary tumor
with sufficient adjacent tissue removed to assess the extent of the intraductal component. In patients without EIC, treatment with radiation therapy including a
boost to the primary site is then considered appropriate without the necessity of
further breast surgery. In patients with EIC, our current practice is to recommend
a re-excision at the primary tumor site. If re-excision results in negative margins,
then treatment by radiation therapy is considered a reasonable option, whereas
patients with positive margins are recommended for mastectomy. This treatment
policy allows for a minimum of breast surgery prior to the initiation of radiation
therapy.

References

Alpert S, Ghossein NA, Stacey P, Migliorelli FA, Efron G, Krishnaswamy V (1978) Primary
management of operable breast cancer by minimal surgery and radiotherapy. Cancer 42:
2054-2058
Amalric R, Santamaria F, Robert F, Seigle J, Altshuler C, Pietra JC, Amalric F, Kurtz JM,
Spitalier JM, Brandone H, Ayme Y, Pollet JF, Bressac C, Fondarai J (1983) Conservative
therapy of operable breast cancer-results at five, ten and fifteen years in 2216 consecutive
cases. In: Harris JR, Hellman S, Silen W (eds) Conservative management of breast cancer. Lippincott, Philadelphia, pp 30-34
Bataini JP, Picco C, Martin M, Calle R (1978) Relation between time-dose and local control
of operable breast cancer treated by tumorectomy and radiotherapy or by radical radio-
therapy alone. Cancer 42: 2059-2065
Bedwinek J, Perez CA, Kramer S, Brady L, Goodman R, Grundy G (1980) Irradiation as
the primary management of stage I and II adenocarcinoma of the breast. Cancer Clin
Trials 3: 11-18
Calle R, Vilcoq JR, Zafrani B, Vielh P, Fourquet A (1986) Local control and survival of
breast cancer treated by limited surgery followed by irradiation. Int J Radiat Oncol Biol
Phys 12: 873-878
Clarke DH, Le MG, Sarrazin D, Lancombe M-J, Fontaine F, Travagli J-P, Françoise M-L,
Contesso G, Arriagada R (1985) Analysis of local-regional relapse in patients with early
breast cancers treated by excision and radiotherapy. Experience of the Institut Gustave-
Roussy. Int J Radiat Oncol Biol Phys 11: 137-145
Connolly JL, Leopold KA, Recht A, Schnitt SJ, Rose MA, Silver B, Harris JR (1987) Results
of conservative surgery and radiation therapy for multiple synchronous cancers of one
breast. Int J Radiat Oncol Biol Phys 13: 160 (Abstract)
Delouche G, Bachelot F, Premont M, Kurtz JM (1987) Conservation treatment of early
breast cancer: Long term results and complications. Int J Radiat Oncol Biol Phys 13:
29-34
Fisher B, Wolmark N, Bauer M, Redmond C, Gebhardt M (1981) The accuracy of clinical

nodal staging and of limited axillary dissection as a determinant of histological nodal status in carcinoma of the breast. Surg Gynecol Obstet 152: 765–772

Fisher B, Bauer M, Margolese R, Poisson R, Pilch Y, Redmond C, Fisher E, Wolmark N, Deutsch M, Montague E, Saffer E, Wickerman L, Lerner H, Glass A, Shibata H, Deckers P, Ketchman A, Oishi R, Russell I (1985) Five-year results of a randomized clinical trial comparing total mastectomy and segmental mastectomy with or without radiation in the treatment of breast cancer. N Engl J Med 312: 665–673

Harris JR, Botnick LE, Bloomer WD, Chaffey JT, Hellman S (1981) Primary radiation therapy for early breast cancer: the experience at the Joint Center for Radiation Therapy. Int J Radiat Oncol Biol Phys 7: 1549–1552

Hünig R, Walther E, Harder F, Almendral AC, Roth J, Torhorst J (1983) The Basel lumpectomy protocol: five-year experience with a prospective study for conservative treatment of breast cancer. In: Harris JR, Hellman S, Silen W (eds) Conservative management of breast cancer. Lippincott, Philadelphia, pp 23–25

Kurtz JM, Spitalier JM, Amalric R (1983) Late breast recurrence after lumpectomy and irradiation. Int J Radiat Oncol Biol Phys 7: 1191–1194

Kurtz JM, Brandone H, Ayme Y, Spitalier JM, Amalric R (1987) Mammary recurrences in women younger than forty. Int J Radiat Oncol Biol Phys 14: 183 (Abstract)

Luini A, Sacchini V, Galimberti V, Farante G, Del Vecchio M, Tana S, Volterrani F, Veronesi U (1987) Conservative treatment of early breast carcinoma: report on 83 T2 patients treated with QU.A.RT. Breast Cancer Res Treat 10: 106 (Abstract)

Muscolino G, Luini A, Bedini AV, Beretta E, Sacchini V (1987) Impact of young age on local recurrence risk in patients with early breast cancer undergone Qu.A.RT. Breast Cancer Res Treat 10: 105 (Abstract)

Nobler MP, Venet L (1985) Prognostic factors in patients undergoing curative irradiation for breast cancer. Int J Radiat Oncol Biol Phys 11: 1323–1331

Osborne MP, Ormiston N, Harmer CL, McKinna JA, Baker J, Greening WP (1984) Breast conservation in the treatment of early breast cancer. Cancer 53: 349–355

Recht A, Silver B, Schnitt S, Connolly J, Hellman S, Harris JR (1985) Breast relapse following primary radiation therapy for early breast cancer. I. Classification, frequency and salvage. Int J Radiat Oncol Biol Phys 11: 1271–1276

Schnitt SJ, Connolly JL, Harris JR, Hellman S, Cohen RB (1984) Pathologic predictors of early local recurrence in Stage I and II breast cancer treated by primary radiation therapy. Cancer 53: 1049–1057

Schnitt SJ, Connolly JL, Khettry U, Mazoujian G, Brenner M, Silver B, Recht A, Beadle G, Harris JR (1987) Pathologic findings on re-excision of the primary site in breast cancer patients considered for treatment by primary radiation therapy. Cancer 59: 675–681

Solin LJ, Fowble B, Martz KL, Pajak TF, Goodman RL (1986) Does residual tumor adversely impact on the outcome of patients undergoing definitive irradiation for early stage breast cancer. Int J Radiat Oncol Biol Phys 12: 91–92 (Abstract)

Solin LJ, Fowble B, Schultz DJ, Goodman RL (1987) Age as a prognostic factor for patients treated with definitive irradiation for early stage breast cancer. Int J Radiat Oncol Biol Phys 14: 184 (Abstract)

Svensson GK, Bjarngard BE, Larson RD, Levene MB (1980) A modified three-field technique for breast treatment. Int J Radiat Oncol Biol Phys 6: 689–694

Valagussa P, Bonadonna G, Veronesi U (1978) Patterns of relapse and survival following radical mastectomy: analysis of 716 consecutive patients. Cancer 41: 1170–1178

van Limbergen E, van der Bogaert W, van der Schueren E, Rijnders A (1987) Tumor excision and radiotherapy as primary treatment of breast cancer. Analysis of patient and treatment parameters and local control. Radiother Oncol 8: 1–9

Veronesi U, Zucali R, Luini A (1986) Local control and survival in early breast cancer: the Milan trial (1986) Int J Radiat Oncol Biol Phys 12: 717–720

Vilcoq JR, Calle R, Stacey P, Ghossein NA (1981) The outcome of treatment by tumorectomy and radiotherapy of patients with operable breast cancer. Int J Radiat Oncol Biol Phys 7: 1327–1332

Critical Review of Problems of Rational Follow-up and Salvage Therapy

D. C. Tormey

Clinical Cancer, Center, Department of Human Oncology K4/632 Clinical Sciences Center, University of Wisconsin, 600 Highland Avenue, Madison, WI 53792, USA

Three general issues discussed during this session seem particularly worthy of comment:

1. The role of radiotherapy in the prevention of local-regional relapse
2. The effectiveness of salvage treatment after recurrence following adjuvant therapy
3. The role of routine postoperative follow-up testing to identify recurrence.

There is no question that the use of routine postoperative radiotherapy will reduce the local-regional recurrence rate. Similar local-regional recurrence rate reductions have been associated with modern systemic adjuvant therapy regimens. This observation has led to attempts to redefine which patients would be most likely to benefit from postoperative radiotherapy combined with systemic chemotherapy. Recently, an analysis of the Eastern Cooperative Oncology Group's (ECOG) postoperative systemic therapy protocols has identified a subset of patients with an isolated local-regional recurrence rate which appears to be similar to the distant recurrence rate (Fowble et al. 1988). Whether treatment of such patients would lead to improved survival will only be learned from randomized trials. Such trials will also need to focus upon issues regarding how best to integrate surgery, radiotherapy, and systemic therapy approaches.

The Milan data continue to show that the survival following therapy for recurrence after either postoperative observation or cyclophosphamide, methotrexate, and 5-fluorouracil (CMF) therapy is similar. This observation appears to be true, even though the response rate among those patients failing within 12 months of completing CMF therapy is very low, whereas the response rate after 12 months is similar to that of patients who have never before received chemotherapy (Valagussa et al. 1986). One explanation for this observation is that patients who relapse early have a cell population which is relatively highly resistant, whereas later relapses have a much lower drug-resistant cell population (Fig. 1). This could explain why patients relapsing early after adjuvant therapy tend to be resistant to chemotherapy, whereas patients relapsing late may have tumors which are sensitive. This interpretation of the data also suggests that current systemic therapy approaches have insufficient cell kill to eliminate drug-resistant populations in a sig-

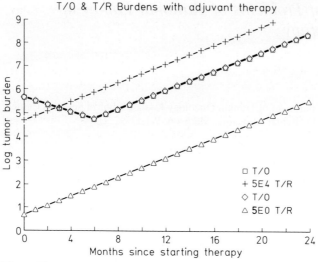

Fig. 1. The total cell population that is chemotherapy sensitive *(T/O)* and chemotherapy resistant *(T/R)* postoperatively, assuming 5E5 residual postoperative cells with a 42-day doubling time, six cycles of postoperative chemotherapy with a cell kill of 0.15 per cycle, and either 5E4 or 5E0 T/R cells postoperatively. The computer output was obtained from a modification of the Goldie/Coldman program using an exponential function for cell growth developed by Harris Lloyd at Southern Research Institute and modified using a probability branching process implemented by Goldstein at the University of Wisconsin. The simulation shows that the patients who relapsed early have a predominantly resistant cell population, whereas the patients relapsing late have a predominance of sensitive cells

nificant proportion of patients. Since the maximal benefit from adjuvant chemotherapy appears to occur with 4–6 months of treatment (Henderson et al. 1986; Tormey, this volume, pp. 106–112), the ratio of sensitive to resistant cells may be ≤ 1.00 after only 4–6 treatment cycles. Allowing for differences in drug action, these considerations are also consonant with the results from the tamoxifen trial reported by the Scottish Group [Report from the Breast Cancer Trials Committee (1987)]. Their results suggest that the first treatment approach, even in the adjuvant setting, is an important determinant of survival.

Many clinical trials have required testing of patients at frequent intervals in order to detect recurrence as early as possible. The theory is that the early detection of a tumor recurrence will be associated with a decreased tumor burden and a decreased probability of cells resistant to further therapy. Thus, the tumor will be more amenable to therapeutic intervention, which will lead to more prolonged survival than if treatment is instituted later. Unfortunately, there is no evidence that this is true with current treatment approaches. It is of considerable concern that no one has convincingly shown that earlier detection of relapse with immediate treatment yields better survival, despite the concept that a major determinant of survival appears to be the first treatment which is utilized. This may be because the current treatment for metastatic disease is palliative rather than potentially curative. The real problem, then, is what tests to use to monitor patients and how often they should be performed. Both the data presented here as well as previously published data suggest that up to 75% of recurrences are detected by the patient or physician. This also suggests that the majority of the remaining recurrences would be detected shortly after the routine tests used in current practice. The problem is, therefore, which tests to use and how often they should be used. It is clear that the retrospective analyses to date have been helpful but that prospective randomization of different follow-up policies for key tests would be very useful to the clinician. In addition, it would be important to know whether a detailed follow-up schedule and early treatment following a standard therapy would lead to an improved survival.

This session has raised serious concerns about how best to integrate radiotherapy with surgery and systemic therapy, the importance of current systemic adjuvant therapy and the role of current follow-up schedules for postoperative patients. Future trials will need to specifically evaluate these problems.

References

Fowble B, Gray R, Gilchrist K, Goodman RL, Taylor S, Tormey DC (1988) Identification of a subgroup of patients with breast cancer and histologically positive axillary nodes receiving adjuvant chemotherapy who may benefit from post-op radiotherapy. J Clin Oncol 6: 1107–1117

Henderson IC, Gelman RS, Harris JR, Canellos GP (1986) Duration of therapy in adjuvant chemotherapy trials. NCI Monogr 1: 95–98

Report from the Breast Cancer Trials Committee (1987) Adjuvant tamoxifen in the management of operable breast cancer: the Scottish trial. Lancet II: 171–175

Valagussa P, Tancini G, Bonadonna G (1986) Salvage Treatment of patients suffering relapse after adjuvant CMF chemotherapy. Cancer 58: 1411–1417

Endocrine Effects of Adjuvant Chemotherapy in Premenopausal Women: Suggestions for the Future*

D. C. Tormey

Clinical Cancer Center, Department of Human Oncology, K4/632 Clinical Sciences Center, University of Wisconsin, 600 Highland Avenue, Madison, WI 53792, USA

Introduction

Controversy continues to exist concerning the reason for an apparently greater therapeutic effect of postoperative chemotherapy in premenopausal Stage 2 patients as compared with postmenopausal patients (Brincker et al. 1987). The two major reasons suggested for the apparent difference have been a lower dose delivery in postmenopausal patients (Bonadonna and Valagussa 1981) and a drug-induced ovarian ablation in premenopausal patients (Pouquier 1978). The dosing hypothesis is not fully supported by other trials such as that of the Eastern Cooperative Oncology Group (ECOG), wherein the results for postmenopausal patients were similar to those of the initial Milan experience (Tormey et al. 1986). Similary, the differences observed in premenopausal patients with postoperative oophorectomy did not always provide a significant effect or appear to be as great as has been observed with postoperative chemotherapy (Cole 1975; Fisher 1971; Meakin 1986). This chapter examines this controversy further and develops a hypothesis to explain the apparently greater therapeutic impact of chemotherapy among Stage 2 premenopausal patients. The hypothesis suggests a treatment approach which could be tested in future premenopausal adjuvant trials.

Materials and Methods

The considerations presented were drawn from previously published data. Special correlations are explained in the text. Calculations of cell kill per course of treatment (Ks) in Stage 4 protocols utilized data only from patients with measurable disease components. Bidimensional measurements were converted to volumes using the formula $v = 4.189 [(a+b)/2]^3$, where v = volume and a and b = bidimensional radii of the lesion. It was then assumed that 1 cc = 1×10^8 cells. Regression curves were fit to the data to arrive at the cell kill observed per course of therapy.

* Supported in part by the National Cancer Institute, National Institutes of Health, USA, grant # PO1-CA20432.

Recent Results in Cancer Research, Vol. 115
© Springer-Verlag Berlin · Heidelberg 1989

Table 1. Impact of postoperative chemotherapy treatment duration upon disease control

Group	Duration	Result	Reference
SWOG	12 vs 24 months	nd	Rivkin et al. 1986
SAKK	6 vs 24 months	nd	Jungi et al. 1984; Senn and Jungi 1984
MILAN	6 vs 12 months	nd	Bonadonna et al. 1986
SECSG	6 vs 12 months	nd	Velez-Garcia et al. 1984
SFCI	15 vs 30 weeks	nd	Henderson et al. 1986

nd, no difference.

The Ks from patients achieving a complete or partial remission were directly calculated. The Ks in patients achieving a stabilization status was calculated to be equivalent to the observed doubling time of the population. For patients with a progressive disease response, Ks was set at zero. The Ks for the population of patients was arrived at by calculating the proportional contributions based upon the known response distributions.

Results and Discussion

Treatment Durations and End Results

A review of published trials suggests that four to five cycles of therapy provide equivalent results to up to 18 cycles spread over 2 years (Table 1). In addition, we have proposed that maintenance tamoxifen following the completion of 12 cycles of chemotherapy further improves the results (Tormey and Jordan 1984, 1987). Based on the clinical data in Table 1, as well as on considerations relating to tumor burden and cell kill (see below), a 1982 Wisconsin trial utilized four cycles of Adriamycin-based chemotherapy followed by maintenance tamoxifen. The early results appear promising, with 3-year relapse free survival rates of 83% overall, 92% with 1–3 N+, 73% with >3 N+, 100% in estrogen receptor positive (ER+), 67% in ER−, 74% in premenopausal, and 96% in postmenopausal patients. In addition, the recently completed randomized ECOG postmenopausal trial shows a significant advantage for the addition of maintenance tamoxifen after 12 months of cyclophosphamide, methotrexate, 5-fluorouracil, prednisone, and tamoxifen (CMFPT) therapy (Falkson 1987, personal communication). One interpretation of these various data sets is that 6 months or less of chemotherapy provides the maximal benefit to be achieved and that tamoxifen should be administered for many years.

Treatment Duration and Menstrual Activity

During the 1982 Wisconsin trial, it was observed that a high proportion of the premenopausal patients continued to have menstrual activity following the completion of 4 months of chemotherapy. This observation led to a re-evaluation of ovarian function and its role in premenopausal patients during chemotherapy combined with tamoxifen and during tamoxifen maintenance. The average time to development of a hormonal postmenopausal state was 4-6 months with chemotherapy alone, but 8-9 months with chemotherapy plus tamoxifen (Jordan et al. 1987). Analysis of patient data from multiple clinical trials performed at Wisconsin also revealed that the development of > 12 months of amenorrhea with chemotherapy regimens occurred in 24 of 43 (55.8%) patients receiving ≥ 12 months of chemotherapy but in only 1 of 12 (8.3%) patients receiving ≤ 6 months (Table 2). The persistence of menstrual activity occurred in 25 of 42 (59.5%) patients, despite the presence of maintenance tamoxifen. As expected, the incidence of amenorrhea was higher in patients over the age of 40; however, the incidence again was less with shorter chemotherapy durations (Table 3).

Hormonal evaluations of these patients revealed that serum estrogen concentrations during tamoxifen maintenance were cyclic and frequently elevated, sometimes to levels five times normal despite the presence of amenorrhea (Fritz et al. 1986; Jordan et al. 1987; Ravdin et al. 1988). These levels are over tenfold the observed maintenance tamoxifen serum levels (Jordan et al. 1987; Tormey and Jordan 1984). The high estrogen levels are disturbing because they are theoretically capable of overriding the achieved serum tamoxifen levels (Ravdin et al. 1988). These data led to a reconsideration of the influence of amenorrhea upon the observed results in postoperative chemotherapy trials.

Table 2. Relationship between treatment duration and the development of > 12 months of amenorrhea in premenopausal patients

Treatment	Duration	Incidence	
		n	(%)
Chemo	12 months	8/13	(61.5)
Chemo + T	12 months + 12 months	9/18	(50.0)
Chemo*T	12 months + years	7/12	(58.3)
Chemo + T	6 months + years	1/12	(8.3)

Chemo, cyclophosphamide + Adriamycin or methotrexate + 5-fluorouracil-based regimens; T, tamoxifen.

Table 3. Relationship between chemotherapy duration and amenorrhea incidence related to patient age at the start of chemotherapy

Treatment	Duration	< 40 years		≥ 40 years	
		n	(%)	*n*	(%)
Chemo	12 months	0/4	(0)	8/9	(89)
Chemo + T	12 months + 12 months	2/9	(22)	7/9	(78)
Chemo + T	12 months + years	3/6	(50)	4/6	(67)
Chemo + T	≤ 6 months + years	0/6	(0)	1/6	(17)

Chemo, cyclophosphamide + Adriamycin or methotrexate + 5-fluorouracil-based regimens; T, tamoxifen.

Impact of Amenorrhea Upon End Results

The relationship between the development of amenorrhea and treatment results in an ECOG premenopausal node-positive trial were first reported in 1984 (Tormey 1984). The ECOG trial randomized patients to receive 12 months of treatment with CMF, CMFP, or CMFPT. There was a relapse-free survival and survival advantage for patients achieving amenorrhea. The advantage was present in both ER-positive and ER-negative patients. A similar effect was also reported using another CMFP regimen (Goldhirsch and Gelber 1986). In another study, no relationship with CMF-induced amenorrhea was observed; however, cyclophosphamide-induced amenorrhea was associated with an improved relapse-free survival rate (Brincker et al. 1987).

Amenorrhea Impact from Cell Kill Estimates

The apparent importance of amenorrhea induction led to a reconsideration of the relative impact of chemotherapy in premenopausal as compared with postmenopausal patients. For this comparison, a data set which provided survival data at 5 or more years for similarly treated premenopausal and postmenopausal patients was required. Further, because of the relationship between CMF-associated amenorrhea and end results, it was desirable to use data from a trial which compared a CMF-based program with a program in which treatment-related amenorrhea did not appear to influence the results. A published data set meeting these criteria consists of a trial of CMF + vincristine and prednisone (CMFVP) vs L-phenylalanine mustard (Osborne et al. 1986). The amenorrhea occurring in patients treated with L-phenylalanine mustard has been reported not to influence treatment end results (Fischer et al. 1979). At 8 years, the survival advantage for CMFVP in this trial was 18% for premenopausal patients and 10% for postmenopausal patients. It could be hypothesized that the apparently greater impact of chemotherapy in the premenopausal patients was due to the impact of CMFVP upon ovarian function. The total cell kill needed to achieve the observed impact of chemotherapy can be estimated from suggested postoperative tumor burden distributions (Skipper 1981) to be 2.93 log for the premenopausal patients and 0.88 log for the postmenopausal patients.

Direct calculations of cell kill per treatment course in Stage 4 measurable disease were obtained from patient records in trials from the ECOG (Tormey et al. 1982, 1983), Cancer and Leukemia Group B (Tormey et al. 1984), National Cancer Institute (Bull et al. 1978; Tormey et al. 1979), and the University of Wisconsin Clinical Cancer Center (Loprinzi et al. 1986). The calculations for these various CMF- and Adriamycin-based regimens suggested an average cell kill per course of 0.15–0.18 log.

Translating this Stage 4 Ks to the postmenopausal Stage 2 patients suggests that the entire chemotherapy impact occurs with 4–6 cycles of therapy (0.88/0.15 or 0.18). This is in keeping with the clinical treatment duration experiences noted above.

The increased apparent cell kill observed in premenopausal patients in this trial appears to be 2.05 log (2.93-0.88). The cytostatic impact of the antiestrogenic effect of a chemotherapy-induced ovarian ablation upon this population could explain the difference in the end results observed between premenopausal and postmenopausal patients.

Currently, there are randomized Stage 2 chemotherapy ± oophorectomy trials maturing in the Southwestern Oncology Group/ECOG and the Ludwig Breast Cancer Study Group. The above considerations would suggest that if sufficient statistical power exists in these trials, they will show an advantage for the combination of chemotherapy plus oophorectomy.

Comment

The results and concepts reviewed in this manuscript suggest that chemotherapy in premenopausal patients causes both direct cell kill and a drug-induced postmenopausal state. The development of the drug-induced postmenopausal state appears to confer a therapeutic advantage. In addition, there is evidence that adjuvant therapy with tamoxifen provides a therapeutic advantage in postmenopausal patients (NIH 1986). These observations support the hypothesis that a distinct therapeutic improvement could be obtained in premenopausal patients by combining chemotherapy with an ovarian ablation and maintenance tamoxifen.

References

Bonadonna G, Valagussa P (1981) Dose-response effect of adjuvant chemotherapy in breast cancer. N Engl J Med 304: 10-15

Bonadonna G, Valagussa P, Tancini G, Rossi A, Brambilla C, Zambetti M, Bignami P, Di Fronzo G, Silvestrini R (1986) Current status of Milan adjuvant chemotherapy trials for node-positive and node-negative breast cancer. NCI Monogr 1: 45-49

Brincker H, Rose C, Rank F, Mouridsen HT, Jakobsen A, Dombernowsky P, Panduro J, Andersen KW (1987) Evidence of a castration-mediated effect of adjuvant cytotoxic chemotherapy in premenopausal breast cancer. J Clin Oncol 5: 1771-1778

Bull JM, Tormey DC, Li S-H, Carbone PP, Falkson G, Blom J, Perlin E, Simon R (1978) A randomized comparative trial of adriamycin versus methotrexate in combination drug therapy. Cancer 41: 1649-1657

Cole MP (1975) A clinical trial of an artificial menopause in carcinoma of the breast. Inserm 55: 143-150

Fisher B (1971) Status of adjuvant therapy: results of the National Surgical Adjuvant Breast Project studies on oophorectomy, postoperative radiation therapy, and chemotherapy. Cancer 28: 1654-1658

Fisher B, Sherman B, Rockette H, Redmond C, Margolese R, Fisher ER (1979) l-Phenylalanine mustard (L-PAM) in the management of premenopausal patients with primary breast cancer: lack of association of disease free survival with depression of ovarian function. Cancer 44: 847-857

Fritz NF, Tormey DC, Jordan VC (1986) Increased ovarian steroidogenesis in premenopausal N + breast cancer patients follows short-term chemotherapy and continuous tamoxifen adjuvant therapy. Breast Cancer Res Treat 8: 89

Goldhirsch A, Gelber R (1986) Adjuvant treatment for early breast cancer: the Ludwig breast cancer studies. NCI Monogr 1: 55-70

Henderson IC, Gelman RS, Harris JR, Canellos GP (1986) Duration of therapy in adjuvant chemotherapy trials. NCI Monogr 1: 95–98

Jordan VC, Fritz NF, Tormey DC (1987) Endocrine effects of adjuvant chemotherapy and long-term tamoxifen administration on node-positive patients with breast cancer. Cancer Res 47: 624–630

Jungi WF, Alberto P, Brunner KW, et al. (1984) Short- or long-term chemotherapy for node-positive breast cancer. LMF 6 versus 18 cycles. SAKK study 27/76. In: Senn HJ (ed) Adjuvant therapy of breast cancer. Springer, Berlin Heidelberg New York Tokyo, pp 175–177 (Recent results in cancer research, Vol 96)

Loprinzi CL, Tormey DC, Rasmussen P, Falkson G, Davis TE, Falkson HC, Chang AYC (1986) Prospective evaluation of carcinoembryonic antigen levels and alternating chemotherapeutic regimens in metastatic breast cancer. J Clin Oncol 4: 46–56

Meakin JW (1986) Review of Canadian trials of adjuvant endocrine therapy for breast cancer. NCI Monogr 1: 111–113

National Institutes of Health consensus development panel on adjuvant chemotherapy and endocrine therapy for breast cancer (1986) Introduction and conclusions. NCI Mongr 1: 1–4

Osborne CK, Rivkin SE, McDivitt RW, Green S, Stephens RL, Costanzi JJ, O'Bryan RO (1986) Adjuvant therapy of breast cancer: Southwest Oncology Group studies. NCI Monogr 1: 71–74

Pouquier H (1978) Adjuvant chemotherapy of breast cancer: is it a direct cytotoxic or has it an indirect hormone effect? Int J Radiat Oncol Biol Phys 4: 917–919

Ravdin PM, Fritz NF, Tormey DC, Jordan VC (1988) Endocrine status of premenopausal node-positive breast cancer patients following adjuvant chemotherapy and long-term tamoxifen. Can Res 48: 1026–1029

Rivkin S, Green S, Metch B, Osborne CK, Knight WA, McDivitt R, Cruz A, Tesh D, Costanzi J, Balcerzak S, Stevens R (1986) Adjuvant chemotherapy for poor prognosis receptor negative Stage II, III breast cancer: one year vs 2 yrs CMFVP. Breast Cancer Res Treat 8: 80

Senn HJ, Jungi WF (1984) Swiss adjuvant trials with LMF(+BCG) in N− and N+ breast cancer patients. In: Jones SE, Salmon SE (eds) Adjuvant therapy of cancer, vol 4. Grune and Stratton, Orlando, Fl, pp 261–270

Skipper HE (1981) Some analyses and trial-and-error simulations of the response of breast cancer to surgery, chemotherapy, and surgery plus chemotherapy. Southern Research Institute Technical Report 18 (Sep 23): 11–16

Tormey DC (1984) Adjuvant systemic therapy in postoperative node positive patients with breast carcinoma: the CALGB trial and the ECOG premenopausal trial. In: Senn HJ (ed) Adjuvant therapy of breast cancer. Springer, Berlin Heidelberg New York Tokyo, pp 155–165 (Recent results in cancer research, vol 96)

Tormey DC, Jordan VC (1984) Long-term tamoxifen adjuvant therapy in node positive breast cancer – A metabolic and pilot clinical study. Breast Cancer Res Treat 4: 297–302

Tormey DC, Jordan VC (1987) Long-term adjuvant tamoxifen study: clinical update. Breast Cancer Res Treat 9: 157–158

Tormey DC, Falkson G, Simon RM, Blom J, Bull JM, Lippman ME, Li S-H, Cassidy J, Falkson HC (1979) A randomized comparison of two sequentially administered combination regimens to a single regimen in metastatic breast cancer. Cancer Clin Trials 2: 247–256

Tormey DC, Gelman R, Band PR, Sears M, Rosenthal SN, DeWys W, Perlia C, Rice MA (1982) Comparison of induction chemotherapies for metastatic breast cancer: an Eastern Cooperative Oncology Group trial. Cancer 50: 1235–1244

Tormey D, Gelman R, Falkson G (1983) Prospective evaluation of rotating chemotherapy in advanced breast cancer: an Eastern Cooperative Oncology Group trial. Am J Clin Oncol 6: 1–189

Tormey DC, Weinberg VE, Leone LA, Glidewell OJ, Perloff M, Kennedy BJ, Cortes E, Silver RT, Weiss RB, Aisner J, Holland JF (1984) A comparison of intermittent vs continuous and of adriamycin vs methotrexate 5-drug chemotherapy for advanced breast cancer: a Cancer and Leukemia Group B study. Am J Clin Oncol 7: 231–239

Tormey DC, Gray R, Taylor SG IV, Knuiman M, Olson JE, Cummings FJ (1986) Postoperative chemotherapy and chemohormonal therapy in women with node-positive breast cancer. NCI Monog 1: 75–80 [and (1987) updated analyses]

Velez-Garcia E, Moore M, Vogel CL, et al. (1984) Postsurgical adjuvant chemotherapy in women with breast cancer and positive axillary nodes: the Southeastern Cancer Study Group (SECSG) experience. In: Jones SE, Salmon SE (eds) Adjuvant therapy of cancer, vol 4. Grune and Stratton, Orlando, pp 273–282

The Milan Experience with Adjuvant Chemotherapy in Premenopausal Breast Cancer*

G. Bonadonna, P. Valagussa, M. Zambetti, and C. Brambilla

Istituto Nazionale Tumori, Via Venezian, 20133 Milano, Italy

Introduction

In spite of the many scientific and clinical debates which have involved adjuvant chemotherapy for high-risk resectable breast cancer, there is general agreement that polydrug regimens, in particular, CMF (cyclophosphamide, methotrexate, and fluorouracil), are effective in improving relapse-free (RFS) and overall survival (OS) rates in premenopausal women (Bonadonna et al. 1977; Bonadonna and Valagussa 1988; Henderson 1987). In this report, we update the results of our two initial prospective randomized trials activated in June 1973 and September 1975 respectively.

Patient Population

A total of 189 premenopausal patients were randomized to two groups of controls (86 cases) and adjuvant CMF for 12 monthly cycles (103 cases). In the subsequent study, 160 premenopausal patients were randomly allocated to receive 12 monthly cycles of CMF, and 164 patients, six cycles of the same drug regimen. Staging and follow-up procedures, as well as type of surgery and drug schedules, have been detailed in previous publications (Bonadonna et al. 1977, Tancini et al. 1983). The median duration of follow-up for the first study is 13 years, for the second study, 10.5 years, respectively. In a third prospective non-randomized trial, CMF was tested for 12 monthly cycles, and the median follow-up of this study is 8 years.

The product-limit method (Kaplan and Meier 1958) was adopted to estimate survival, which was measured from the date of surgery. Disease relapse and contralateral breast cancer were taken as the end point for RFS, whereas death from all causes was taken as the end point for OS. The log-rank test (Peto et al. 1977) was used to assess the differential effect of treatments.

---

* Supported in part by Contract NO1-CM-07338 with the Division of Cancer Treatment, National Cancer Institute, National Institutes of Health.

Table 1. First CMF program: comparative median duration in months in premenopausal women

		Control	CMF
RFS,	Total	32	141
	Nodes ($n = 1$–3)	63	144
	Nodes ($n > 3$)	20	44
OS,	Total	96	NR
	Nodes ($n = 1$–3)	130	NR
	Nodes ($n > 3$)	77	89

NR, not reached.

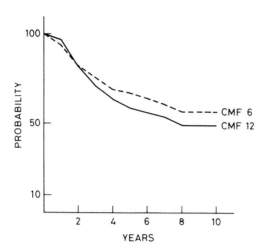

Fig. 1. Second CMF program: Comparative RFS for premenopausal breast cancer. *CMF 6*, six cycles of CMF therapy; *CMF 12*, 12 cycles of CMF therapy

Results

Table 1 compares the median duration in months of RFS and OS between the control and CMF-treated groups in the first study. The benefit from adjuvant chemotherapy is evident in all nodal subsets. It is important to stress that the median duration of OS was not reached in the entire case series and in the subset with one to three positive axillary nodes.

Figures 1 and 2 compare RFS and OS for patients treated with 12 as opposed to six cycles of adjuvant CMF. The initial trend in favor of CMF administered for six cycles remains at the 10-year analysis. A full explanation for this difference has not yet been found even when a retrospective analysis of dose intensity has been performed (Hryniuk et al. 1987). As previously reported, in about half of patients the estrogen receptor (ER) status was available for comparative analysis. Also at 10 years from surgery, there was no difference in RFS and OS between women whose tumors were classified as either ER positive or ER negative.

Figure 3 compares the RFS experience of three consecutive premenopausal study groups treated at the Milan Cancer Institute with adjuvant CMF, the control

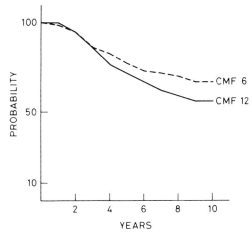

Fig. 2. Second CMF program: Comparative OS for premenopausal breast cancer. *CMF 6,* six cycles of CMF therapy; *CMF 12,* 12 cycles of CMF therapy

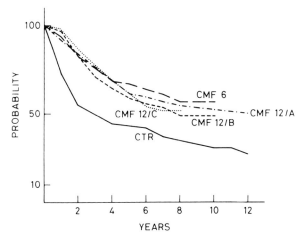

Fig. 3. RFS in various study protocols (*CTR,* control group; *CMF 6,* six cycles of CMF therapy, second trial; *CMF 12/A,* 12 cycles of CMF therapy, first trial; *CMF 12/B,* second trial; *CMF 12/C,* third trial)

group being that of our first randomized trial. The consistency in the observed findings in patients selected, treated, and followed up with identical methods is quite evident.

Conclusions

Our updated results with adjuvant CMF in premenopausal women are consistent and confirm our initial premises (Bonadonna et al. 1976). The greatest effect of

CMF was observed in women with one to three positive lymph nodes. Our findings support the concepts relating to the cause of primary tumor cell resistance (Goldie and Coldman 1984), and thus adjuvant CMF does not need to be administered for 12 monthly cycles. Provided full – dose chemotherapy is administered as frequently as technically feasible, six monthly cycles of CMF will probably achieve the maximum therapeutic benefit. However, as stressed by Valagussa et al. (this volume, pp. 69), retreatment with CMF can result in about 50% complete plus partial remission in patients whose primary treatment failure following adjuvant CMF occurs after a disease-free period in excess of 12 months from the end of adjuvant therapy.

The above-mentioned findings concerning the efficacy of salvage CMF, the therapeutic activity of surgical castration in women who became amenorrheic following CMF chemotherapy (Valagussa et al., this volume, pp. 69), the similarity of RFS in our patients regardless of amenorrhea and, last but not least, the significant improvement of the 5-year RFS and OS in node-negative receptor-negative women (Bonadonna and Valagussa 1988), run counter to the hypothesis that the therapeutic activity of adjuvant CMF is mediated in part through chemical castration.

Available results, including those recently published by the Ludwig Breast Cancer Study Group (1985) and the Danish Breast Cancer Cooperative Group (Brincker et al. 1987) are also difficult to interpret because the steroid receptor was not assayed for all study women given adjuvant chemotherapy. We cannot exclude a priori that, within the complex mosaic of breast cancer patient subsets do exist (e.g., with histologic grade 1, low percentage of S-phases, high steroid receptor content), who will benefit almost exclusively by adjuvant endocrine treatment. Whatever the biological explanation is and within the limits of interseries comparison, we believe that in premenopausal node-positive women full-dose adjuvant combination chemotherapy has so far yielded long-term results which are superior to adjuvant castration or adjuvant tamoxifen.

References

Bonadonna G, Brusamolino E, Valagussa P, Rossi A, Brugnatelli L, Brambilla C, De Lena M, Tancini G, Bajetta E, Musumeci R, Veronesi U (1976) Combination chemotherapy as an adjuvant treatment in operable breast cancer. N Engl J Med 294: 405–410

Bonadonna G, Rossi A, Valagussa P, Banfi A, Veronesi U (1977) The CMF program for operable breast cancer with positive axillary nodes: Updated analysis on the disease-free interval, site or relapse and drug tolerance. Cancer 39: 2904–2915

Bonadonna G, Valagussa P (1988) The contribution of medicine to the primary treatment of breast cancer. Cancer Res 48: 2314–2324

Brincker H, Rose C, Rank F, Mouridsen HT, Jakobsen A, Dombernowsky P, Panduro J, Andersen KW on behalf of the Danish Breast Cancer Cooperative Group (1987) Evidence of a castration-mediated effect of adjuvant cytotoxic chemotherapy in premenopausal breast cancer. J Clin Oncol 5: 1771–1778

Goldie JH, Coldman AJ (1984) The genetic origin of drug resistance in neoplasms: Implications for systemic therapy. Cancer Res 44: 3643–3653

Henderson IC (1987) Adjuvant systemic therapy for early breast cancer. Curr Probl Cancer 11: 125–207

Hryniuk WM, Bonadonna G, Valagussa P (1987) The effect of dose intensity in adjuvant chemotherapy. In: Salmon SE (ed) Adjuvant therapy of cancer, vol 5. Grune and Stratton, Orlando, pp 13–23

Kaplan EL, Meier P (1958) Non-parametric estimation from incomplete observations. J Am Stat Assoc 53: 457–481

Ludwig Breast Cancer Study Group (1985) A randomized trial of adjuvant combination chemotherapy with or without prednisone in premenopausal breast cancer patients with metastases in one to three axillary lymph nodes. Cancer Res 45: 4454–4459

Peto R, Pike MC, Armitage P, Breslow NE, Cox DR, Howard SV, Mantel N, McPherson K, Peto J, Smith PG (1977) Design and analysis of randomized clinical trials requiring prolonged observation of each patient. II. Analysis and examples. Br J Cancer 35: 1–39

Tancini G, Bonadonna G, Valagussa P, Marchini S, Veronesi U (1983) Adjuvant CMF in breast cancer: comparative 5-year results of 12 versus 6 cycles. J Clin Oncol 1: 2–10

Adjuvant Chemo- and Endocrine Therapy Alone or in Combination in Premenopausal Patients (GABG Trial 1)*

M. Kaufmann, W. Jonat, and U. Abel

Abteilung für Gynäkologie und Geburtshilfe, Universität Heidelberg, Voßstraße 9, 6900 Heidelberg, FRG

Introduction

The natural history of operable breast cancer can be affected by adjuvant treatment (Lippman 1986; Salmon 1987). Adjuvant combination chemotherapy, e.g., cyclophosphamide, methotrexate, and 5-fluorouracil (CMF) results in a significant prolongation of disease-free (DFS) and overall survival (OS) in *premenopausal* node-positive patients. These data were mainly obtained by overview analyses of randomized trials with treatment groups as compared with no adjuvant therapy (control) after mastectomy.

The most important known prognostic factors in primary breast cancer are the axillary lymph node and the hormone receptor status (Kaufmann 1983; Wilson et al. 1984). To date, no randomized trial has been conducted which separtely randomized patients in a prospective way according to these clinically important prognostic factors. Also until now, no long-term follow-up data which compare endocrine treatment alone with cytotoxic therapy in prospectively defined subgroups of node-positive (N+) primary breast cancer have been available.

This paper reports the *premenopausal* data of two risk-adapted randomized prospective adjuvant trials conducted in West-Germany between January 1981 and January 1988 by 13 university and larger regional hospitals (see Appendix A). Patient entry was closed in May 1986. (For postmenopausal data, see Jonat et al., this volume).

In the low-risk situation ($n = 1$-3 involved axillary nodes *and* hormone receptor-positive tumors) patients entered the trial to receive tamoxifen (TAM) or CMF chemotherapy. In the high-risk situation ($n > = 4$ involved nodes *or* $n = 1$-3 nodes and hormone receptor-negative tumors), patients were treated with adriamycin and cyclophosphamide (AC) alone or in combination with TAM. The aim of the study was to analyze adjuvant endocrine, cytotoxic, and chemoendocrine therapy in defined subsets ($< = 49$ years) of women with N+ breast cancer.

---

* This work was partially supported by grants from ICI-Pharma, Plankstadt, FRG, and Farmitalia Carlo Erba, Freiburg, FRG.

Recent Results in Cancer Research, Vol. 115
© Springer-Verlag Berlin·Heidelberg 1989

Table 1. GABG 1: Patient characteristics

		Low-risk n (%)		High-risk n (%)	
		TAM	CMF	AC	AC + TAM
Age	< = 49 years	49 (36)	70 (51)	116 (49)	96 (41)
	> = 50 years	89 (64)	68 (49)	121 (51)	138 (59)
Tumor size	T 1	34 (25)	35 (25)	34 (14)	36 (15)
	T 2	92 (67)	93 (67)	158 (67)	151 (65)
	T 3	12 (8)	10 (7)	45 (19)	47 (20)
Node histology	1	72 (52)	60 (44)	21 ⎱	19 ⎱
	2	44 (32)	50 (36)	22 ⎰ (22)	9 ⎰ (17)
	3	22 (16)	28 (20)	10 ⎰	12 ⎰
	4–9			116 (49)	143 (61)
	> = 10			68 (29)	51 (22)
Receptor status	ER +	129 (93)	124 (90)	92 (39)	108 (46)
	ER −	9 (7)	14 (10)	145 (61)	126 (54)
	unknown	0	0	0	0
	PR +	104 (75)	106 (77)	73 (31)	90 (38)
	PR −	30 (22)	19 (14)	140 (59)	119 (51)
	PR unknown	4 (3)	13 (9)	24 (10)	25 (11)
	Total	138	138	237	234

Patients and Methods

Patients

Women < = 49 years old with histologically invasive T 1–3 tumors treated by modified radical mastectomy and axillary lymph node dissection (levels I and II ± III) entered this trial. No postoperative radiotherapy was used. Only women with a least ten biopsied and analyzed nodes and known hormone receptor status [estrogen (ER) and/or progesterone receptor (PR)] were randomized. Treatment was started within 3 weeks of surgery. In total, 747 of 774 patients were evaluable for both trials according to the defined entry criteria.

Table 1 summarizes the distribution of patient and tumor characteristics for both trials and for each therapy group (pre- and postmenopausal patients).

Adjuvant Treatment

A total of 119 *low-risk* patients ($n = 1$–3, ER + or PR +) were randomized after mastectomy to TAM (30 mg/day orally continuously for 2 years) or CMF (Bonadonna et al. 1976) i.v. for six cycles every 4 weeks. Full doses of C (500 mg/m^2), M (40 mg/m^2), and F (600 mg/m^2) were given on days 1 and 8. A total of 212 *high-risk* patients ($n > = 4$, or $n = 1$–3, ER − and PR −) were randomized to AC (Salmon and Jones 1979) i.v. alone or AC + TAM. At intervals of 3 weeks, full doses of eight cycles of A (30 mg/m^2) were given on day 1 and of C (300 mg/m^2) on days 1 and 8. TAM was also administered for 2 years.

Hormone Receptor Analysis

ER and PR were determined by the EORTC standard method using dextran-coated charcoal (EORTC 1973). All primary tumor specimens were assayed at least for ER. Tumors were defined as receptor positive at levels of $> =20$ fmols/mg cytosol protein. Interlaboratory quality control studies were conducted twice a year (Kaufmann et al. 1985).

Follow-up Studies

Clinical and hemtologic assessment was carried out before each i.v. cytotoxic drug administration every 3 months for 2 years and thereafter every 6 months. Liver ultrasound examinations, bone scans, and chest X-rays were repeated every 6 months and after 2 years, annually.

Randomization and Statistical Methods

Randomization was conducted by each hospital with centrally distributed envelopes. The method of Kaplan and Meier (1958) and a log-rank test with values of significance (Peto et al. 1977) were used to estimate DFS and OS from the date of surgery.

Results

With respect to DFS and OS, the Kaplan Meier curves give for all 747 (pre- and postmenopausal) low- and high-risk patients significant ($P=0.00001$) differences after 6 years of follow-up. DFS and OS are also directly related to the number of involved nodes ($n=1$–3 and ER+, $n=1$–3 and ER−, $n> =4$–9, $n> =10$).

For 331 premenopausal patients, the rate of first recurrences and deaths after 6 years is demonstrated in Table 2. For TAM and CMF treatment, locoregional failure is only 18.4% and 4.3% respectively, while in the AC and AC+TAM

Table 2. GABG 1 Study: Recurrence and death after 6 years for premenopausal patients ($n=331$)

Type	Low risk (%)		High risk (%)	
	TAM	CMF	AC	AC+TAM
Locoregional	18.4	4.3	20.7	16.7
Distant (+combination)	32.7	11.4	36.2	34.4
Total	51.1	15.7	56.9	51.1
Death	20.4	4.3	30.2	31.3

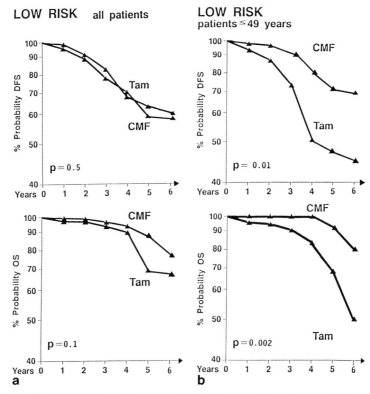

Fig. 1a, b. DFS and OS by treatment for **a** all 276 low-risk patients and **b** all 119 low-risk premenopausal patients

group, it is 20.7% as opposed to 16.7%. Distant and locoregional failures are higher for the TAM arm in the low-risk group and identical for the AC ± TAM treatment in the high-risk group. In total, death rates are less for CMF than for TAM treatment. No significant differences exist in the high-risk groups. Life table analysis showed no significant differences by treatment for all 747 low (Fig. 1a) and high (Fig. 2a) risk patients. In these defined subgroups, endocrine treatment (TAM) produces results equal to cytotoxic CMF treatment, and chemoendocrine combination therapy is not significantly superior to cytotoxic combination therapy alone. In the low-risk premenopausal situation, CMF is significantly superior to TAM for DFS ($P=0.01$) and OS ($P=0.002$) (Fig. 1b). No differences were yielded in the high-risk collective for chemo- or chemoendocrine therapy (Fig. 2b). However, AC alone tends to be superior to the endocrine-cytotoxic combination for this subgroup.

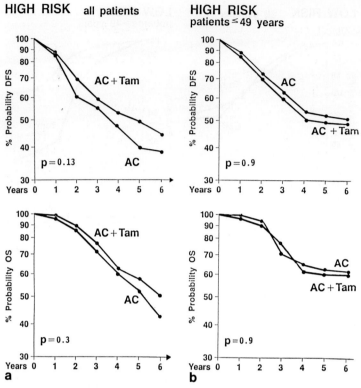

Fig. 2a, b. DFS and OS by treatment for **a** all 471 high-risk patients and **b** all 212 high-risk premenopausal patients

Discussion

Our study design was prospectively based and randomized according to lymph node and hormone-receptor status for a so-called low- and high-risk situation. All N+ premenopausal patients treated at the participating institutions were included in the trial. (For postmenopausal patients, see Jonat et al. this volume). In a defined low-risk subset ($n = 1$–3 nodes, ER+ or PR+ status), a comparison between TAM alone and cytotoxic chemotherapy alone was conducted. TAM was given for 2 years and CMF i.v. for 6 months. In a defined high-risk subset ($n > = 4$ nodes, or negative receptor status) the efficacy of cytotoxic combination chemotherapy was compared with that of chemoendocrine treatment. AC was given i.v. for eight cycles in 6 months along with TAM for two years.

For low-risk situations, the question of whether endocrine treatment is as effective as cytotoxic therapy arises, whereas for high-risk situations there is some theoretical rationale for combined chemoendocrine treatment (Bonadonna and Valagussa 1986; Fisher et al. 1981, 1986). In accordance with our earlier reports (Kaufmann et al. 1984, 1985), again no significant differences between the two various aggressive therapies for all low-risk patients can be demonstrated for DFS and OS after 6 years. However, for all high-risk patients neither DFS nor OS were significantly superior for chemoendocrine therapy as compared with chemotherapy alone. However, subset analyses yielded interesting results which correspond to conclusions stated at the 1985 Consensus Development Conference (1985) and support the idea of defining prognostic subgroups of patients with primary breast cancer before starting adjuvant systemic treatment.

Premenopausal low-risk women (≤ 49 years) benefit from 6 months chemotherapy, e.g., CMF. Combined chemoendocrine (AC + TAM) treatment did not improve results for DFS or OS in premenopausal patients. No significant improvement was observed by adding TAM to cytotoxic treatment. In both trials, endocrine therapy mainly affects hormone-receptor-positive tumors, as reported by other study groups (Fisher et al. 1987; Hubay et al. 1980; Ludwig Breast Cancer Study Group 1984; Rose et al. 1985).

None of the published reports have documented a significant survival benefit in premenopausal patients from endocrine treatment alone – the NATO and Scottish trial excluded (NATO 1985; Scottish Cancer Trial 1987). Both of these trials found an improvement in survival, independent of nodal and menopausal status, this observation needs further clarification (anonymous 1987).

At present, despite clear recommendations given by the NIH Consensus Development Conference that TAM should be used only in postmenopausal women with N + and receptor-positive tumors, it remains unclear whether combined chemoendocrine treatment is superior to TAM given alone and irrespective of nodal and receptor status. It is surprising that TAM treatment alone is ineffective in the adjuvant premenopausal situation and effective in the palliative treatment of premenopausal women. Several controversial reports have been made on the relation of ovarian function and cytotoxic adjuvant treatment (Bonadonna and Valagussa 1985; Padmanabhan et al. 1987). Chemotherapy-induced amenorrhea is often combined with permanent castration, and DFS or OS may be improved in this way. Adjuvant ovarian ablation delays recurrence and prolongs survival (Meakin 1986). However, in the Ludwig Trial (1985), no advantage was seen when oophorectomy was combined with CMF.

Our results confirm that lymph node and receptor status are per se prognostic factors. Low- and high-risk situations also exist after first failure; this seems to be due to the natural histories of primary breast cancer. New methodologies, e.g., new quality-of-life-oriented end points for the assessment of adjuvant therapy are needed to assist in the selection of therapeutic approach (Gelber and Goldhirsch 1986).

The design of new randomized trials must take into consideration risk-adapted treatment modalities in defined subsets of patients with operable breast cancer in order to improve further survival and quality of life.

Acknowledgment. We thank all participating institutions for their excellent cooperation and also wish to acknowledge the essential contributions of the many clinicians, pathologists, and laboratory workers who made this collaborative study possible.

124   M. Kaufmann et al.

Appendix A
Gynecological Adjuvant Breast Cancer Group, FRG (GABG 1)

Main investigator	Institution
M. Kaufmann, F. Kubli[a]	University of Heidelberg
W. Jonat, H. Maass	University of Hamburg
H. Caffier, K. H. Wulf	University of Würzburg
R. Kreienberg, V. Friedberg	University of Mainz
J. Hilfrich, J. Schneider	University of Hannover
W. Kleine, A. Pfleiderer	University of Freiburg
M. Neises, F. Melchert	University of Mannheim/Heidelberg
M. Mahlke, P. Knapstein	Städtische Frauenklinik Krefeld
G. Trams	Städtische Frauenklinik Bremen
K. Brunnert, J. Schermann, P. Dördelmann	Städtische Frauenklinik Karlsruhe
U. Stosiek, K. Gumbrecht	Diakonissen Krankenhaus Karlsruhe
R. Stigelmeyer, F. Seeger, O. Fettig	Vincentius Krankenhaus Karlsruhe
U. Abel	Tumorzentrum Heidelberg

References

Anonymous (1987) Adjuvant tamoxifen in early breast cancer. Lancet ii: 191–192

Bonadonna G, Brusamolino E, Valagussa P et al. (1976) Combination chemotherapy as an adjuvant treatment in operable breast cancer. N Engl J Med 294: 405–410

Bonadonna G, Valagussa P (1985) Adjuvant systemic therapy for resectable breast cancer. J Clin Oncol 3: 259–275

Bonadonna G, Valagussa P (1986) Adjuvant chemoendocrine therapy in breast cancer. J Clin Oncol 4: 451–454

Consensus Conference (1985) Adjuvant chemotherapy for breast cancer. JAMA 254: 3461–3463

EORTC: Breast Cancer Cooperative Group (1973) Standards for the assessment of estrogen receptors in human breast cancer. Eur J Cancer Clin Oncol 9: 379–381

Fisher B, Redmond C, Brown A et al. (1981) Treatment of primary breast cancer with chemotherapy and tamoxifen. N Engl J Med 305: 1–6

Fisher B, Redmond C, Brown A et al. (1986) Adjuvant chemotherapy with and without tamoxifen in the treatment of primary breast cancer: 5-year results from the National Surgical Adjuvant Breast and Bowel Project Trial. J Clin Oncol 4: 459–471

Fisher ER, Sass R, Fisher B et al. (1987) Pathologic findings from the National Surgical Adjuvant Breast Project: Correlations with concordant and discordant estrogen and progesterone receptors. Cancer 59: 1554–1559

Gelber RD, Goldhirsch A for the Ludwig Breast Cancer Study Group (1986) A new endpoint for the assessment of adjuvant therapy in postmenopausal women with operable breast cancer. J Clin Oncol 4: 1772–1779

Hubay C, Pearson OH, Marshall US et al. (1980) Antiestrogen, cytotoxic chemotherapy and bacillus Calmette-Guérain vaccination in stage II breast cancer: a preliminary report. Surgery 87: 494–501

Kaplan EL, Meier P (1958) Nonparametric estimation from incomplete observations. J Am Statis Assoc 53: 457–481

Kaufmann M (1983) Biochemische prognostische Faktoren beim Mamma-Karzinom. In: Kubli F, Nagel GA, Kadach U, Kaufmann M (eds) Neue Wege in der Brustkrebsbehandlung. Zuckschwerdt, Munich, pp 46–61 (Aktuelle onkologie, vol 8)

---

[a] Deceased.

Kaufmann M, Jonat W et al. (GABG) (1984) Risk adapted adjuvant chemo-hormonother-
    apy in operable nodal positive breast cancer. In: Jones SE, Salmon SE (eds) (1984) Adju-
    vant therapy of cancer, vol 4. Grune and Stratton, New York, pp 369-378
Kaufmann M, Jonat W, Caffier H, Hilfrich J, Melchert F, Mahlke M, Abel U, Maass H,
    Kubli F for the Gynecological Adjuvant Breast Cancer Group (1985) Adjuvant chemo-
    hormonotherapy selected by axillary node and hormone receptor status in node-positive
    breast cancer. Reviews Endocrine-Related Cancer 17: [Suppl] 57-63
Meakin JW (1986) Review of Canadian Trials of adjuvant endocrine therapy for breast can-
    cer. NCI Monogr 1: 111-113
Lippman ME (ed) (1986) NIH Consensus Development Conference on adjuvant chemo-
    therapy and endocrine therapy breast cancer 1985. NCI Monogr 1
Ludwig Breast Cancer Study Group (1984) Randomized trial of chemo-endocrine therapy,
    endocrine therapy and mastectomy alone in postmenopausal patients with operable
    breast cancer and axillary node metastases. Lancet i: 1256-1260
Ludwig Breast Cancer Study Group (1985) Chemotherapy with or without oophorectomy
    high-risk premenopausal patients with operable breast cancer. J Clin Oncol 3: 1059-1067
Nolvadex Adjuvant Trial Organization (NATO) (1985) Controlled trial of tamoxifen as sin-
    gle adjuvant agent in management of early breast cancer. Analysis at six years. Lancet i:
    836-840
Padmanabhan N, Wang DY, Moore JW, Rubens RD (1987) Ovarian function and adjuvant
    chemotherapy for early breast cancer. Eur J Cancer Clin Oncol 23: 745-748
Peto R, Pike MC, Armitage P et al. (1977) Design and analysis of randomized clinical trials
    requiring prolonged observation of each patient. Analysis and examples. Br J Cancer 35:
    1-39
Rose C, Thorpe S, Anderson KW et al (1985) Beneficial effect of adjuvant tamoxifen thera-
    py in primary breast cancer patients with high oestrogen receptor value. Lancet i: 16-19
Salmon SE (ed) (1987) Adjuvant therapy of cancer, vol 5. Grune and Stratton, New York
Salmon SE, Jones SE (1979) Studies of the combination of adriamycin and cyclophospham-
    ide (alone or with other agents) for the treatment of breast cancer. Oncology 36: 40-44
Scottish Cancer Trial (1987) Adjuvant tamoxifen in the management of operable breast can-
    cer: The Scottish Trial. Lancet ii: 171-175
Wilson RE, Donegan WL, Mettlin C et al. (1984) The 1982 national survey of carcinoma of
    the breast in the United States. Surg Gynecol Obstet 159: 309-318

Scottish Adjuvant Breast Cancer Trials: Results in Pre-menopausal Patients

H. J. Stewart

Scottish Cancer Trials Office (MRC), The Medical School, Edinburgh, EH8 9AG, Great Britain

Introduction

In 1980, with support from the Medical Research Council of Great Britain, the Scottish Cancer Trials Office was established principally to conduct four parallel adjuvant therapy trials in primary breast cancer.

Trial A

The first of these, Trial A, remains open and is only for pre-menopausal patients with proven involvement of axillary lymph nodes. We were stimulated to undertake this trial by reports of benefit in the pre-menopausal subgroups of the Milan CMF trial by Bonnadonna et al. (1977) and the Toronto ovarian ablation trial by Meakin et al. (1977), as well as the suggestion from others (Rose and Davis 1977; Hubay et al. 1980) that the beneficial effect of CMF might in part be mediated through functioning ovaries. Randomisation in Trial A is thus for either CMF chemotherapy or ovarian ablation each with or without long-term prednisone therapy, 7.5 mg daily for 5 years (Fig. 1). Oestrogen-receptor (ER) information is recorded when available but plays no part in the randomisation procedure. Initially, local therapy was by mastectomy with either an axillary lymph node clearance or a sampling procedure and post-operative radiotherapy. Subsequently, in the hope of increasing accrual, initial therapy by breast conservation for those patients with lesions of less than 4 cm was also allowed. Accrual to this trial has been disappointing, as has compliance with allocated option (Table 1). The low referral rate (257 in 8 years) is not only because of the inherent small size of the patient group under study but also because of the reluctance of many otherwise supportive clinicians to accept one or other of the therapy options. This non-participation has increased with time, some clinicians no longer being prepared to ignore ER status when considering adjuvant therapy.

A watching brief with interim analysis has been kept on the results, but although some subgroups appear to be doing slightly better than others, the numbers are too small for these differences to be meaningful. Between the major treatment arms, there is as yet no significant difference in outcome.

Recent Results in Cancer Research, Vol. 115
© Springer-Verlag Berlin · Heidelberg 1989

SCOTTISH TRIAL A

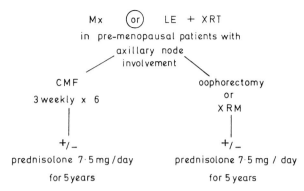

Fig. 1. Flow chart for Scottish pre-menopausal poor-prognosis adjuvant therapy trial (Trial A). *Mx*, total mastectomy; *LE*, wide local excision of primary breast cancer; *XRT*, postoperative radical X-ray therapy given either (a) after Mx and axillary node sample to chest wall and regional nodes, or (b) to residual breast tissue, but only to nodal areas as well if a sample is performed; *XRM*, X-ray menopause; *CMF*, cyclophosphamide 750 mg/m², methotrexate 50 mg/m² and 5-fluorouracil 600 mg/m², all given intravenously

Table 1. For each of the four randomised options, the intake during the first 8 years to the Scottish pre-menopausal poor prognosis trial (Trial A), with the proportions compliant within each group for the first 200 patients randomised within the trial

	Prednisone 7.5 mg per day for 5 years	No prednisone
Ovarian ablation		
8 year entry	62	64
fraction (%) compliant out of first 200 randomisations	40/49 (82%)	45/52 (87%)
CMF IV 3 weekly for 6–8 courses		
8 year entry	65	66
fraction (%) compliant out of first 200 randomisations	32/50 (64%)	34/49 (69%)

Our belief in the importance of the objectives of the trial led to acceptance by our statistician of three modifications to the original protocol, namely the reduction of chemotherapy courses from 12 to six, the inclusion, as already stated, of conservation therapy as an acceptable alternative to mastectomy and the admission of patients referred from Guy's Hospital in addition to the Scottish intake. Although the latter has been extremely valuable, the future of the trial remains uncertain, and premature closure is currently under consideration. The patients remain on follow-up and hopefully, at some time in the future, trial data will contribute to worthwhile combined analyses.

Adjuvant Tamoxifen: Trials B, C and D

Tamoxifen therapy, 20 mg daily, was the randomised adjuvant treatment option for all other Scottish trial referrals up until September 1984. Although administered as separate trials, the data obtained have been handled as if belonging to one. Data from 1312 patients, of whom 242 (18.4%) are pre-menopausal (being within 12 months of menstruation at entry), are available for analysis. Special features of these trials which make them different from most other adjuvant tamoxifen trials are the 5 years' duration of therapy and the comparison of this treatment with tamoxifen given in the management of the first relapse. The results available represent the effect of an average of 47 months' therapy for those in the tamoxifen arm and a 93% incidence of tamoxifen, for a minimum of 6 weeks, for those with recurrent disease in the control arm. In addition, the level of ER in the primary tumour is known for 742 patients (57%).

With over 90 surgeons taking part in the tamoxifen trials, it would have been unreasonable to ask for a single form of local management. Consequently, surgeons were expected to adhere to one or other of two management policies, namely, mastectomy and axillary node clearance or mastectomy, axillary node sample and, only if this confirmed involvement, post-operative radiotherapy. Patients were stratified according to this initial therapy, as well as according to the region of referral and the menopausal and nodal status.

Overall results (anonymous 1987) have indicated a highly significant prolongation of disease-free survival (DFS) ($P < 0.0001$) similar to that in the NATO trial (anonymous 1985). When one looks at this effect within the three separate trials for node-negative, node-positive and node-undetermined cases, it would seem that adjuvant tamoxifen delays relapse in all three nodal categories (Table 2). The majority of these patients, however, are post-menopausal, there being no pre-menopausal patients in the node-positive trial, and only 28% pre-menopausal patients in each of the node-negative and node-undetermined trials.

The ratio of the rates at which any end point is occurring within the two treatment arms is termed the hazard ratio. When this ratio is unity, the treatments being compared have similar end results, while the further it is away from unity, the greater is the difference between the treatments under study. The size of the 95% confidence interval is a measure of the reliability of this statistical estimate of true difference.

Table 2. Relapse rates by nodal subgroups in Scottish adjuvant trials based on follow-up duration of 2.5–8 years (median number of nodes examined per patient, 5; range, 0–45)

	Adjuvant tamoxifen (%)	Observation (%)
Node-negative	20	33
Node status undetermined	30	37
Node-positive, fewer than 5 examined	44	69
1–3 positive nodes, 5 or more examined	26	50
4 or more positive nodes, 5 or more examined	59	82

Table 3. The comparison of treatment and control arms for different groups of patients expressed as hazard ratios over total period of follow-up with 95% confidence intervals

	Hazard ratio	95% Confidence interval
Distant DFS	0.64	0.53–0.79
Total survival	0.71	0.58–0.89
Survival in pre-menopausal patients	0.57	0.27–1.19
Survival in node-negative patients	0.73	0.51–1.04

In an adjuvant trial in which initial local control may vary with the treatment given, the relevance of distant relapse is increased. Table 3 gives the hazard ratios with confidence intervals for this and for overall survival (OS), as well as for total survival within the pre-menopausal and node-negative subgroups. While the first two sets of results represent a statistically significant benefit from adjuvant tamoxifen ($P < 0.0001$ and $P = 0.002$ respectively), it is not surprising that at this stage in the follow-up process the confidence intervals for the good prognosis subgroups are too wide for reliable conclusions to be made. Nonetheless, a detectable difference is present and is in the expected direction.

Although stratification by age was not carried out, the pre-menopausal treatment groups are well balanced for age, the range being 30–55 years (mean, 44.2 ± 5.5 years) for the adjuvant arm and 27–56 years (mean, 43.8 ± 5.9 years) for the control arm patients. A total of 110 patients under the age of 45 and 32 of 45 years or more were randomised. Both groups show benefit from adjuvant tamoxifen, but there was found to be no significant interaction between treatment and age in these pre-menopausal patients ($\chi^2 = 2.83$, $P = 0.09$) despite the apparently greater effect in the older group.

Estimates of the ER content of the primary tumour were carried out on 742 (57%) of the total entrants to the trials, but once again the pre-menopausal subgroup suffers from being small (141). Conclusions for them will only be possible, after further follow-up, from detailed multivariate analyses. The overall picture, however, is one of fewer breast cancer events as a result of adjuvant tamoxifen for those with ER-poor tumours (values of 0–19 fmol per mg protein), as well as for those with ER-rich tumours (ER levels of 20 fmol or more).

Secondary Randomisation

Since 1985, patients who are free from recurrence after 5 years on tamoxifen have been randomised to stop as originally planned or to continue indefinitely until relapse or death. As this is ongoing, no formal assessment can be made, but details of the current rate of acceptance of the randomisation procedure can be given. Out of 277 patients eligible by the end of 1987, 29 (11%) have refused randomisation, 22 because they wished to continue and only seven because they elected to stop. No patient has refused to continue, while 12 have refused to stop when requested to do so; thus, the overall option acceptance rate is running at 85%. For the pre-menopausal subgroup, this is 88% (59/67).

Table 4. Entry to Scottish Conservation trial by stratification sub-groups and randomised therapy from 1 April 1985 to 29 February 1988 (Receptor-poor tumours have an ER level of 19 fmol per mg protein or less

	Pre-menopausal node negative		Postmenopausal	
	XRT	No XRT	XRT	No XRT
Receptor rich (adjuvant tamoxifen)	21	20	70	72
Receptor absent or poor (adjuvant CMF)	19	19	33	32
Receptor not assayed (adjuvant tamoxifen)	9	9	12	13
Total	49	48	115	117

XRT, radiotherapy.

Conservation Trial

From April 1985, after the closure of the adjuvant tamoxifen trials, pre-menopausal patients with no spread to axillary lymph nodes and willing to accept breast-conserving therapy have been eligible for inclusion in the Scottish Conservation trial. In this trial, all patients receive systemic therapy determined by the ER level found on assay of the locally excised primary cancer. If the ER level is less than 20 fmol, chemotherapy is initiated (CMF, IV 3 weekly, ×6). All other patients referred for inclusion are prescribed tamoxifen, 20 mg/day for 5 years in the first instance. Randomisation within this trial is for or not for radical irradiation to the residual breast tissue. Axillary irradiation is also given if an axillary lymph node clearance has not been performed.

Entry to this trial to date is shown in Table 4. The proportion of those without lymph node involvement who are pre-menopausal (38%) is higher than in the earlier post-mastectomy tamoxifen trials. However, the overall accrual rate is less, fewer clinicians agreeing to participate. Specialist units excepted, there is still in Scotland a strong belief in the benefit of routine local radiotherapy, some reluctance to accept the toxicity of CMF chemotherapy and a residual faith in mastectomy even for young women with early disease.

References

Anonymous (1985) Controlled trial of tamoxifen as single adjuvant agent in management of early breast cancer. Analysis of six years by Nolvadex Adjuvant Trial Organisation. Lancet I: 836–840

Anonymous (1987) Adjuvant tamoxifen in the management of operable breast cancer. The Scottish Trial. Lancet II: 171–175

Bonadonna G, Rossi A, Valagussa P, Banfi A, Veronesi U (1977) The CMF program for operable breast cancer with positive axillary nodes. Updated analysis in the disease-free interval, site of relapse and drug tolerance. Cancer 39: 2904–2915

Hubay CA, Pearson OH, Marshall JS, Rhodes RS, Debanne SM, Mansour EG, Hermann RE, Jones JC, Flynn WJ, Eckert C, McGuire WL and 27 participating investigators (1980) Adjuvant chemotherapy, anti-estrogen therapy and immunotherapy for Stage II breast cancer. In: Mouridsen HT, Palshof T (eds) Breast cancer - experimental and clinical aspects. Proceedings of the second EORTC breast cancer working conference. Eur J Cancer Supplement 1

Meakin JW, Allt WEC, Beale FA, Brown TC, Bush RS, Clark RM, Fitzpatrick PJ, Hawkins NV, Jenkins RDT, Pringle JF, Rider WD, Hayward JL, Bulbrook RD (1977) Ovarian irradiation and prednisone following surgery for carcinoma of the breast. In: Salmon SE, Jones SE (eds) Adjuvant therapy of cancer. North-Holland, New York, pp 95-99

Rose DP, Davis TE (1977) Ovarian function in patients receiving adjuvant chemotherapy for breast cancer. Lancet I: 1174-1176

Critical Review of Adjuvant Therapy in Premenopausal Patients

H. T. Mouridsen

Department of Oncology ONA, Finsen Institute, Copenhagen, Denmark

Introduction

There is now substantial evidence that adjuvant systemic chemotherapy is associated with an improved prognosis in premenopausal node-positive patients. Thus, the overview analysis reveals a highly significant reduction (approximately 25%) in the odds of death (Early Breast Cancer Trials Collaborative Group 1988). The same overview analysis has also demonstrated the lack of benefit from adjuvant tamoxifen in premenopausal patients. The value of chemotherapy and tamoxifen in premenopausal patients as estimated from this indirect comparison has been confirmed in one prospective randomized trial conducted by the Gynecological Adjuvant Breast Cancer Group (CABC) in Germany (Kaufmann, this volume, pp. 118–125).

Some important unanswered questions in the area of systemic treatment of premenopausal patients, which were discussed in this session of the Third International Conference on Adjuvant Therapy of Primary Breast Cancer include the relationship between treatment outcome and the induction of menopause by the chemotherapy, the role of endocrine therapy added to the chemotherapy, the role of treatment dose and duration, and the role of anthracyclines.

Medical Castration by Chemotherapy

The fact that adjuvant systemic therapy reduces mortality in patients under 50 years old, in contrast to patients 50 years or older, has given rise to the hypothesis that the chemotherapy works by inducing a medical castration.

Trials utilizing adjuvant castration by ovarian irradiation or oophorectomy were initiated 10–15 years before the major trials of adjuvant chemotherapy. All but one of these trials demonstrated an improvement in survival, which as statistically significant in two of the trials (Goldhirsch et al. 1987).

It was apparent in all these studies that the difference in favor of the treated group appeared late. However, this may be explained by rather small numbers of patients in the individual trials. Also, the patients were not selected according to receptor status, as receptor determinations had not yet been introduced when the trials were initiated, and finally the trials included a significant fraction of patients with node-negative tumors (Henderson 1987). The fact that all these trials demonstrated some degree of prevention of relapse and death has provided evidence that the suppression of ovarian function is beneficial, and in view of this, the role of endocrine approaches in the adjuvant treatment of premenopausal patients has retained its clinical relevance.

Cytotoxic drugs, especially alkylating agents, may cause suppression of the endocrine function of the ovary, the suggestion being that this is due to the direct effect of the drugs upon hormone-producing cells (Koyama et al. 1977; Rose and Davis 1980). Analyzing the ECOG data, Tormey (this volume, pp. 106–112) argued that at least part of the efficacy of cytotoxic therapy might be mediated via medical castration. Other trials have analyzed the effect of amenorrhea during adjuvant chemotherapy (Goldhirsch et al. 1987). In these trials 61%–87% of the patients experienced amenorrhea during therapy, and all but one trial (Bonadonna et al. 1985) concluded in agreement with Tormey. In this context, it is noteworthy that the effect of amenorrhea was observed exclusively in the subpopulations of patients with tumors which were hormone-receptor positive (Padmanabhan et al. 1986; Brincker et al. 1987: Ludwig Breast Cancer Group 1985a). Although for methodological reasons these retrospective analyses may be subject to bias, as discussed previously (Goldhirsch et al. 1987), the relative effectiveness of adjuvant castration and adjuvant chemotherapy in premenopausal patients deserves further study in randomized trials utilizing modern methods of patient selection.

Chemotherapy in Combinaton with Endocrine Therapy

The combination of adjuvant chemotherapy with concomitant endocrine therapy has been studied in several trials (Goldhirsch et al. 1987, Dombernowsky et al. 1988), one of which is presented in this volume (Tormey, this volume, p. 106). In all but one of these trials (Everson et al. 1986), there has been no significant advantage for the chemotherapy plus endocrine therapy as compared with chemotherapy alone. Indeed, in the NSABP trial (Fischer et al. 1986), a retrospective subgroup analysis revealed a difference in favor of the chemotherapy alone in patients who were receptor-negative, and in the Danish trial early data of survival indicated that the chemoendocrine group did significantly worse than those treated with cyclophosphamide, methotrexate, 5-fluorouracil (CMF) chemotherapy alone or with CMF in combination with radiotherapy (Dombernowsky et al. 1987).

Two trials compared chemotherapy alone with chemotherapy plus oophorectomy in premenopausal patients (Ludwig Breast Cancer Group 1985b; Osborne et al. 1986). Also in these trials, no significant benefit was observed with the combinations.

Later data from the ongoing trials are needed to draw final conclusions, but at present it would seem that adding endocrine therapy to chemotherapy offers no benefit in premenopausal patients.

Drug Dose and Duration of Therapy

The importance of drug dose is discussed in another section of this volume. Bonadonna et al. (this volume, p. 113) presented a follow-up of the 6 versus 12 months CMF trial, and it appeared that the prolonged schedule offers no advantage in terms of recurrence-free survival and overall survival. Another six trials have randomized patients to two different durations of therapy with the same regimen as reviewed by Henderson (1987). Only one of these trials has demonstrated a significant difference in recurrence-free survival, but half of the studies have shown a trend towards improved survival with the shorter course of therapy. Based on these results it seems unlikely that any benefit will be achieved by employing programs exceeding 6 months of therapy.

The Role of Anthracyclines

This subject was discussed in detail by Fischer and Redmond (1988). In advanced disease, the anthracyclines doxorubicin/epirubicin are probably the most active single agents. However, there are only limited data from randomized comparisons about their role in the adjuvant setting. Owing to the potential risk of inducing cardiac failure, the anthracyclines should be restricted to patients with a high risk of developing recurrent disease.

Conclusion

Adjuvant cytotoxic therapy reduces the odds of death in premenopausal patients, but so far the optimal regimen is unknown. With the drugs and methods available today, a number of questions are still open and should be addressed in clinical trials. These should also be designed with the aim of improving our knowledge about the biology of the disease and how it is influenced by adjuvant systemic therapies, with the ultimate goal of improving the therapeutic outcome.

References

Bonadonna G, Valagussa P, Rossi A, Tancini G, Brambilla C, Zambetti M, Veronesi U (1985) Ten-year experience with CMF-based adjuvant chemotherapy in resectable breast cancer. Breast Cancer Res Treat 5: 95–115

Brincker H, Rose C, Rank F, Mouridsen HT, Jacobsen A, Dombernowsky P, Panduro J, Andersen KW (1987) Evidence of a castration-mediated effect of adjuvant cytotoxic chemotherapy in premenopausal breast cancer. J Clin Oncol 5: 1771–1778

Dombernowsky P, Mouridsen HT, Brincker H, Hansen M, Jacobsen A, Andersen KW, Zedeler K (1987) Adjuvant treatment with CMF + radiotherapy versus CMF versus CMF + tamoxifen in pre- and menopausal high-risk breast cancer patients. Proceedings of the 4th EORTC Breast Cancer Working Conference, London, June 30–July 3, 1987, abstract C2D.14

Dombernowsky P, Brincker H, Hansen M, Mouridsen HT, Overgård M, Panduro J, Rose C, Axelson CK, Andersen J, Andersen KW (1988) Adjuvant therapy of pre- and menopausal high-risk breast cancer patients: Present status of the Danish Breast Cancer Cooperative Group trials 77-b and 82-b. Acta Oncol 27: 691-699

Early Breast Cancer Trialist Collaborative Group (1988) Effects of adjuvant tamoxifen and of cytotoxic therapy on mortality in early breast cancer: An overview of 61 randomized trials among 28, 896 women. New Engl J Med 319: 1681-1692

Everson LK, Ingle JN, Vieand HS, Martin JK, Votava HJ, Fitzgibbons RG, Weiland LH, Krook JE, Ahmann DL, Cullinan SA (1986) Randomized trials of adjuvant therapy with cyclophosphamide, 5-fluorouracil, prednisone with or without tamoxifen following mastectomy in premenopausal women with node positive breast cancer. Proc Am Soc Clin Oncol 5: 63

Fischer B, Redmond C, Brown A, Fischer ER, Wolmark N, Bowman D, Plotkin D, Wolter J, Bornstein R, Legault-Poisson S, Saffer EA (1986) Adjuvant chemotherapy with and without tamoxifen in the treatment of primary breast cancer: 5-year results from the National Surgical Adjuvant Breast and Bowel Project Trial. J Clin Oncol 4: 459-471

Goldhirsch A, Mouridsen HT (1987) Adjuvant chemotherapy in premenopausal patients: A more complicated form of oophorectomy. In: Cavalli F (ed.) Endocrine therapy of breast Cancer II. Current developments and new methodologies. Springer, Berlin Heidelberg New York London Paris Tokyo, pp 11-19

Henderson C (1987) Adjuvant cystemic therapy for early breast cancer. Curr Probl Cancer 11: 129-207

Koyama H, Wada T, Nishzawa Y, Takeshi I, Aoki Y, Terasawa T, Kosaki G, Yamamoto T, Wada A (1977) Cyclophosphamide-induced ovarian failure and its therapeutic significance in patients with breast cancer. Cancer 39: 1403-1409

Ludwig Breast Cancer Study Group (1985a) A randomized trial of adjuvant combination chemotherapy with or without prednisone in premenopausal breast cancer patients with metastases in 1 to 3 axillary lymph nodes. Cancer Res 45: 4454-4459

Ludwig Breast Cancer Study Group (1985b) Chemotherapy with or without oophorectomy in high-risk premenopausal patients with operable breast cancer. J Clin Oncol 3: 1059-1067

Osborne CK, Rivkin SE, McDivitt RW, Green S, Stephens RL, Costanzi JJ, O'Bryan R (1986) Adjuvant therapy of breast cancer: Southwest Oncology Group studies. NCI Monogr 1: 71-74

Padmanabhan N, Howell A, Rubens RD (1986) Mechanism of action of adjuvant chemotherapy in early breast cancer. Lancet II: 411-414

Rose DP, Davis TE (1980) Effects of adjuvant chemo-hormonal therapy on the ovarian and adrenal function of breast cancer patients. Cancer Res 40: 4043-4047

The Role of Adjuvant Endocrine Therapy in Primary Breast Cancer

M. Baum and S. R. Ebbs

Department of Surgery, King's College School of Medicine and Dentistry, London, Great Britain

Introduction

Women accept the toxicity imposed by adjuvant chemotherapy in a trade-off for the expectation of a prolonged disease-free interval and a longer life. However, a recent review of the results of randomised controlled trials of adjuvant chemotherapy suggests that whilst a 30% reduction in the risk of dying over the first 5 years may be achieved following the treatment of pre-menopausal women with node-positive disease, the benefits for post-menopausal women are, to say the least, marginal (Goldhirsch et al. 1986). It also appears that, whatever combination regimen is used, there is likely to be a significant delay in the time to first relapse.

The intriguing difference between the behaviour of pre- and post-menopausal women deserves some explanation. A possible alternative explanation for this differential effect might be that the cytotoxic drugs are mediating their effect by a chemical castration. This hypothesis has already won some support, following studies of ovarian and pituitary function in women receiving adjuvant chemotherapy (Rose and Davis 1977; Cole 1970). It follows, therefore, that to test the hypothesis generated by the trials of adjuvant chemotherapy, one should conduct trials of adjuvant endocrine therapy designed to interfere at some point in the complex balance between the breast cancer cell and its hormonal environment.

Trials of Adjuvant Endocrine Therapy

A more acceptable mode of therapy is not to interfere with the ovarian and extra-ovarian synthesis of sex steroids by either surgical or medical ablation, but to modulate the interaction between the carcinoma and the endogenous hormone. Tamoxifen, by binding to the specific oestrogen-receptor (ER) protein found in many breast cancer cells, is a relatively non-toxic drug that achieves this end. In 1977, the Nolvadex Adjuvant Trial Organisation (NATO) launched a study to investigate whether tamoxifen (Nolvadex) would have any benefit for women undergoing mastectomy for early breast cancer (NATO 1983).

Recent Results in Cancer Research, Vol. 115
© Springer-Verlag Berlin · Heidelberg 1989

Approximately 1300 patients were recruited over a period of 2½ years. These consisted predominantely of post-menopausal women but also included pre-meno-pausal node-negative cases. Following local therapy, women were randomised to receive tamoxifen, 10 mg twice daily for 2 years, or to an untreated control group. A second-order hypothesis suggested that the women most likely to benefit were those whose primary tumour was rich in ER content. Therefore, as a parallel study, attempts were made to collect samples of the tumours from all patients entered into the trial. However, for logistic reasons, this was only possible in about 50% of the cases. The published data have demonstrated a significantly prolonged disease-free interval in the treated group as a whole, which has recently been translated into a 30% reduction in the risk of dying within the first 5 years following treatment (NATO 1985a).

Current Status of NATO Trial

An updated analysis of the NATO trial at a maximum follow-up of 8 years has demonstrated no material difference with the already published data. Table 1 describes an analysis of survival broken down into sub-groups according to meno-pausal and nodal status. It can be seen that the hazard ratios are very close to each other in all three groups, as with previous analysis, and the benefit for both pre-menopausal and post-menopausal women appears equal.

Analysis of event-free survival or actual survival according to oestradiol receptor content of the primary tumour, using cut-off points between 5 and 30 fmol/mg cytosolic protein, have failed to demonstrate a sub-group that is qualitatively different in its response to adjuvant tamoxifen. For example, Table 2 illustrates the analysis for survival using 30 fmol (which is close to the median value for this study), with the observed/expected ratios in both the receptor and the receptor-poor group being remarkably similar.

An analysis performed for the first time within this trial describes the log hazard ratios for both events and death in 2-year blocks, within the 8 years of this study.

Table 1. NATO trial analysis of survival: comparison of treatment groups by menopausal and nodal status (after recurrence audit)

Group	Number in group	Observed events (n)	Expected events (n)	Ratio of observed to expected events
Premenopausal node positive				
Nolvadex	72	28	33.9	0.83
No treatment	57	30	24.1	1.24
Postmenopausal node negative				
Nolvadex	300	55	66.1	0.83
No treatment	305	77	65.9	1.17
Postmenopausal node positive				
Nolvadex	181	77	90.4	0.85
No treatment	190	99	85.6	1.16

Table 2. NATO trial analysis of survival: comparison of treatment groups by oestrogen receptor status (after recurrence audit)[a]

Group	Number in group	Observed events (n)	Expected events (n)	Ratio of observed to expected events
ER unknown				
'Nolvadex'	296	90	98.3	0.92
No treatment	296	103	94.7	1.09
ER <30				
'Nolvadex'	138	40	51.9	0.77
No treatment	122	56	44.1	1.27
ER >30				
'Nolvadex'	119	30	40.0	0.75
No treatment	134	47	37.0	1.27

[a] Cut-off point, 30 fmol per mg protein.

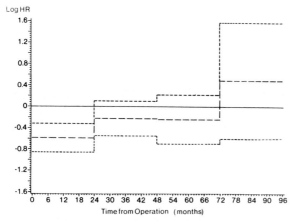

Fig. 1. NATO events to 8 years. Log ratio of hazard rates (with 95% confidence limits)

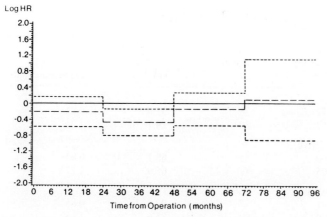

Fig. 2. NATO deaths to 8 years. Log ratio of hazard rates (with 95% confidence limits)

These analyses are illustrated in Fig. 1 and Fig. 2. It is clearly demonstrated that the significant reduction in the number of events appears only in the first 2 years, during which time the patients are on tamoxifen, whereas the significant reduction in the number of deaths occurs only in the 3rd and 4th years in the period immediately after cessation of treatment. There is no suggestion of a rebound phenomenon after withdrawal of therapy.

The Cancer Research Campaign Trial

Once recruitment into the NATO trial had been completed and long before any significant differences had emerged, the Cancer Research Campaign launched a new multi-centre trial within the United Kingdom to repeat both the NATO study and the Scandinavian multi-centre trial of adjuvant chemotherapy. This was a 2×2 factorial design for both pre- and post-menopausal women of either negative or positive axillary nodal status. Measurements of ER were not a prerequisite for entry into this trial.

Half the patients in the study received tamoxifen, 20 mg daily for 2 years, and half were randomised to receive peri-operative cyclophosphamide, 5 mg/kg for 6 days commencing within 24 h of surgery. Figure 3 illustrates the factorial design of this study, and Table 3 describes the numbers of patients of each sub-group entered into the study.

It should be noted that approximately one-third of the 2300 patients randomised were pre-menopausal. As the median follow-up of the patients in this new study is still less than 3 years, the main effect analysis of peri-operative cyclophosphamide will not be reported. However, it was felt worthwhile to report an analysis of event-free survival for the tamoxifen main effect, since it was at this stage that the NATO trial first demonstrated the benefit of adjuvant tamoxifen. Figures 4 and 5 show life-table analyses for the pre- and post-menopausal patients, and it can be seen that there is a highly significant reduction in the rate of events in both groups receiving adjuvant tamoxifen. Although no significant survival advantages have been demonstrated to date, an analysis of the site of first recurrence (Table 4) would suggest that the delay in occurrence of distant metastases could well be followed by a significant prolongation of survival.

Table 3. CRC adjuvant breast trial: control and tamoxifen groups[a]

	Control $n=948$		Tamoxifen $n=942$	
	(n)	$(\%)$	(n)	$(\%)$
Premenopausal	259	(27.3)	280	(29.7)
Postmenopausal	442	(46.6)	405	(43.0)
Node negative	469	(49.5)	446	(47.3)
Node positive	367	(38.7)	396	(42.0)

[a] Missing patients have unknown menstrual or nodal status.

CONTROL (no adjuvant therapy)	TAMOXIFEN (20mg bd)
CYCLOPHOSPHAMIDE (5mg/kg/day iv for 6 days post-op)	COMBINATION (Tamoxifen + Cyclophosphamide)

Fig. 3. Cancer Research Campaign (CRC) trial: 2×2 factorial design

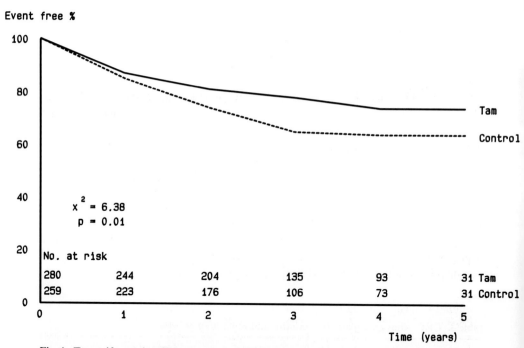

Fig. 4. Tamoxifen main effects analysis – first event, premenopausal patients in CRC Adjuvant Breast trial. In this and subsequent figures the numbers at risk represent the number of patients event free at entry and annually thereafter. This number decreases in the latter years since there are fewer patients with relevant times

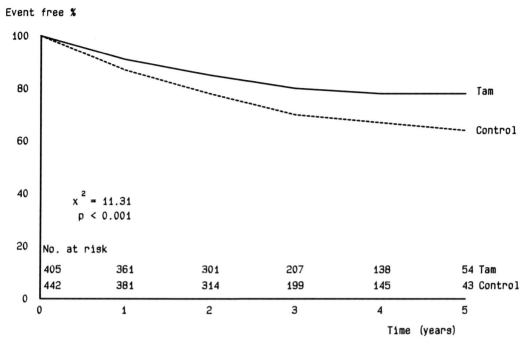

Fig. 5. Tamoxifen main effects analysis – first event, postmenopausal patients in CRC Adjuvant Breast trial

Table 4. Initial recurrence in control and tamoxifen groups

	Control $n=948$		Tamoxifen $n=942$	
	(n)	(%)	(n)	(%)
Recurrences	263		182	
Local				
Flaps/scar	65	(24.7)	52	(28.6)
Ipsilateral axilla	39	(14.8)	23	(12.6)
Distant				
Supraclavicular	25	(9.5)	21	(11.5)
Opposite axilla	6	(2.3)	2	(1.1)
Bone	80	(30.4)	52	(28.6)
Lungs	34	(12.9)	27	(14.8)
Liver	28	(10.7)	22	(12.1)
Brain	5	(1.9)	6	(3.3)
Other	15	(5.7)	6	(3.3)

The Scottish Trial

A trial conducted in Scotland recruiting between 1978 and 1984 has recently been reported (Breast Cancer Trials Committee 1987). Women under the age of 80 with early breast cancer were studied, although unlike the NATO trial, pre-menopausal node-positive cases were excluded. A total of 1312 eligible patients were randomised either to adjuvant tamoxifen for 5 years or to the control group which had tamoxifen reserved for the treatment of first relapse. The early results after a mean duration of tamoxifen therapy of 47 months reinforces the findings of the NATO study, with a highly significant delay in relapse for the adjuvant-treated group and the maintenance of a benefit in the overall survival comparisons. Like NATO, the benefit was independent of nodal, menopausal and ER status.

Discussion

The data presented in this paper would reinforce the recommendation to the NIH Consensus Development Conference that tamoxifen should be considered as worthwhile adjuvant therapy in post-menopausal women. It also suggests that the question of tamoxifen in pre-menopausal women is an open one. The undoubted benefit of adjuvant tamoxifen in this younger age group once again reinforces the hypothesis that, at least in some part, the benefits of adjuvant systemic chemotherapy could be mediated via an endocrine mechanism.

The log hazard ratio analysis for events and survival from the NATO trial also provides an interesting pointer for the future, suggesting that the maintained long-term benefit of adjuvant tamoxifen is a result of the delay in recurrence amongst the patients whilst receiving the drug. This would indicate that a policy of dosage with tamoxifen for more than 2 years would produce an improved cumulative reduction in mortality.

Potentially of greater interest is the suggestion that the ER status of the primary tumour does not predict the likelihood of response to adjuvant tamoxifen. As such an outcome fails to reinforce popular prejudice, there would naturally be the temptation to ignore or reject these data. It has been suggested already that the measurement of ER in a multi-centre trial with inter- and intra-laboratory variation will produce many false-negative results. Indeed, this may be the case, but it remains unquestionable that in this study the assay of ER has indicated something of biological relevance about the primary cancers, as there is a powerful correlation between the ER status and prognosis, and between ER status and histological grade, irrespective of adjuvant therapy (NATO 1985b). Rather than ignore these data, it would be more fruitful to try to incorporate them within a modified hypothesis. There is little doubt that the major pathway mediating the anti-tumour effect of tamoxifen in advanced breast cancer is via the oestradiol receptor; however, the observations from the NATO trial raise the question of whether tamoxifen exerts some of its effect on microscopic foci of the disease by another pathway.

Recent experimental work suggests that anti-oestrogens might be better thought of as affecting growth factors and their receptors, which appear to be an expression of oncogene amplification. The stromal environment of micro-metastases may also be an important determinant of hormone responsiveness in addition to the malignant cells themselves (Anonymous 1987).

Acknowledgements. We gratefully acknowledge the working parties and participants of the NATO and CRC clinical trials groups, without whose active support all this would have been impossible. We also acknowledge with gratitude the hard work of the CRCCTC Data Centre staff, and thank the Cancer Research Campaign for generous financial support.

References

Anonymous (1987) The role of adjuvant tamoxifen in the management of early breast cancer. Lancet II: 191

Breast Cancer Trials Committee (1987) Adjuvant tamoxifen in the management of operable breast cancer: The Scottish trial. Lancet II: 171–175

Cole MP (1970) Prophylactic compared with therapeutic X-ray artificial menopause. 2nd Tenovus Workshop on Breast Cancer. Alpha-Omega, Cardiff, pp 2–11

Goldhirsch A, Gelber RD, Davis BW (1986) Adjuvant chemotherapy trials in breast cancer: an appraisal and lessons for patient care outside the trials. In: Forbes JG (ed) Breast disease. Churchill Livingstone, Edinburgh pp 123–138

Nolvadex Adjuvant Trial Organisation (NATO) (1983) Controlled trial of tamoxifen as single adjuvant agent in management or early breast cancer. Interim analysis at 4 years by NATO. Lancet I: 257–261

Nolvadex Adjuvant Trial Organisation (NATO) (1985a) Controlled trial of tamoxifen as single adjuvant agent in management of early breast cancer. Analysis at 6 years by NATO. Lancet II: 836–840

Nolvadex Adjuvant Trial Organisation (NATO) (1985b) Six year results of a controlled trial of tamoxifen as single adjuvant agent in management of early breast cancer. World J Surg 9: 756–764

Rose DP, Davis TE (1977) Ovarian function in patients receiving adjuvant chemotheray for brest cancer. Lancet I: 1174–1176

How to Improve Adjuvant Treatment Results in Postmenopausal Patients

H. T. Mouridsen

Department of Oncology ONA, Finsen Institute/Rigshospitalet, 49 Standboulevarden, 2100 Copenhagen Ø, Denmark

Overall Estimates of Reduction in Mortality

The most widely tested adjuvant systemic therapies in postmenopausal breast cancer patients have included tamoxifen (TAM) and various cytotoxic agents, given singly or in combination.

A clinically important but statistically insignificant result may well be overlocked in the individual trials, owing to a limited number of patients.

In the overview analysis conducted by Peto in collaboration with The Early Breast Cancer Trials Collaborative Group (1988), each trial provides an estimate of the magnitude of treatment effect that is summated with estimates from other trials to provide an overview measure. As it is based on much larger patient samples, this measure is less subject to random variation than any of the individual trial data alone, and thus the overview analysis will be able to detect smaller real differences in treatment effects.

The results of the overview analysis were initially presented at the NIH consensus development conference on adjuvant chemotherapy for breast cancer (CDCR 1985). Brief summaries and references to the data and methodology have been published (Lippman 1985; Meeting Report 1984), and a full report of the analysis will be published in the near future (EBCTCG 1988).

By August 1985, about 9000 patients had been randomized in trials of adjuvant chemotherapy. These included 33 trials in which patients were randomized to either chemotherapy or no chemotherapy or to either chemotherapy plus TAM or TAM only. There were approximately 16000 women randomized in 28 trials of TAM; these included either trials in which patients were randomized to TAM or to no systemic treatment or trials with randomization to TAM plus chemotherapy or to chemotherapy alone.

The estimates of reduction in odds of death from the overview are presented in Table 1. It appears that for postmenopausal patients a reduction of 20% in the odds in death can be achieved with adjuvant TAM, whereas for the same patient group no survival gain can be observed with chemotherapy.

In conclusion, the adjuvant treatment of choice for postmenopausal patients is TAM. Specific subgroups of patients may benefit more or less from the therapy

Recent Results in Cancer Research, Vol. 115
© Springer-Verlag Berlin · Heidelberg 1989

Table 1. Overview estimate of reduction in odds of death ($\% \pm SE$)

Comparison	Age < 50 years	Age = 50 + years
TAM vs. nil	− 1 ± 8	20 ± 3
CT, single vs. nil	11 ± 10	− 4 ± 10
CT, multiple vs. nil	26 ± 7	8 ± 6

TAM, tamoxifen; CT, chemotherapy.

(Mouridsen and Rose 1988) but an analysis of these subgroups will not be included in this report.

This manuscript will briefly discuss some potential approaches to be tested in the adjuvant situation. These include approaches within the area of endocrine therapy, chemotherapy, and diphosphonates, with special emphasis on endocrine therapy, which seems more specifically relevant for the postmenopausal patient group.

Duration of TAM Therapy

Among the major trials of adjuvant TAM, treatment duration varied from 1 year (Ludwig Breast Cancer Study Group 1984; Ribeiro and Palmer 1983; Rose et al. 1983) to 2 years (NATO 1983, Pritchard et al. 1984; Wallgren 1982) and 5 years (SCTO 1987). So far, significantly improved survival has been demonstrated in only three of these trials (Mouridsen et al. 1988; NATO 1985; SCTO 1987). These differences may be ascribed to statistical reasons (small number of end points, different follow-up times), to an uneven distribution of prognostic variables in the different trials, as discussed in more detail recently (Mouridsen and Rose 1988), to different treatment policies after recurrence, or to the variations in the duration of adjuvant TAM. The important question of possible improvement of the treatment results with prolonged TAM is awaiting an answer from randomized trials of different treatment durations.

Combined Endocrine Therapy

With the exception of TAM combined with prednisolone, a series of randomized trials in advanced disease have demonstrated similar therapeutic gain with TAM compared with TAM in combination with other endocrine agents (Mouridsen 1986).

However, the alternating endocrine approach (i.e., treatment with one endocrine agent followed by treatment with another endocrine agent) should be applied in the adjuvant setting. The rationale for this approach is the demonstration of partial cross-sensitivity and partial non-cross-resistance between treatment with TAM and other endocrine agents (Table 2). Thus, in patients having responded to first-line TAM, the chance of subsequent response to another endocrine agent is 42%, and in patients failing to respond to first-line therapy with TAM, approxi-

Table 2. Definitions of cross-sensitivity/resistance and non-cross-sensitivity/resistance

Second-line ET	First-line ET	
	+ response	− response
+ response	cross-sensitivity	non-cross-resistance
− response	non-cross-sensitivity	cross-resistance

ET, endocrine therapy.

mately 15% will respond to second-line endocrine therapy (Rose and Mouridsen 1986).

So far, alternating treatment with TAM and medroxyprogesterone-acetate (MPA) has been analyzed in four published trials (Bruno et al. 1983; Kvinnsland 1986; Mauriac et al. 1986; Pouillart et al. 1984). In three of the trials (Bruno et al. 1983; Mauriac et al. 1986; Pouillart et al. 1984), TAM and MPA were alternated every second week. The rate of response and other treatment end points in these three trials were similar both for the combination and for TAM alone. Since the half-life of TAM supersedes 2 weeks, it can be argued that the lack of an additive effect of the alternating approach is due to pharmacodynamic interaction at the receptor level. Recently, preliminary results from a trial in advanced breast cancer comparing TAM alone with TAM alternating with MPA every 8 weeks have been presented (Kvinnsland 1986). A total of 119 patients, known to be estrogen-receptor positive have been included in the trial, and so far 95 patients are evaluable. The response rates are 68% and 45% in TAM/MPA- and TAM-treated patients respectively. It is noteworthy that the increased overall response rate is due to an increase in the rate of complete remission. These results encourage a further exploration of alternating endocrine modalities in the adjuvant setting and the questions to be addressed include durations, numbers, and sequences of the different endocrine therapies.

Intermittant Endocrine Therapy

Hormone deprivation of hormone-dependent tumors may enhance the process of dedifferentiation to autonomy. This is suggested by several experiments (Kim and Depowski 1975; Noble 1977; Sluyser and van Nier 1974) in which estrogen-dependent breast tumors rapidly became autonomous when transplanted in an estrogen-free host. The most interesting experiments in this context are those of Noble (1977) and Bruchowsky et al. (1978), who showed that partial replacement of estrogens or androgens after deprivation of these hormones in experimental hormone-dependent mammary or prostatic cancer, slowed down the progression to autonomy.

The intermittant approach is now beeing tested in a randomized EORTC trial in advanced disease (Beex et al. 1987) but should also be tested in primary disease to answer the important question of the possible postponement of development from hormone dependency to hormone independency.

Table 3. Randomized studies comparing TAM with TAM plus chemotherapy in postmenopausal patients

Study	Reference	(n)	Median follow-up (years)	Chemo-therapy	RFS improved with chemotherapy ($P \leq 0.05$)
Ludwig III	16	463[a]	4	CMFP	Yes
Case Western	19	94	3	CMFVP	Yes
SWOG	37	600+[b]		CMFVP	Yes
DBCG 82 C	32	1347[c]	2	CMF	Yes

[a] One-third of patients randomized to control group.
[b] One-third of patients randomized to chemotherapy.
[c] One-third of patients randomized to TAM plus radiotherapy.

Combined Endocrine and Chemotherapy

Simultaneous Treatment

Four major trials have been published which randomized the patients to either TAM or to TAM plus chemotherapy. A brief review of the results is presented in Table 3. In all these studies, a significant increase of relapse-free survival (RFS) was observed with chemotherapy. Follow-up is short in all the studies, and so far only one study has provided survival data (Mouridsen et al. 1988) which were identical in the two treatment groups.

More mature data from ongoing trials must be generated to make possible final conclusions.

Recruitment

Estrogen and some other hormones and growth factors can induce recruitment of quiescent cells into the proliferative phase of the cell cycle, causing the cells to be more sensitive to subsequent administration of cytotoxic drugs (Clarke et al. 1985; Hug et al. 1986; Osborne 1987: Weichselbaum et al. 1978). Five clinical studies involving such hormonal manipulation in patients with advanced disease have been published (Allegra 1983, Conte et al. 1987, Eisenhauer et al. 1984, Lippman et al. 1984, Paridaens et al. 1987), two of which were randomized (Conte et al. 1987; Lippman et al. 1984).

In the initial study (Allegra 1983), a remarkably high response rate (72%) was achieved with sequential TAM and conjugated estrogens (Premarin) combined with methotrexate and 5-fluorouracil. However, with the same treatment regimen, Eisenhauer et al. (1984) observed only three responders among 30 patients.

In the two randomized studies, a trend towards a higher rate of complete remission was observed in the group of patients randomized to intermittant estrogen than in the control group. However, overall respone rate and other major end points were similar.

Although the available data in advanced disease has been disappointing so far, this approach should be further exploited in advanced disease and in primary disease in patients with a high risk of recurrence. The questions to be addressed in these studies include the choice of any other growth-stimulatory agent to be used other than estrogen, the optimal dosage of the stimulatory agent, the duration of the stimulation period, and the time interval from stimulation to administration of chemotherapy. More information should also be gained about the effect of stimulation on the cellular uptake of the cytotoxic agents.

Chemotherapy

It has been argued that the lack of effect of chemotherapy in post-menopausal patients may be ascribed to the administration of reduced doses to the postmenopausal patients. Indeed, Bonadonna and Valagussa (1981) described a positive relationship between the administered dose and RFS for premenopausal and postmenopausal patients as well. However, retrospective analyses may well be biased by factors not related to the dose level as such, but rather, to the fact that patients at greatest risk of recurrence are less able to tolerate the drugs. Henderson (1987) recently summarized the results of several adjuvant trials which retrospectively analyzed RFS in relation to dose levels, and none of these trials could confirm the results of the Milan trial.

Hryniuk and Levine (1986) argued that RFS is positively related to the dose intensity. However, their analyses are based upon a number of presumptions which may invalidate the conclusions. As an example, the dose intensities in the DBCG 77 B trial, calculated according to Hryniuk and Levine, were 0.34 for cyclophosphamide and 0.74 for cyclophosphamide, methotrexate, 5-fluorouracil (CMF). Toxicities with the two regimens were similar. In spite of the fact that the dose intensities were significantly different, the RFS at 3 and 8.5 years and the survival at 8.5 years were similar with the two regimens (Dombernowsky et al. 1988; Mouridsen et al. 1984).

In conclusion, prospective trials with groups of different dose intensities are necessary to elucidate this important question. Other areas of interest in chemotherapy include the introduction of new drugs and combinations, as well as the alternating approach with two or more non-cross-resistant regimens.

Diphosphonates

In advanced breast cancer, approximately 60% of the patients will suffer from lytic bone metastases caused by an increase of osteoclastic bone resorption, probably occurring in response to factors secreted by the tumor cells. Diphosphonates reduce the bone turn-over (Fleisch et al. 1969; Miller and Jess 1977; Schenk et al. 1973), and it is currently believed that they exert their effects by a combined effect on crystal behavior and osteoclastic function (Fleisch 1980).

The first studies in patients with bone metastases from breast cancer were published by Elomaa et al. (1983, 1985). Seventeen patients received CL2MDP,

1600 mg/day for 12 months. These patients experienced fewer episodes of hypercalcemia, had fewer new bone metastases and bone fractures, and required smaller doses of analgetics than 17 control patients treated with placebo. Also, after 1 and 2 years of observation, fewer deaths were reported in the treated group than in the control group. The frequency of new nonosseous metastases was identical in the two groups.

Similar results were presented recently (van Holten-Verzantvoort et al. 1987). In this study, patients with bone metastases were randomized to treatment with and without diphosphonate (amidronate = APD, 150 mg twice daily). Within the time of observation, significantly fewer episodes of hypercalcemia, fractures, and deaths were observed in the APD-treated group.

Further studies should be undertaken with diphosphonate in advanced disease and should also be considered for the treatment of primary disease in patients with a high risk of developing bone metastases. These studies should also be designed with the aim of defining the optimal dose, schedule, and duration of therapy and to analyze the long-term effects.

Conclusion

Adjuvant tamoxifen reduces mortality in postmenopausal patients with primary breast cancer. However, it is evident from the available data that the therapeutic results achieved so far represent only a minor step towards a dramatic improvement of the prognosis. However, some newer approaches are now available and should be tested in advanced disease and in primary disease in patients with high risk of recurrence.

References

Allegra JC (1983) Methotrexate and 5-fluorouracil following tamoxifen and premarin in advanced brest cancer. Semin Oncol 10, [Suppl 2]: 23–28

Beex LVAM, Rose C, Sylvester R, Rotmensz N (1987) Continuous tamoxifen versus intermittent tamoxifen versus alternating tamoxifen and medroxyprogesterone acetate (MPA). First line endocrine therapy for post-menopausal patients with advanced breast cancer, a phase III study (trial 10863). 4th EORTC breast cancer working conference, London, June 30–July 3, 1987, abstract no 1.14

Bonadonna G, Valagussa P (1981) Dose-response effect of adjuvant chemotherapy in breast cancer. N Engl J Med 304: 10–15

Bruchowsky N, Rennie P, Van Doorn E, Noble R (1978) Pathological growth of androgen sensitive tissue resulting from latent actions of steroid hormones. J Toxicol Environ Health 4: 391–408

Bruno M, Roldan E, Diaz B (1983) Sequential vs. simultanous administration of tamoxifen and medroxyprogesterone acetate in advanced breast cancer. J Steroid Biochem 19: 87 S, abstract 261

Clarke R, Berg HW van der, Kennedy DJ, Murphy RF (1985) Estrogen receptor status and the response of human breast cancer cell lines to a combination of methotrexate and $17\text{-}\beta$ oestradiol. Br J Cancer 51: 365–369

Consensus Development Conference Report (1985) Adjuvant chemotherapy for breast cancer. JAMA 254: 3461–3463

Conte PF, Pronzato P, Rubagotti A, Alanea A, Amadori D, Demicheli R, Gardin G, Gentili-
ni P, Jacomuzzi A, Lionetto R, Monzeglio C, Nicolin A, Rosso R, Sismondi P, Sussio M,
Santi L (1987) Conventional versus cytokinetic polychemotherapy with estrogenic recruitment in metastatic breast cancer: Results of a randomized cooperative trial. J Clin Oncol
5: 339-347

Dombernowsky P, Brincker H, Hansen M, Mouridsen HT, Overgård M, Panduro J, Rose C,
Axelsson CK, Andersen J, Andersen KW (1988) Adjuvant therapy of pre- and menopausal high-risk breast cancer patients: Present status of the Danish Breast Cancer Cooperative Group Trials 77-b and 82-b. Acta Oncologica. 27: 691-699

Early Breast Cancer Triallist Collaborative Group (1988) Effects of adjuvant tamoxifen and
of cytotoxic therapy on mortality in early breast cancer: an overview of 61 randomized
trials among 28, 896 women. N Engl J Med. 319: 1681-1692

Eisenhauer EA, Bowman D, Pritchard KI (1984) Tamoxifen and conjugated estrogens
(premarin) followed by sequenced methotrexate and 5-FU in refractory advanced breast
cancer. Cancer Treat Rep 68: 1421-1422

Elomaa I, Blomqvist C, Grohn P, Porkka L. Kairento A-L, Selander K, Lamberg-Allardt C,
Holmstrøm T (1983) Long-term controlled trial with diphosphonate in patients with
osteolytic bone metastases. Lancet I: 146-149

Elomaa I, Blomqvist C, Porkka L. Holmstrøm T, Taube T, Lamberg-Allardt C, Borgstrøm
GH (1985) Diphosphonates for osteolytic metastases. Lancet II: 1155-1156

Fleisch H (1980) Experimental basis for the clinical use of diphosphonates in Paget's disease of bone. Arthritis Rheum 23: 1162-1171

Fleisch H, Russell RGG, Francis MD (1969) Diphosphonates inhibit hydroxyapatite disso-
lution in vitro and bone resorption in tissue culture in vivo. Science 165: 1262-1264

Goldhirsch A, Gelber R (1986) Adjuvant treatment for early breast cancer: The Ludwig
Breast Cancer Studies. NCI Monogr 1: 55-71

Henderson C (1987) Adjuvant systemic therapy for early breast cancer. Curr Probl Cancer
11: 129-207

Hryniuk W, Levine MN (1986) Analysis of dose intensity for adjuvant chemotherapy trials
in stage II breast cancer. J Clin Oncol 4: 1162-1170

Hubay CA, Pearson OH, Gordon NH, Marshall JS, Crowe J, Guyton S, Arafah BM,
McGuire WL (1986) Randomized trial of endocrine versus endocrine plus cytotoxic
chemotherapy in women with stage II, estrogen receptor positive breast cancer. ASCO 63:
245

Hug V, Johnston D, Finders M, Hortobagyi G (1986) Use of growth stimulatory hormones
to improve the in vitro therapeutic index of doxorubicin for human breast tumors. Cancer
Res 46: 147-152

Kim U, Depowski M (1975) Progression from hormone dependence to autonomy in mammary tumors as an in vivo manifestation of sequential clonal selection. Cancer Res 35:
2068-2077

Kvinnsland S (1986) Alternating sequences of tamoxifen and medroxyprogesterone acetate
in postmenopausal women with advanced breast cancer. Symposium on MPA in malignant tumors, Copenhagen, Sept 9, 1986, Abstract

Lippman ME (1985) The NIH consensus development conference on adjuvant chemotherapy for breast cancer - A commentary. Breast Cancer Res Treat 6: 195-200

Lippman ME, Cassidy J, Wesley M, Young RC (1984) A randomized attempt to increase the
efficacy of cytotoxic chemotherapy in metastatic breast cancer by hormonal synchronization. J Clin Oncol 2: 28-36

Ludwig Breast Cancer Study Group (1984) Randomized trial of chemo-endocrine therapy,
endocrine therapy and mastectomy alone in postmenopausal patients with operable
breast cancer and axillary node metastasis. Lancet I: 1256-1260

Mauriac L, Durand M, Chauvergne J, Bonichon F (1986) Randomized trial comparing alternating sequences of tamoxifen and medroxyprogesterone acetate with successive applications in metastatic breast cancer. International Symposium on Hormonal Manipulation
of Cancer, Rotterdam, June 4-6, 1986, Abstract 101

Meeting Report London (1984) Review of mortality results in randomized trials in early breast cancer. Lancet II: 1205

Miller SC, Jee WSS (1977) The comparative effects of dichloromethylene diphosphonate (C12MDP) and ethane-1-hydroxy-1,1-diphosphonate (EHDP) on growth and modeling of the rat tibia. Calcif Tissue Res 23: 207–214

Mouridsen HT (1986) Endocrine treatment of advanced breast cancer. Endocrine mechanism and treatment for brest cancer. In: Cavalli F (ed) Endocrine therapy of breast cancer, Springer, Berlin Heidelberg New York Tokyo pp 79-90

Mouridsen HT, Rose C (1988) Attempting to understand differences between the results of the main trials of adjuvant tamoxifen in primary breast cancer. Bresciani F, King RJB, Lippmann ME, Raynaud JP (eds) Progress in cancer research and therapy, vol 35, Raven, New York, pp 417–422

Mouridsen HT, Rose C, Brincker H, Thorpe SM, Rank F, Fischerman K, Andersen KW on behalf of the Danish Breast Cancer Cooperative Group (1984) Adjuvant systemic therapy in high risk breast cancer. Danish Breast Cancer Cooperative Group Trials of cyclophosphamide or CMF in premenopausal and tamoxifen in postmenopausal patients. In: Senn HJ (ed) Adjuvant chemotherapy of breast cancer. Springer, Berlin Heidelberg New York Tokyo, pp 117-128 (Recent results in cancer research, vol 96)

Mouridsen HT, Rose C, Overgaard M, Dombernowsky P, Panduro J, Thorpe S, Rasmussen BB, Blichert-Toft M, Andersen KW (1988) Adjuvant treatment of postmenopausal patients with high risk primary breast cancer. Results from the Danish studies DBCG 77 C and 82 C. Acta Oncol. 27: 699–707

Noble R (1977) Hormonal control of growth and progression in tumors of Nb rats and a theory action. Cancer Res 37: 82-94

Nolvadex Adjuvant Trial Organisation (1983) Controlled trial of tamoxifen as adjuvant agent in management of early brest cancer. Lancet I: 257-261

Nolvadex Adjuvant Trial Organisation (NATO) (1985) Controlled trial of tamoxifen as single adjuvant agent in management of early breast cancer. Lancet I: 836-840

Osborne CK (1987) Hormonal manipulation of tumour cells in combination with chemotherapy. In: Klijn JGM, Paridaens R, Foekens JA (eds) Hormonal manipulation of cancer: peptides, growth factors and new (anti)steroidal agents. Raven, New York, pp 469-476 (EORTC monograph series)

Osborne CK, Rivkin SE, McDivitt RW, Green S, Stephens RL, Costanzi JJ, O'Bryan R (1986) Adjuvant therapy of breast cancer: Southwest oncology group studies. NCI Monogr 1: 71-75

Paridaens R, Julien JP, Klijn J, van Zyjl J, Piccart M, Margreiter R, Rotmensz N, Sylvester RJ (1987) Assessment of cyclic combination chemotherapy with estrogenic recruitment in advanced breast cancer: a phase III double trial of the EORTC Breast Cancer Cooperative Group (trial 10835). 4th EORTC breast cancer working conference, London, June 30-July 3, 1987, abstract no 1.10

Pouillart P, Jouve M, Palangie T, Garcia-Giralt E, Bretaudeau B, Magdalenat H, Asselaen B (1984) Disseminated brest cancer: sequential administration of tamoxifen and medroxyprogesterone acetate. Results of a controlled trial. In: Robustelli Della Cuna G, Pannuti F, Pouillart P, Jonat W, Pellegrini A (eds) Role of medroxyprogesterone in endocrine-related tumors, Raven, New York, pp 141-155

Pritchard KI, Meakin JW, Boyd NF, Ambus U, De Boer G, Dembo AJ, Paterson AGH, Sutherland DJA, Wilkinson RH, Bassett AA, Evans WK, Beale FA, Clarck RM, Keane TJ (1984) A prospective randomized controlled trial of adjuvant tamoxifen in postmenopausal women with axillary node positive breast cancer. In: Jones SE, Salmon SE (eds) Adjuvant therapy of cancer, vol 4. Orlando, Grune and Stratton, pp 339-347

Ribeiro G, Palmer MK (1983) Adjuvant tamoxifen for operable carcinoma of the breast: report of clinical trial by the Christie Hospital and Holt Radium Institute. Br Med J 286: 827-830

Rose C, Mouridsen HT (1986) Combined endocrine treatment of postmenopausal patients with advanced breast cancer. The Danish experience. In: Senn HJ (ed) Tumor diagnostics and therapy 8. Thieme, Stuttgart, pp 279-281

Rose C, Thorpe SM, Mouridsen HT, Andersen JA, Brincker H, Andersen KW (1983) Antiestrogen treatment of postmenopausal women with primary high risk breast cancer: 36 months of life table analysis and steroid hormone receptor status. Breast Cancer Res Treat 66: 2081–2083

Schenk R, Merz WA, Muhlbauer R, Russell RGG, Fleisch H (1973) Effects of ethane-1-hydroxy-1,1-diphosphonate (EHDP) and dichloromethylene diphosphonate (C12MDP) on the calcification and resorption of cartilage and bone in the tibial epiphysis and metaphysis of rats. Calcif Tissue Res 11: 196–214

Scottish Cancer Trials Office (1987) Adjuvant tamoxifen in the management of operable breast cancer: The Scottish trial. Lancet II: 171–175

Sluyser M, van Nier R (1974) Estrogen receptor content and hormone responsive growth of mouse mammary tumors. Cancer Res 34: 3253–3257

van Holten-Verzantvoort A, Harinck H, Hermans J, Bijvoet O, Cleton F (1987) Supportive APD treatment reduces skeletal morbidity in breast cancer. 4th EORTC breast cancer working conference, London, June 30–July 3, 1987, Abstract no F 5.2

Wallgren A (1982) Treatment with Nolvadex alone and in combination with chemotherapy in postmenopausal women. Rev Endocr Rel Cancer 12: 15–20

Weichselbaum RR, Hellman S, Piro AJ, Nove JJ, Little JB (1978) Proliferation kinetics of a human breast cancer cell line in vitro following treatment with 17-β-estradiol and 1-β-D-arabinofuranosylcytosine. Cancer Res 38: 2339–2342

Adjuvant Chemo-Endocrine Therapy or Endocrine Therapy Alone for Postmenopausal Patients: Ludwig Studies III and IV

A. Goldhirsch and R. D. Gelber*

Ludwig Institut für Krebsforschung, Inselspital, 3010 Bern, Switzerland

Introduction

The use of adjuvant endocrine therapy in operable breast cancer was based upon observations made in patients with advanced disease. The first randomized trial of ovarian ablation (Cole 1975) was conducted before the formulation of the current theories concerning the necessity of controlling micrometastatic disease. An overview of the results of trials on ovarian ablation (either by ovarian radiation or by oophorectomy) showed an overall reduction of relapses and prolonged survival (Henderson 1987). The only study showing a significant survival benefit for the adjuvant-treated patients was the Toronto trial (Meakin et al. 1979). Premenopausal women (45 years old or older) who received both ovarian radiation and low-dose continuous prednisone for the duration of 5 years had a significantly better outcome than patients who received no adjuvant therapy.

The Ludwig Group's choice of the endocrine therapy regimen for postmenopausal women with operable breast cancer (Goldhirsch and Gelber 1986) was based on the efficacy of tamoxifen for the control of advanced disease and the significant results of the combined ovarian ablation and low-dose prednisone.

Recently, the combination of tamoxifen and prednisone (p + T) has been compared with tamoxifen alone in randomized trials. The response rate, response duration, and survival were increased by the combination of the two agents (Stewart et al. 1982; Rubens and Knight 1985). Adjuvant chemotherapy has been shown to reduce the relapse rate and prolong survival, especially in premenopausal women with operable breast cancer (Bonadonna et al. 1977; Fisher et al. 1979). An overview of available results from adjuvant trials has shown that combination chemotherapy also reduced early mortality in postmenopausal women (Meeting Report 1984). The combination of chemoendocrine therapy in the adjuvant setting for postmenopausal patients was used in an attempt to improve the results of both modalities.

---

* On behalf of the Ludwig Breast Cancer Study Group.

Recent Results in Cancer Research, Vol. 115
© Springer-Verlag Berlin·Heidelberg 1989

This report describes the findings from the two Ludwig trials in postmenopausal women and indicates future directions of research, which derive from the analysis at a median follow-up of 7 years, with special emphasis on the advantages derived from the use of combined chemoendocrine therapy.

Patients, Materials, Methods

From 1978 to 1981, 783 evaluable postmenopausal women with axillary node involvement were randomized into Ludwig Studies III and IV (Table 1). General eligibility criteria, conduct of the trials, statistical methods, and results at median observation times of 3 and 4 years have already been described (Goldhirsch and Gelber 1986, 1987; Ludwig Breast Cancer Study Group 1984).

Special aspects of Ludwig III related to the life quality of patients treated with the different therapies were also described (Gelber and Goldhirsch 1986; Gelber et al. 1987).

The analysis of endocrine therapy alone versus observation was performed comparing the p + T patient groups of trials III and IV ($n=320$) with their respective observation groups ($n=309$). For this comparison, all analyses were stratified by trial (i.e., age ≤ 65 or age $= 66-80$ years). Patient characteristics for this comparison are described in Table 2.

The randomized comparison between adjuvant chemoendocrine therapy with either endocrine therapy alone or no adjuvant therapy was the subject of trial III. Patient characteristics for this study are listed in Table 3.

Table 1. Ludwig studies III and IV in postmenopausal women with node-positive breast cancer (783 evaluable patients randomized 1978-81)

					Evaluable patients (n)
Ludwig III	Surgery	postmenopausal N+	R A N D O M	Observation	156
				p + T × 12 months	153
		65 years old or less		CMFp + T × 12 cycles	154
Ludwig IV	Surgery	postmenopausal N+	R A N D O M	Observation	153
		66-80 years old		p + T × 12 months	167

N+, node positive; C, cyclophosphamide (100 mg/m² orally, days 1-14); M, methotrexate (40 mg/m² i.v., days 1,8, q 4 weeks); F, 5-fluorouracil (600 mg/m² i.v., days 1,8); p, prednisone (7.5 mg/day orally (5 mg each morning; 2.5 mg each evening); T, tamoxifen (20 mg/day orally); p + T, given continuously.

Table 2. Patient characteristics for Ludwig trials III and IV: endocrine therapy (p+T) vs no adjuvant therapy (observation)

	Total	Treatment	
		p+T	Observation
Patients *(n)*	629	320	309
Ludwig III (≦65 years)	309	153	156
Ludwig IV (66–80 years)	320	167	153
Positive nodes (%)			
1–3	58	58	58
≧4	42	42	42
Hormone receptor status (%)			
ER+ (≧10 fmol)	32	32	32
ER− (0–9 fmol)	16	16	16
ER unknown	52	52	52

ER, estrogen receptor.

Table 3. Patient characteristics for Ludwig III: chemoendocrine therapy (CMFp+T) *vs* endocrine therapy alone (p+T) vs no adjuvant therapy (observation)

	Total	Treatment		
		CMFp+T	p+T	Observation
Patients *(n)*	463	154	153	156
Positive nodes (%)				
1–3	56	58	54	55
≧4	44	42	46	45
Hormone receptor status (%)				
ER+ (≧10 fmol)	33	38	29	34
ER− (0–9 fmol)	18	12	20	21
ER unknown	49	50	51	45

Results

At a median follow-up of 7 years, disease-free survival (DFS) was significantly longer for the p+T patients than for those in the observation group (Fig. 1); overall survivals (OS) were similar (Fig. 2). The 7-year DFS and OS percentages are described in Table 4. The patterns of first event are shown in Table 5 and indicate that treatment with p+T for 1 year reduced local, contralateral breast, and regional relapses, but not failures in distant sites.

The results of Ludwig III at a median follow-up of 7 years are displayed in Figs. 3 (DFS) and 4 (OS), as well as in Table 6. The prolonged overall survival for the cyclophosphamide, methotrexate, 5-fluorouracil, and p+T (CMFp+T) group as compared with both the observation group ($P=0.04$) and the p+T group ($P=0.08$) appeared only after 7 years of median observation time.

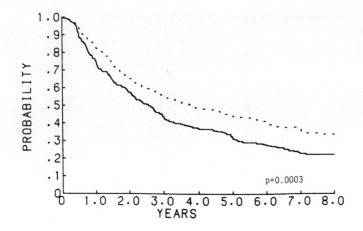

Treatment	NED	FAIL	TOTAL	7-YR % ± s.e.
—— Obs	73	236	309	23 ± 3
- - - p + T	116	204	320	36 ± 3

Fig. 1. Ludwig III and IV: DFS for 629 postmenopausal patients randomized to receive either p + T or no adjuvant treatment. *NED,* No evidence of disease

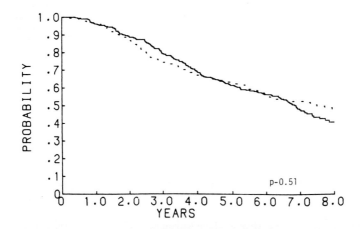

Treatment	ALIVE	DEAD	TOTAL	7-YR % ± s.e.
—— Obs	145	164	309	48 ± 3
- - - p + T	167	153	320	53 ± 3

Fig. 2. Ludwig III and IV: OS for 629 postmenopausal patients randomized to receive either p + T or no adjuvant treatment

Table 4. Ludwig III and IV: Results at 7 years' median follow-up (7-year DFS and OS percentages $\pm$ s.e. for patients in p + T or in the observation group)

	DFS (%)		P value[a]	OS (%)		P value[a]
	p + T	Observation		p + T	Observation	
Overall	36 ± 3	23 ± 3	0.0003	53 ± 3	48 ± 3	0.51
Ludwig III	36 ± 4	24 ± 3	0.02	51 ± 4	47 ± 4	0.81
Ludwig IV	36 ± 4	22 ± 4	0.005	54 ± 4	49 ± 4	0.49
Nodes involved						
1–3	45 ± 4	32 ± 4	0.004	61 ± 4	58 ± 4	0.80
≧ 4	23 ± 4	10 ± 3	0.02	41 ± 4	34 ± 4	0.47
ER status						
ER + (≧ 10 fmol)	36 ± 5	23 ± 5	0.01	57 ± 5	51 ± 6	0.88
ER − (0–9 fmol)	19 ± 6	21 ± 6	0.41	33 ± 7	39 ± 7	0.25
ER unknown	41 ± 4	23 ± 3	0.0004	56 ± 4	48 ± 4	0.13

[a] 2-Sided logrank test stratified by study.

Table 5. Ludwig III and IV: Patterns of first event as percentage of total patients in each treatment group at 7 years' median follow-up[a]

	Relapsed		Died	
	p + T	Observation	p + T	Observation
Total patients (n)	320 (167)	309 (153)	320 (167)	309 (153)
Events	64[b] (62)	76[b] (77)	48 (47)	53 (54)
Local or contralateral breast alone	11 (9)	20 (19)	5 (3)	8 (9)
Regional ± local	7 (6)	15 (17)	7 (6)	12 (13)
Distant ± other	36 (34)	36 (33)	27 (25)	28 (24)
Second neoplasia (not breast)	3 (2)	2 (1)	2 (2)	2 (1)
Deaths without relapse	7 (11)	3 (7)	7 (11)	3 (7)

[a] Percentages for trial IV alone are in parentheses (patients 66–80 years old).
[b] Including death without recurrence.

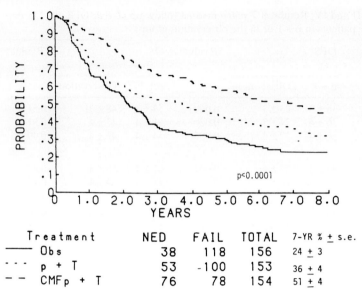

Treatment	NED	FAIL	TOTAL	7-YR % ± s.e.
—— Obs	38	118	156	24 ± 3
- - - p + T	53	-100	153	36 ± 4
– – CMFp + T	76	78	154	51 ± 4

Fig. 3. Ludwig III: DFS for 463 postmenopausal patients 65 years old or younger randomized to receive either CMFp + T, p + T, or no adjuvant treatment

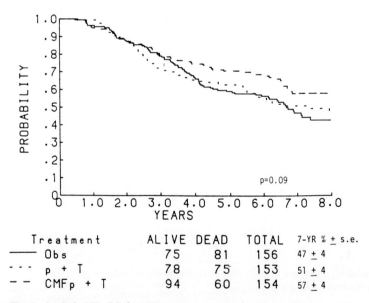

Treatment	ALIVE	DEAD	TOTAL	7-YR % ± s.e.
—— Obs	75	81	156	47 ± 4
- - - p + T	78	75	153	51 ± 4
– – CMFp + T	94	60	154	57 ± 4

Fig. 4. Ludwig III: OS for 463 postmenopausal patients 65 years old or younger randomized to receive either CMFp + T, p + T, or no adjuvant treatment

Table 6. Ludwig III: results at 7 years' median follow-up (7-year DFS and OS percentages ± s.e.)[a]

	DFS (%)			OS (%)		
	CMFp + T	p + T	Observation	CMFp + T	p + T	Observation
Overall	51 ± 4**	36 ± 4	24 ± 3	57 ± 4	51 ± 4	47 ± 4
Nodes involved						
1–3	64 ± 5*	48 ± 6	30 ± 5	71 ± 5	63 ± 6	60 ± 6
≧4	33 ± 6	23 ± 5	15 ± 4	39 ± 7	37 ± 6	31 ± 6
ER status						
ER +	52 ± 7	39 ± 8	26 ± 6	61 ± 7	57 ± 8	59 ± 7
ER −	52 ± 12**	20 ± 7	21 ± 7	55 ± 12	37 ± 9	38 ± 9
ER unknown	50 ± 6	41 ± 6	23 ± 5	55 ± 6	53 ± 6	42 ± 6

[a] CMFp + T vs p + T: differences evaluated by 2-sided logrank test.
* P value between 0.05–0.01.
** P value < 0.01.

Table 7. Ludwig III: patterns of first event as percentage of total patients in each treatment group at 7 years' median follow-up (postmenopausal women 65 years old or younger)

	Relapsed			Died		
	CMFp + T	p + T	Observation	CMFp + T	p + T	Observation
Total patients (n)	154	153	156	154	153	156
Events	51[a]	65[a]	76[a]	39[a]	49[a]	52[a]
Local or contra-lateral breast	7	13	21	2	8	8
Regional ± local	6	8	13	4	7	10
Distant ± other	29	40	38	24	30	31
Second neoplasia (not breast)	2	2	3	2	2	2
Death without relapse	(7)	(2)	(1)	7	2	1

[a] Including death without recurrence.

This might be because only a moderate reduction of relapses in distant sites was observed even for the combined CMFp + T regimens (Table 7) and because there was a higher mortality rate *without* signs of malignant disease in the CMFp + T-treated group.

Discussion

The use of adjuvant therapy for the prolongation of DFS and for the reduction of mortality in breast cancer patients of almost all ages, especially those at high risk for relapse, has become common practice. Adjuvant endocrine therapy with tamoxifen for at least 5 years' duration has shown its efficacy in reducing mortality even when compared with the systematic use of the same drug upon appearance of relapse in the control group (Scottish Breast Cancer Trials Committee 1987). One of the first trials in which 20 mg/day of adjuvant tamoxifen was given for 1 year (Ribeiro and Swindell 1985) showed no statistically significant improvement in either DFS or OS in 588 patients included in the trial. The higher dosage (30 mg/day for 1 year) used in the Danish trial (Rose et al. 1985) in 1650 patients was hypothesized by investigators of the Scottish trial (Scottish Breast Cancer Trials Committee 1987) to result in a significant DFS advantage.

The two British trials (Scottish Breast Cancer Trials Committee 1987; Baum for NATO 1985) in which the exposure to tamoxifen was prolonged (2 years for the NATO trial and 5 years for the Scottish trial) have also shown a significantly prolonged OS. The use of low-dose prednisone together with tamoxifen, 20 mg/day for 1 year only, resulted in a significant reduction of relapse rates. Prolonged use of this combination of endocrine agents might be a way of improving the outcome of adjuvant endocrine therapy in postmenopausal women.

Ludwig III clearly demonstrates the superiority of the CMFp + T combination over no adjuvant treatment or endocrine therapy alone in controlling disease and reducing mortality for postmenopausal patients. Improvement of the therapeutic index for combined chemoendocrine adjuvant treatment is an area for future research. Prolonged exposure to tamoxifen with an initial short course of chemotherapy might provide some additional cell kill and hence prolong DFS and OS in these patients. Studies currently accruing patients will eventually increase our knowledge about this issue (Goldhirsch and Gelber 1987).

Appendix A
Ludwig Breast Cancer Study Group: Participants and Authors

Ludwig Institute for Cancer Research, Inselspital, Bern, Switzerland	A. Goldhirsch *(Study Coordinator)*, B. Davis, R. Bettelheim, W. Hartmann, M. Neville *(Study Pathologists)*, M. Castiglione, A. Pedrazzini, D. Zava, C. Wiedmer
Harvard School of Public Health and Dana-Farber Cancer Institute, Boston, U.S.A.	R. D. Gelber *(Study Statistician)*, K. Price, K. Stanley, K. Larholt, N. Snudden, M. Zelen
Frontier Science and Technology Research Foundation, Buffalo, New York, U.S.A.	M. Isley, M. Parsons, L. Szymoniak
Auckland Breast Cancer Study Group, Auckland, New Zealand	R. G. Kay, J. Probert, B. Mason, H. Wood, E. G. Gifford, J. F. Carter, J. C. Gillmann, J. Anderson, L. Yee, I. M. Holdaway, G. C. Hitchcock, M. Jagusch
Spedali Civili e Fondazione Beretta, Brescia, Italy	G. Marini, E. Simoncini, P. Marpicati, U. Sartori, A. Barni, L. Morassi, P. Grigolato, D. Di Lorenzo, A. Albertini, G. Marinone, M. Zorzi
Groote Schuur Hospital, Cape Town, Republic of South Africa	A. Hacking, D. M. Dent, J. Terblanche, A. Tiltmann, A. Gudgeon, E. Dowdle, R. Sealy, P. Palmer, P. Helman

University of Essen, West German Tumor Center, Essen, Federal Republic of Germany
University of Düsseldorf, Düsseldorf, Federal Republic of Germany
West Swedish Breast Cancer Study Group, Göteborg, Sweden

C.G.Schmidt, K.Höffken, F.Schüning, L.D.Leder, H.Ludwig, R.Callies, A.E.Schindler
P.Faber, H.G.Schnürch, H.Bender, H.Bojar
C.-M.Rudenstam, J.Säve-Söderbergh, E.Cahlin, L.O.Hafström, S.Holmberg, C.Johansén, S.Nilsson, J.Fornander, H.Salander, C.Andersson, O.Ruusvik, G.Ostberg, L.Mattsson, C.G.Bäckström, S.Bergegardh, G.Ekelund, Y.Hessman, S.Holmberg, O.Nelzén, S.Dahlin, G.Wallin, L.Ivarsson, O.Thorem, L.Lundell, U.Ljungquist

The Institute of Oncology, Ljubljana, Yugoslavia

J.Lindtner, J.Novak, D.Erzen, M.Sencar, J.Cervek, O.Cerar, B.Stabuc, R.Golouh, J.Lamovec, J.Jancar, S.Sebek

The Royal Free Hospital, London, England

S.Parbhoo, K.Hobbs, E.Boessen, D.Skeggs, B.Stoll, F.Sennanayake, B.Scott, K.Griffiths

Madrid Breast Cancer Group, Madrid, Spain

H.Cortés-Funes, F.Martinez-Tello, F.Cruz Caro, M.L.Marcos, M.A.Figueras, F.Calero, A.Suarez, F.Pastrana, R.Huertas, C.Guzman

Anti-Cancer Council of Victoria, Melbourne, Australia

J.Collins, R.Snyder, R.Bennett, W.I.Burns, J.Forbes, J.Funder, T.Gale, L.Harrison, S.Hart, V.Humenuik, P.Jeal, P.Kitchen, R.Lovell, R.Mclennan, R.Reed, I.Russell, M.Schwarz, L.Sisely, P.Williams, H.Ritchie

Sir Charles Gairdner Hospital Nedlands, Western Australia

M.Byrne, P.M.Reynolds, H.J.Sheiner, S.Levitt, D.Kermode, K.B.Shilkin, R.Hähnel, G.van Hazel

SAKK (Swiss Group for Clinical Cancer Research)
Inselspital, Bern, Switzerland

K.Brunner, G.Locher, E.Dreher, K.Buser, H.Cottier, K.Bürki, M.Walther, R.Joss, H.Bürgi, M.Spreng, U.Herrmann, R.Kissling

Kantonsspital, St. Gallen, Switzerland

H.J.Senn, W.F.Jungi, R.Amgwerd, U.Schmid, Th.Hardmeier, E.Hochuli, U.Haller, O.Schildknecht

Ospedale San Giovanni, Bellinzona, Switzerland

F.Cavalli, H.Neuenschwander, W.Müller, C.Sessa, P.Luscieti, E.S.Passega, M.Varini, G.Losa

Kantonsspital, Basel, Switzerland

J.P.Obrecht, F.Harder, H.Stamm, U.Laffer, A.C.Almendral, U.Eppenberger, J.Torhorst

Hôpital Cantonal Universitaire, Geneva, Switzerland

P.Alberto, F.Krauer, R.Egeli, M.Aapro, R.Mégevand, M.Forni, P.Schäfer, E.Jacot des Combes, A.M.Schindler, F.Misset

CHUV, Lausanne, Switzerland
Hôpital des Cadolles, Neuchâtel, Switzerland
Kantonsspital, Luzern, Switzerland
Kantonsspital, Zürich, Switzerland

S.Leyvraz
P.Siegenthaler, V.Barrelet, R.P.Baumann

H.J.Schmid
G.Martz

Ludwig Institute for Cancer Research and
Royal Prince Alfred Hospital, Sydney,
Australia

Wellington Hospital, Wellington,
New Zealand

M. H. N. Tattersall, R. Fox, A. Coates,
D. Hedley, D. Raghavan, F. Niesche,
R. West, S. Renwick, D. Green, J. Donovan,
P. Duval, A. Ng, T. Foo, D. Glenn, T. J. Nash,
R. A. North, J. Beith, G. O'Connor
J. S. Simpson, E. C. Watson, C. T. Collins,
A. J. Gray, J. W. Logan, J. J. Landreth,
W. Brander, P. Cairney, L. Holloway,
I. M. Holdaway, C. Unsworth

References

Baum M (1985) Nolvadex Adjuvant Trial Organisation: controlled trial of tamoxifen as single adjuvant agent in management of early breast cancer: analysis at 6 years. Lancet I: 836–839

Bonadonna G, Rossi A, Valagussa T (1977) The CMF program for operable breast cancer with positive axillary nodes: update analysis of disease-free interval, site of relapse and drug tolerance. Cancer 39: 2904–2915

Cole MP (1975) A clinical trial of an artificial menopause in carcinoma of the breast. INSERM 55: 143–150

Fisher B, Sherman B, Rockette H, et al. (1979) L-phenylalanine mustard (L-PAM) in the management of premenopausal patients with primary breast cancer. Cancer 44: 847–857

Gelber RD, Goldhirsch A (1986) A new endpoint for the assessment of adjuvant therapy in postmenopausal women with operable breast cancer. J Clin Oncol 4: 1772–1779

Gelber RD, Goldhirsch A, Castiglione M et al. (1987) Time without symptoms of toxicity (TWiST): A quality-of-life-oriented endpoint to evaluate adjuvant therapy. In: Salmon SE (ed) Adjuvant therapy of cancer, vol 5. Grune and Stratton, Orlando, pp 455–466

Goldhirsch A, Gelber RD, for the Ludwig Breast Cancer Study Group (1986) Adjuvant treatment for early breast cancer: The Ludwig Breast Cancer Studies. CI Monogr 1: 55–70

Goldhirsch A, Gelber RD, for the Ludwig Breast Cancer Study Group (1987) Adjuvant therapy for breast cancer: The Ludwig Breast Cancer Trials 1987, In: Salmon SE (ed) Adjuvant therapy of cancer, vol 5. Grune and Stratton, Orlando, pp 279–309

Henderson IC (1987) Adjuvant systemic therapy of early breast cancer. In: Harris JR, Hellman S, Henderson IC, Kinne PW (eds) Breast diseases. Lippincott, Philadelphia, pp 324–353

Ludwig Breast Cancer Study Group (1984) Randomized trial of chemo-endocrine therapy, endocrine therapy, and mastectomy alone in postmenopausal patients with operable breast cancer and axillary node metastasis. Lancet I: 1256–1260

Meakin JW, Allt WEC, Beale FA et al. (1979) Ovarian irradiation and prednisone following surgery and radiotherapy for carcinoma of the breast. Can Med Assoc J 120: 1221–1231

Meeting Report, London (1984) Review of mortality results in randomized trials in early breast cancer. Lancet II: 1205

Scottish Breast Cancer Trials Committee (1987) Adjuvant tamoxifen in the management of operable breast cancer: The Scottish trial. Lancet II: 171–175

Stewart JS, Rubens RD, King RJE et al. (1982) Contribution of prednisolone to the primary endocrine treatment of advanced breast cancer. Eur J Cancer Clin Oncol 18: 1307–1309

Ribeiro G, Swindell R (1985) The Christie Hospital tamoxifen (Nolvadex) adjuvant trial for operable breast cancer – 7-year results. Eur J Cancer Clin Oncol 21: 897–900

Rose C, Anderson KW, Mouridsen HT et al. (1985) Beneficial effect of adjuvant tamoxifen in primary breast cancer patients with high estrogen receptor values. Lancet I: 16–19

Rubens RD, Knight RK (1985) The contribution of prednisolone to primary endocrine therapy in advanced breast cancer. Proc Am Soc Clin Oncol 4: 53

Chemo- or Endocrine Adjuvant Therapy Alone or Combined in Postmenopausal Patients (GABG Trial 1)*

W. Jonat, M. Kaufmann, and U. Abel

Abteilung für Gynäkologie und Geburtshilfe, Universitätsklinik Hamburg, Martinistraße 52, 2000 Hamburg 20, FRG

Introduction

The natural history of operable breast cancer can be altered by adjuvant treatment (Lippmann 1986; Salmon 1987). Adjuvant combination chemotherapy (AC), e.g., cyclophosphamide, methotrexate, and 5-fluorouracil (CMF) results in a significant prolongation of disease-free (DFS) and overall survival (OS) in *premenopausal* node-positive patients. *Postmenopausal* node-positive patients seem to benefit from endocrine therapy. These data were mainly obtained by overview analysis of randomized trials with treatment groups compared with groups receiving no adjuvant therapy (control) after mastectomy.

The most important known prognostic factors in primary breast cancer are the axillary lymph node and the hormone receptor status (Kaufmann 1983; Wilson et al. 1984). To date, no randomized trial has been conducted including separate prospective randomization of patients according to these clinically important prognostic factors. Also until now, no long-term follow-up data which compare endocrine treatment with cytotoxic therapy in prospectively defined subgroups of node-positive primary breast cancer have been available.

This paper reports the *postmenopausal* data of two risk-adapted randomized prospective adjuvant trials conducted in West Germany between January 1981 and January 1988 by 13 university and larger regional hospitals (see Appendix A). Patient entry was closed in May 1986. (For premenopausal data, see Kaufmann et al., this volume). In the low-risk situation ($n = 1-3$ involved axillary nodes *and* hormone-receptor–positive tumors), patients were entered in the trial to receive tamoxifen (TAM) or CMF chemotherapy. In the high-risk situation ($n > = 4$ involved nodes or n 1–3 nodes and hormone-receptor–negative tumors), patients were treated with Adriamycin and cyclophosphamide (AC) alone or in combination with TAM.

The aim of the study was to analyze adjuvant endocrine, cytotoxic, and chemo-endocrine therapy in defined subsets ($> = 50$ years) of women with node-positive breast cancer.

* This work was partially supported by grants from ICI-Pharma, Plankstadt, FRG, and Farmitalia Carlo Erba, Freiburg, FRG.

Table 1. GABG 1: Patient characteristics

		Low-risk n (%)		High-risk n (%)	
		TAM	CMF	AC	AC+TAM
Age	< = 49 years	49 (36)	70 (51)	116 (49)	96 (41)
	> = 50 years	89 (64)	68 (49)	121 (51)	138 (59)
Tumor size	T 1	34 (25)	35 (25)	34 (14)	36 (15)
	T 2	92 (67)	93 (67)	158 (67)	151 (65)
	T 3	12 (8)	10 (7)	45 (19)	47 (20)
Node histology	1	72 (52)	60 (44)	21	19
	2	44 (32)	50 (36)	22	9
	3	–	–	10	12
	4-9	–	–	116 (49)	143 (61)
	> = 10	–	–	68 (29)	51 (22)
Receptor status	ER +	129 (93)	124 (90)	92 (39)	108 (46)
	ER −	9 (7)	14 (10)	146 (61)	126 (54)
	unknown	0	0	0	0
	PR +	104 (75)	106 (77)	73 (31)	90 (38)
	PR −	30 (22)	19 (14)	140 (59)	119 (51)
	PR unknown	4 (3)	13 (9)	24 (10)	25 (11)
	Total	138	138	237	234

Patients and Methods

Patients

Women over 50 years old with histologically invasive T 1-3 tumors treated by modified radical mastectomy and axillary lymph node dissection (level I and II ± III) entered in these trials. No post-operative radiotherapy was used. Only women with a least ten biopsied analyzed nodes and known hormone-receptor status [estrogen (ER) - and/or progesterone receptor (PR)] had been randomized. Treatment was started within 3 weeks of surgery.

In total, 747 of 774 patients were evaluable for both trials (premenopausal patients, see Kaufmann et al., this volume) according to the defined entry criteria.

Table 1 summarizes the distribution of patient and tumor characteristics for both trials and for each therapy group (pre- and postmenopausal patients).

Adjuvant Treatment

A total of 157 *low-risk* postmenopausal patients ($n=1$-3, ER + or PR +) were randomized after mastectomy to TAM (30 mg/day orally continuously for 2 years) or CMF (Bonadonna et al. 1976) i.v. for 6 cycles every 4 weeks. Full doses of C (500 mg/m^2), M (40 mg/m^2), and F (600 mg/m^2) were given on days 1 and 8.

Of the *high-risk* postmenopausal patients, 259 ($n > =4$, or $n=1$-3 and ER − and PR −) were randomized to AC (Salmon and Jones 1979) i.v. alone or

AC + TAM. Full doses in eight cycles at 3-weekly intervals of A ($30 \, mg/m^2$) on day 1 and of C $300 \, mg/m^2$ on days 1 and 8 were given. TAM was also administered for 2 years.

Hormone Receptor Analysis

ER and PR were determined by the EORTC dextran-coated charcoal standard method (EORTC 1973). All primary tumor specimens were analyzed at least for ER. Tumors were defined as receptor positive at levels of $> = 20 \, fmol/mg$ cytosol protein. Interlaboratory quality control studies were conducted twice a year (Kaufmann et al. 1985).

Follow-up Studies

Clinical and hematologic assessment was carried out before each i.v. cytotoxic drug administration, every 3 months for 2 years, and thereafter every 6 months. Liver ultrasound, bone scans, and chest X-rays were repeated every 6 months, and after 2 years, annually.

Randomization and Statistical Methods

Randomization was conducted by each hospital with centrally distributed envelopes. The method of Kaplan and Meier (1958) and a logrank test with values of significance (Peto et al. 1977) were used to estimate DFS and OS from the date of surgery.

Results

A total of 416 postmenopausal patients referred by 13 institutions were randomized. The 157 low-risk patients received TAM or CMF, and the 259 high-risk patients were allocated to receive AC or AC + TAM. As shown in Table 1, the major patient and tumor variables are evenly distributed between the treatment arms, although a slightly higher proportion of patients received TAM (alone or in combination with AC). The patterns of first relapse or event by treatment group are reported in Table 2. Moreover, the percentage of deaths is given for all subgroups.

To date, recurrent disease has developed in 39 of 157 (24.8%) low-risk patients and 161 of 259 (62.2%) high-risk patients. This shows that adjuvant TAM alone or in combination has delayed the onset of the major types of recurrences in both defined subgroups.

Patients without recorded relapse for low-risk patients number 76 in the TAM group and 42 in the CMF arm and, for high-risk patients, 66 in the AC + TAM group compared with 32 in the AC arm.

In the *low-risk* subgroup, five (5.6%) of the 89 in the TAM arm and six (8.8%) in the CMF arm have died so far. In the *high-risk* subgroup, mortality amounts to 40

Table 2. GABG 1 study: Recurrence and death after 6 years in postmenopausal patients ($n=416$)

Type	Low risk (%)		High risk (%)	
	TAM	CMF	AC	AC+TAM
Loco-regional	6.7	16.2	27.3	16.7
Distant (+combination)	7.9	22.1	46.3	35.5
Total	14.6	38.3	73.6	52.2
Death	5.6	8.8	38.8	29.0

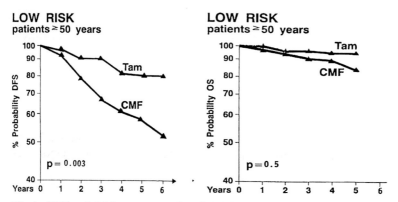

Fig. 1. DFS and OS by treatment for all 157 low-risk postmenopausal patients

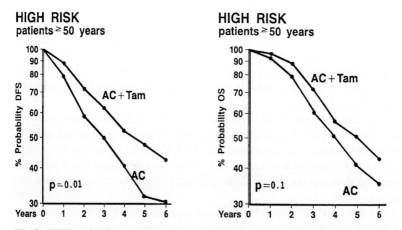

Fig. 2. DFS and OS by treatment for all 259 high-risk postmenopausal patients

(29%) of 138 patients in the AC + TAM group and 47 (38.8%) of 121 patients in the AC arm.

Figures 1 and 2 demonstrate the life table analyses for DFS and OS for low- and high-risk patients. Each figure shows a significant benefit regarding DFS for those treated with TAM therapy compared with chemotherapy alone or in combination with TAM. P levels were 0.003 for low-risk and 0.01 for high-risk patients. The OS analyses have not yet reached a significant level, but there is a trend in favor of TAM-treated patients for both *low-risk* and *high-risk* patients.

Regarding hormone receptor levels, there is a consistent trend in favor of positive and/or high ER levels. In the low-risk group, patients with tumors showing ER levels of 100 fmol/mg protein or more had the best DFS ($P = 0.003$), while in the high-risk group, women with ER-positive levels of $> = 20$ fmol/mg protein showed the best DFS.

Discussion

At present, despite clear recommendations given by the NIH Consensus Development Conference that TAM should be used in postmenopausal women with node-positive and receptor-positive tumors, it remains unclear whether chemotherapy given at full dosage or combined chemoendocrine treatment is equal or superior to TAM given alone and irrespective of nodal and receptor status. In our study, we have tried to answer these questions in specially defined subsets of postmenopausal breast cancer patients.

Our study design was prospectively based and randomized according to lymph node and hormone-receptor status for a so-called low- and high-risk situation. All node-positive postmenopausal patients treated at the participating institutions were included in the trial. (Regarding premenopausal patients, see Kaufmann et al., this volume). In a defined low-risk subset ($n = 1$–3 nodes, ER- or PR-positive status) a comparison between TAM alone and cytotoxic chemotherapy alone was conducted. TAM was given for 2 years and CMF i.v. for 6 months. In a defined high-risk subset ($n > = 4$ nodes, or ER- and PR-negative status) the efficacy of cytotoxic combination chemotherapy was compared with chemoendocrine treatment. AC was given i.v. for eight cycles over 6 months, TAM, in addition to which was continued for 2 years.

In accordance with earlier reports (Kaufmann et al. 1984, 1985), subset analyses yielded interesting results which correspond to conclusions stated at the Consensus Conference 1985 and support the idea of defining prognostic subgroups of patients with primary breast cancer before starting adjuvant systemic treatment. Postmenopausal low-risk women ($> = 50$ years) show benefits from TAM given for 2 years compared with those derived from chemotherapy alone. Combined chemoendocrine (AC + TAM) treatment improves results significantly for DFS and slightly for OS.

In both trials, endocrine therapy mainly affects hormone receptor-positive tumors, as reported by other study groups (Fisher et al. 1987; Hubay et al. 1980; Ludwig Breast Cancer Study Group 1984; Rose et al. 1985).

In contrast, however, to the clinical importance of the results of the Danish Breast Cancer Cooperative Group's trial (Rose et al. 1985) and the Scottish Cancer trial (1987), the crude analyses of our data do not support the conclusion that a benefit from adjuvant TAM therapy becomes significant for patients with ER levels of > 100 fmol/mg protein. Significant levels for DFS and a positive trend for OS were found for levels greater than 20 fmol/mg protein. Our results confirm the fact that lymph node and receptor status are per se prognostic factors. Low- and high-risk situations also exist after the first failure; this seems to be due to the natural histories of primary breast cancer.

New methods, e.g., new quality-of-life-oriented end points for the assessment of adjuvant therapy are needed to assist in the selection of therapeutic approach (Gelber and Goldhirsch 1986).

The design of new randomized trials have to take into consideration risk-adapted treatment modality in defined subsets of patients with operable breast cancer to improve further survival and quality of life.

Acknowledgement. We thank all participating institutions for their excellent cooperation and also wish to acknowledge the essential contributions of the many clinicians, pathologists, and laboratory workers who made this collaborative study possible.

Appendix A
Gynecological Adjuvant Breast Cancer Group, FRG GABG I

Main Investigator	*Institution*
M. Kaufmann, F. Kubli	University of Heidelberg
W. Jonat, H. Maass	University of Hamburg
H. Caffier, K. H. Wulf	University of Würzburg
R. Kreienberg, V. Friedberg	University of Mainz
J. Hilfrich, J. Schneider	University of Hannover
W. Kleine, A. Pfleiderer	University of Freiburg
M. Neises, F. Melchert	University of Mannheim/Heidelberg
M. Mahlke, P. Knapstein	Städtische Frauenklinik Krefeld
G. Trams	Städtische Frauenklinik Bremen
K. Brunnert, J. Schermann, P. Dördelmann	Städtische Frauenklinik Karlsruhe
U. Stosiek, K. Gumbrecht	Diakonissen Krankenhaus Karlsruhe
R. Stigelmeyer, F. Seeger, O. Fettig	Vincentius Krankenhaus Karlsruhe
U. Abel	Tumorzentrum Heidelberg

References

Bonadonna G, Brusamolino E, Valagussa P, et al. (1976) Combination chemotherapy as an adjuvant treatment in operable breast cancer. N Engl J Med 294: 405–410

Consensus Conference (1985) Adjuvant chemotherapy for breast cancer. JAMA 254: 3461–3463

EORTC: Breast Cancer Cooperative Group (1973) Standards for the assessment of estrogen receptors in human breast cancer. Eur J Cancer 9: 379–381

Fisher ER, Sass R, Fisher B, et al. (1987) Pathologic findings from the National Surgical Adjuvant Breast Project: Correlations with concordant and discordant estrogen and progesterone receptors. Cancer 59: 1554–1559

Gelber RD, Goldhirsch A, for the Ludwig Breast Cancer Study Group (1986) A new endpoint for the assessment of adjuvant therapy in postmenopausal women with operable breast cancer. J Clin Oncol 4: 1772–1779

Hubay C, Pearson OH, Marshall US (1980) Antiestrogen, cytotoxic chemotherapy and bacillus Calmette-Guérain vaccination in stage II breast cancer: a preliminary report. Surgery 87: 494–501

Kaplan EL, Meier P (1958) Nonparametric estimation from incomplete observations. J Am Statis Assoc 53: 457–481

Kaufmann M (1983) Biochemische prognostische Faktoren beim Mamma-Karzinom. In: Kubli F, Nagel GA, Kadach U, Kaufmann M (eds) Neue Wege in der Brustkrebsbehandlung Zuckschwerdt, München, pp 46–61 (Aktuelle Onkologie, vol 8)

Kaufmann M, Jonat W (GABG) (1984) Risk adapted adjuvant chemo-hormonotherapy in operable nodal positive breast cancer. In: Jones SE, Salmon SE (eds): Adjuvant therapy of cancer, vol 4. Grune and Stratton, New York, pp 369–378

Kaufmann M, Jonat W, Caffier H, Hilfrich J, Melchert F, Mahlke M, Abel U, Maass H, Kubli F for the Gynecological Adjuvant Breast Cancer Group (1985) Adjuvant chemo-hormonotherapy selected by axillary node and hormone receptor status in node-positive breast cancer. Reviews Endocrine-Related Cancer Supp 17: 57–63

Lippmann ME (ed) (1986) NIH Consensus Development Conference on adjuvant chemotherapy and endocrine therapy for breast cancer 1985. NCI Monogr

Ludwig Breast Cancer Study Group (1984) Randomized trial of chemo-endocrine therapy, endocrine therapy and mastectomy alone in postmenopausal patients with operable breast cancer and axillary node metastases. Lancet I: 1256–1260

Peto R, Pike MC, Armitage P et al. (1977) Design and analysis of randomized clinical trials requiring prolonged observation of each patient: Analysis and examples. Br J Cancer 35: 1–39

Rose C, Thorpe S, Anderson KW et al (1985) Beneficial effect of adjuvant tamoxifen therapy in primary breast cancer patients with high estrogen receptor value. Lancet I: 16–19

Salmon SE, Jones SE (1979) Studies of the combination of adriamycin and cyclophosphamide (alone or with other agents) for the treatment of breast cancer. Oncology 36: 40–44

Salmon SE (ed) (1987) Adjuvant therapy of cancer, vol 5. Grune and Stratton, New York

Scottish Cancer Trial (1987) Adjuvant tamoxifen in the management of operable breast cancer: the Scottish trial. Lancet II: 171–175

Wilson RE, Donegan WL, Mettlin C (1984) The 1982 national survey of carcinoma of the breast in the United States. American College of Surgeons. Surg Gynecol Obstet 159: 309–318

Prognostic Factors and Treatment for Node-Negative Patients

Prognosis in Breast Cancer*

W. L. McGuire and G. M. Clark

Department of Medicine, Division of Oncology, University of Texas Health Science Center, 7703 Floyd Curl Drive, San Antonio, TX 78284-7884, USA

Only one-half of patients presenting with primary breast cancer are cured by local therapy. It is thus desirable to have a method to predict which patients are likely to have a recurrence so that systemic therapy can be instituted to delay, or even prevent, such recurrences. For many years, our laboratory in San Antonio has been measuring factors in human breast cancer patients which have been hypothesized to correlate with clinical outcome. Our efforts have dealt primarily with the prognostic factors listed in Table 1. We will briefly review each of these prognostic factors and provide the essential data which correlates each factor with clinical outcome. In this summary of San Antonio efforts, we will not attempt to review the literature or detail the work of others.

Table 1. Prognostic factors

1. Axillary nodal status
2. Steroid receptors
3. Proliferative rate
4. Ploidy
5. Oncogene amplification

Axillary Nodal Status

It has been known for many years from a variety of clinical trials that axillary node status is the most important factor predicting for recurrence and survival in breast cancer. Our own efforts in this regard complement previous work and serve to validate recurrence and survival data in our own patient population. We have studied the disease-free survival (DFS) in almost 4000 patients according to the number of positive axillary lymph nodes, as determined by pathological examination. We find a remarkable inverse correlation between the probability of DFS and

---

* This work was supported by grant number NIH CA30195.

Table 2. Multivariate analysis of survival prediction by receptors and other factors in axillary node-negative breast cancer (1647 patients, San Antonio receptor database)

	Disease-free survival P	Survival P
ER	<0.0001	0.0003
Size	0.0002	0.0041
Age	NS	NS
PR	NS	NS

NS, not significant.

the number of involved lymph nodes. We find the same relationship between absolute survival and the number of involved nodes. The results leave little doubt that axillary lymph node involvement is the gold standard with which all other prognostic factors must be compared.

Steroid Receptors

Many years ago, we were the first to show that estrogen receptor (ER) measurements could identify patients at high risk for recurrence (Knight et al. 1977). A more recent update of 1647 patients revealed that ER and size are the most important factors for predicting recurrence in axillary node-negative patients. The results shown in Table 2 indicate by multivariate analysis that the two factors provide independent prognostic information. In Stage II breast cancer (axillary node positive), we have found that progesterone receptor (PR) assessment is superior to other measured prognostic factors and appears equivalent to the number of positive axillary lymph nodes for predicting recurrence (Clark et al. 1983). We conclude that ER and PR are firmly established prognostic factors for early recurrence and survival in both Stage I and Stage II breast cancer.

Tumor Cell Proliferative Activity and Ploidy

Pathologists have known for a long time that the more mitotic figures in a tumor specimen, the more likely the tumor would be to exhibit aggressive behavior, with subsequent shortening of the patient's survival. More recently, the thymidine labeling index has been used as a quantitative measure of tumor cells engaging in DNA synthesis. Several separate studies provide independent confirmation that the higher the proliferative rate of a tumor as measured by the thymidine labeling index, the more likely a patient is to have a breast cancer recurrence (Meyer 1986; Silvestrini et al. 1986; Tubiana et al. 1984; McGuire et al. 1985; McGuire and Dressler 1985).

Since the thymidine labeling index requires fresh tissue, we turned to flow cytometric methods on frozen pulverized breast tumors to measure the proliferative

Table 3. S-Phase, ploidy, and receptor status

ER	PR	(n)	Median	
			S-phase fraction	Aneuploid fraction
−	−	153	12.7	70
			P=0.0001	P=0.006
+	−	364	6.4	54
			P=0.0001	P=0.08
+	+	552	4.6	48

Table 4. Risk factors for relapse in axillary node-negative breast cancer

1. Negative ER/PR
2. High S-phase
3. Aneuploidy
4. Large tumor (>2 cm)

rate as the percentage of cells in S-phase, and also to determine ploidy. We find that diploid tumors have a median S-phase of 2.6%, significantly lower than the median S-phase of 10.3% in the aneuploid population. Even more important is the wide range of S-phase values in both populations, suggesting that it is not sufficient to know merely whether a tumor is diploid or aneuploid.

The relationship of ploidy, S-phase fraction, and receptor status are illustrated in Table 3. Receptor-negative tumors are much more likely to be aneuploid and to have a high median S-phase than receptor-positive tumors. In our axillary node-negative patients, we have data to indicate that both S-phase fraction and ploidy are significant prognostic factors for relapse. Thus, the factors listed in Table 4 might be used to select axillary node-negative patients at high risk for relapse, who might therefore be candidates for adjuvant treatment. As yet, we do not know the precise combination of these factors which should be used in a clinical setting, but their importance is undeniable.

Oncogene Amplification

In a collaborative study with Slamon and colleagues at UCLA and Ullrich at Genentech, we studied the frequency of HER-2/*neu* oncogene amplification in our San Antonio breast cancer patients (Slamon et al. 1987). The HER-2/*neu* oncogene is a member of the erb B-like family and is related to, but distinct from, the epidermal growth factor (EGF) receptor. Its amino acid sequence suggests a probable receptor function, although a ligand has not yet been identified. We were unable to find any correlation with HER-2/*neu* gene amplification and ER, PR, or tumor size. There was a modest association with age, but a highly significant correlation with the number of involved axillary lymph nodes. Based on this finding, we studied a subset of 86 Stage II (axillary node positive) patients with com-

Table 5. HER-2/*neu* gene amplification, recurrence, and survival stage II breast cancer patients, $n=86$

Factor	Relapse P	Survival P
Number of positive nodes	0.001	0.0003
HER-2/*neu*	0.001	0.02
PR	NS	NS
Size of tumor	NS	NS
ER	NS	NS
Age	NS	NS

NS, not significant.

plete recurrence and survival follow-up data. Using a multivariate analysis, HER-2/*neu* gene amplification was more predictive of shorter survival than PR, tumor size, or ER (Table 5). Amplification of the HER-2/*neu* gene is a significant independent predictor of both recurrence and survival in node-positive breast cancer.

Conclusion

We have presented an overview of our data regarding lymph node status, receptors, proliferative rate, aneuploidy, and oncogene amplification. We believe that these factors are not just a group of unrelated items, but rather can be connected to provide a coherent picture of how the factors affect recurrence and survival. We know that approximately 58% of primary breast tumors are aneuploid. We have demonstrated that aneuploidy is correlated with receptor-negative tumors. It is easy to understand that receptor-negative tumors would not respond to endocrine therapy, either in the adjuvant setting or for metastatic disease. This of course would result in increased recurrence and poor survival. Aneuploidy is also related to an increased median S-phase in breast tumors. This higher proliferative capacity of the tumor could cause tumors to recur earlier and shorten patient survival times. The amplification of the HER-2/*neu* gene, which can be thought of as microaneuploidy, could lead to increased recurrence and poor patient survival because the tumor has overexpressed a receptor for a putative growth factor which is driving the tumor at a higher proliferative rate. It is therefore easy to see how all of these factors in concert influence recurrence and survival. A more detailed understanding of this pathophysiology will lead to more rational treatment programs.

References

Clark GM, McGuire WL, Hubay CA, Pearson OH, Marshall JS (1983) Progesterone receptors as a prognostic factor in Stage II breast cancer. N Eng J Med 309: 1343–1347

Knight WA III, Livingston RB, Gregory EJ, McGuire WL (1977) Estrogen receptor as an independent prognostic factor for early recurrence in breast cancer. Cancer Res 37: 4669–4671

McGuire WL, Dressler LG (1985) Emerging impact of flow cytometry in predicting recurrence and survival in breast cancer patients. J Natl Cancer Inst 75: 405–410

McGuire WL, Meyer JS, Barlogie B, Kute TE (1985) Impact of flow cytometry on predicting recurrence and survival in breast cancer patients. Breast Cancer Res Treat 5: 117–128

Meyer JS (1986) Cell kinetics in selection and stratification of patients for adjuvant therapy of breast carcinoma, NCI Monogr 1: 25–28

Silvestrini R, Daidone MG, De Fronzo G, Morabito A, Valagussa P, Bonadonna G (1986) Prognostic implication of labeling index versus estrogen receptors and tumor size in node-negative breast cancer. Breast Cancer Res Treat 7: 161–169

Slamon DJ, Clark GM, Wong SG, Levin WJ, Ullrich A, McGuire WL (1987) Amplification of the HER-2/*neu* oncogene correlates with relapse and survival in human breast cancer. Science 235: 177–182

Tubiana M, Pejovic MH, Chavaudra N, Contesso G, Malaise EP (1984) The long-term prognostic significance of the thymidine labelling index in breast cancer. Int J Cancer 33: 441–445

Adjuvant Chemotherapy for Node-Negative Breast Cancer Patients*

G. Bonadonna, M. Zambetti, and P. Valagussa

Istituto Nazionale Tumori, Via Venezian, 1, 20133 Milano, Italy

Introduction

Recent results have confirmed that adjuvant systemic therapies increase the relapse-free survival (RFS) and overall survival (OS) of patients with resectable
breast cancer (Bonadonna and Valagussa 1988; Early Breast Cancer Trialists Collaborative Group 1988). Most of the available adjuvant results at 5 or more years
are based on prospective trials designed for node-positive (N+) patients. For
many years, the reluctance of research physicians to mount adjuvant trials on
node-negative (N−) women was due to the uncertainty about reproducible prognostic variables upon which patient selection could be based. In fact, it should
first be recalled that 15%–20% of all N− patients relapse during the first 5 years
after local-regional therapy, while in the subsequent 5 years another 5–10% relapse. Therefore, the number of analyzable events are indeed few, unless specific
criteria for selection of patients with a high risk of early relapse are utilized.

   In this brief review, we will summarize the essential results reported in the medical literature with adjuvant chemotherapy in N− women treated within the context of prospective randomized trials with local-regional therapy (surgery with or
without radiotherapy) alone as a control group.

Treatment Results

Table 1 provides a synopsis of published results with adjuvant single agent and
combination chemotherapy. It should be stressed that patient selection, i.e., primary local-regional therapy and in particular the extent of axillary node dissection, as well as duration and intensity of drug treatment, differ considerably from
series to series. No consistent RFS and OS advantage was detectable in the first
five trials listed in the table. In contrast, the last three trials have shown significant

* Supported in part by Contract NO1-CM-07338 with the Division of Cancer Treatment,
National Cancer Institute, National Institutes of Health.

Table 1. Synopsis of published results in N− breast cancer

Research Group	Patients (*n*)	Follow-up (years)	Trial design	RFS (%)
NSABP (Fisher et al. 1987)	382	10	Placebo vs short course perioperative thiotepa	76 vs 73
Scandinavian (Nissen-Meyer et al. 1987)	609	20	Control vs short course perioperative cyclo-phosphamide	55 vs 63
Osako (Senn et al. 1987)	123	10	Control vs LMF + BCG × 6	62 vs 68
Midlands (Morrison et al. 1987)	543	5	Control vs LMF × 8	74 vs 75
Mainz (Caffier et al. 1984)	175	5	Radiotherapy vs CMF × 12	72 vs 82
Wien (Jakesz et al. 1987)	128	6	Control vs CMFVP ± immunostimulants × 4→2→2 cycles	77 vs 84
Cardiff (Williams et al. 1987)	52[a]	3	Control vs AVC × 6	71 vs 83
Milan (present series)	90[a]	5	Control vs iv CMF × 12	45 vs 87

[a] Receptor-negative tumors.

L, Leukeran (chlorambucil); M, methotrexate; F, fluorouracil; C, cyclophosphamide; V, vinblastine; A, Adriamycin; BCG, bacillus Calmette-Guérin.

benefit from adjuvant combination chemotherapy. In particular, the Vienna group (Jakesz et al. 1987) reported a significant OS advantage in the absence of significant RFS differences following combination chemotherapy (with or without immunostimulants) administered for 3 years. The Cardiff group (Williams et al. 1987) reported a significant RFS difference in favor of the chemotherapy treatment group in a subset of 52 N− women selected on the basis of receptor-negative tumors.

In December 1980, the Milan Cancer Institute started a prospective randomized trial for N− and estrogen-receptor-negative (ER−) tumors. The criteria for patient selection were based on prior findings indicating the unfavorable prognosis of N− women whose ER were negative (Crowe et al. 1982; Valagussa et al. 1984). Within 1 month of local-regional therapy, patients were randomly allocated to receive no further therapy or intravenous cyclophosphamide, methotrexate, and fluorouracil (CMF) for a total of 12 courses. The doses of i.v. CMF were as follows: C and F, 600 mg/m^2 and M, 40 mg/m^2. Adjuvant treatment was delivered as much as possible at full-dose regimen, and in the presence of myelosuppression on day 21, the dose of CMF was delayed for 7–14 days rather than reduced by 50%. Four of 45 women allocated to receive CMF refused to continue adjuvant therapy after the first treatment cycle.

Table 2 summarizes the comparative treatment results. The actuarial 5-year RFS for the entire series of 90 women was 45% for the control group versus 87% for the treatment group ($P < 0.001$). OS was 65% versus 90%, respectively ($P = 0.02$). There were no remarkable differences between pre- and postmenopausal patients.

Table 2. Milan adjuvant trial in N− breast cancer

	Total patients (n)	Failures (n)	Deaths (n)
Control group	45	21	12
Premenopausal	27	12	7
Postmenopausal	18	9	5
CMF group	45	4	3
Premenopausal	27	2	2
Postmenopausal	18	2	1

Many relapsing women presented new disease manifestations in viscera (11 of 25, or 44%) and, despite prompt institution of salvage therapies, 15 patients died from progressive disease within 1 year of relapse (range, 4–19 months).

Discussion

At present, there is no standard adjuvant systemic treatment for N− breast cancer. For this reason, clinical and biological research in this patient subset should continue. However, certain prognostic findings are gradually being confirmed, and they are expected to improve patient selection for appropriate adjuvant trials as well as for treatment of high-risk patients.

First of all, clinicians should be confident that they are really dealing with a N− tumor. Full axillary lymph node dissection and a thorough histopathologic examination of the axillary content should be carried out (Fisher et al. 1981), as adjuvant treatment based on surgical sampling of the axilla will only provide misleading results. The recent results published by Mansi et al. (1987) also suggest that occult bone marrow metastases can be identified by immune-cytochemical methods.

ER status has been firmly established to be a good prognostic indicator for early recurrence and survival in resectable breast cancer (McGuire 1987). Furthermore, our own findings reported in this paper confirm that ER-negative tumors are associated with poor prognosis when treated only with a local-regional modality. The concomitance of both ER and progesterone receptor (PR) negativity will probably make possible the more accurate selection of very high-risk patients.

In recent years, the value of histologic grade as an indicator of outcome following adjuvant therapy has been reported by a number of investigators (Fisher et al. 1983; Davis et al. 1986; Contesso et al. 1987). Despite considerable differences in the classification of histologic grade, all authors agree that the RFS and OS rates were significantly influenced by tumor grade, and patients with highly undifferentiated tumors were those exhibiting the most favorable response to adjuvant chemotherapy, including postmenopausal women (Fisher et al. 1987). Since ER and PR are markers to tumor differentiation, their influence on outcome has recently been evaluated by the NSABP Group (Fisher et al. 1986) along with nuclear grade. The retrospective study clearly indicated that ER, PR, and nuclear grade have independent influences on outcome and that a more accurate assessment of outcome was obtained when more than one marker was employed.

More recent studies have taken tumor cell proliferative activity and ploidy into consideration. At least four separate studies (Meyer 1986; Silvestrini et al. 1986; Tubiana et al. 1984; Hery et al. 1987) have shown that the higher the proliferative rate of a tumor, as measured by the thymidine labeling index (LI), the higher the risk of a breast cancer recurrence. In particular, the studies of Silvestrini et al. (1986) and of Hery et al. (1987) have provided independent confirmation that LI is the best prognostic factor for N− breast cancer. A higher frequency of grade III tumors was also noted in patients with an LI above the median value. Flow cytometric methods on frozen pulverized breast tumors were utilized particularly by the San Antonio group (McGuire 1987; Merkel et al. 1987) to measure the proliferative rate as the percentage of cells in S-phase and also to determine ploidy. Receptor-negative tumors were found to be more often aneuploid and to have a high median S-phase than receptor-positive tumors. Furthermore, in N− women preliminary findings indicated that the percentage of both S-phase and ploidy were significant prognostic factors for early relapse.

In conclusion, several prognostic indicators are now available to identify N− patients as a high risk for relapse. Since we do not at present know the precise combination of the indicators that could be used in a clinical setting, information should be obtained on as many markers as possible. It is quite possible, in fact, that a more accurate assessment of outcome will be obtained when more than one marker is employed.

References

Bonadonna G, Valagussa P (1988) The contribution of medicine to the primary treatment of breast cancer. Cancer Res 48: 2314–2324

Caffier H, Rotte K, Haeggqwist O (1984) Adjuvant chemotherapy versus postoperative irradiation in node negative breast cancer. In: Jones SE, Salmon SE (eds) Adjuvant therapy of cancer, vol 4. Grune and Stratton, Orlando, FL, pp 417–424

Contesso G, Mouriesse H, Friedman S, Genin J, Sarrazin D, Rouessé J (1987) The importance of histologic grade in long-term prognosis of breast cancer. A study of 1010 patients, uniformly treated, at the Institute Gustave Roussy. J Clin Oncol 5: 1378–1386

Crowe JP, Hubay CA, Pearson OH, Marshall JS, Rosenblatt J, Mansour EG, Hermann RE, Jones JC, Flynn WJ, McGuire WL, and Participating Investigators (1982) Estrogen receptor status as a prognostic indication for stage I breast cancer patients. Breast Cancer Res Treat 2: 171–176

Davis BW, Gelber RD, Goldhirsh A, Hartmann WH, Locher GW, Reed R, Golauh R, Save-Soderbergh J, Holloway L, Russel I, Rudenstam CM, for the Ludwig Breast Cancer Study Group (1986) Prognostic significance of tumor grade in clinical trials of adjuvant therapy for breast cancer with axillary lymph node metastasis. Cancer 58: 2662–2670

Early Breast Cancer Trialists Collaborative Group (1988) The effects of adjuvant tamoxifen and of cytotoxic therapy on mortality in early breast cancer: an overview of 61 randomized trials among 28,896 women. N Engl J Med 319: 1681–1692

Fisher B, Wolmark N, Bauer M, Redmond C, Gebhardt M (1981) The accuracy of clinical nodal staging and of limited axillary dissection as a determinant of histologic nodal status in carcinoma of the breast. Surg Gynecol Obstet 152: 765–772

Fisher ER, Redmon C, Fisher B, and participating NSABP Investigators (1983) Pathologic findings from the National Surgical Adjuvant Breast Project. VIII. Relationship of chemotherapeutic responsiveness to tumor differentiation. Cancer 51: 181–191

Fisher B, Fisher ER, Redmond C, Brown A, and Contributing NSABP Investigators (1986) Tumor nuclear grade, estrogen and progesterone receptors: their value alone or in combination as indicators of outcome following adjuvant therapy for breast cancer. Breast Cancer Res Treat 7: 147–160

Fisher B, Redmond CK, Wolmark N, and NSABP Investigators (1987) Long term results from NSABP trials of adjuvant therapy for breast cancer. In: Salmon SE (ed) Adjuvant therapy of cancer, vol 5. Grune and Stratton, Orlando, pp 283–295

Hery M, Gioanni J, Lelanne CM, Namer M, Courdi A (1987) The DNA labelling index: a prognostic factor in node-negative breast cancer. Breast Cancer Res Treat 9: 207–211

Jackez R, Kolb R, Reiner G, Schemper M, Rainer H, Dittrich C, Reiner A (1987) Adjuvant chemotherapy in node-negative breast cancer patients. In: Salmon SE (ed) Adjuvant therapy of cancer, vol 5. Grune and Stratton, Orlando, pp 223–231

Mansi JL, Berger U, Easton D, McDonnell T, Redding WH, Gazet JC, McKinna A, Powles TJ, Coombes RC (1987) Micrometastases in bone marrow in patients with primary breast cancer: evaluation as an early predictor of bone metastases. Br Med J 295: 1093–1096

McGuire WL (1987) Prognostic factors for recurrence and survival in human breast cancer. Breast Cancer Res Treat 10: 5–9

Merkel DE, Dressler LG, McGuire WL (1987) Flow cytometry, cellular DNA content, and prognosis in human malignancy. J Clin Oncol 5: 1690–1703

Meyer JS (1986) Cell kinetics in selection and stratification of patients for adjuvant therapy of breast carcinoma. NCI Monogr 1: 25–28

Morrison JM, Howell A, Grieve RJ, Monnypenny IJ, Walker R, Kelly KA, Waterhouse JA (1987) The West Midlands Oncology Association Trials of adjuvant chemotherapy for operable breast cancer. In: Salmon SE (ed) Adjuvant therapy of cancer, vol 5. Grune and Stratton, Orlando, pp 311–318

Nissen-Meyer R, Host H, Kjellgren K, Mansson B, Norin T (1987) Neoadjuvant chemotherapy in breast cancer: as single perioperative treatment and with supplementary long-term chemotherapy. In: Salmon SE (ed) Adjuvant therapy of cancer, vol 5. Grune and Stratton, Orlando, pp 253–261

Senn HJ, Barett-Mahler R, for the OSAKO and SAKK Groups (1987) Update of Swiss adjuvant trials with LMF and CMF in operable breast cancer. In: Salmon SE (ed) Adjuvant therapy of cancer, vol 5. Grune and Stratton, Orlando, pp 243–252

Silvestrini R, Daidone MG, Di Fronzo G, Morabito A, Valagussa P, Bonadonna G (1986) Prognostic implication of labeling index versus estrogen receptors and tumor size in node-negative breast cancer. Breast Cancer Res Treat 7: 161–169

Tubiana M, Pejovic MH, Chavaudra N, Contesso G, Malaise EP (1984) The long-term prognostic significance of the thymidine labelling index in breast cancer. Int J Cancer 33: 441–445

Valagussa P, Bignami P, Buzzoni R, Di Fronzo G, Andreola S, Rilke F, Bonadonna G, Veronesi U (1984) Are estrogen receptors alone a reliable prognostic factor in node negative breast cancer? In: Jones SE, Salmon SE (eds) Adjuvant therapy of cancer, vol 4. Grune and Stratton, Orlando, pp 407–415

Williams CJ, Buchanan RB, Hall V, Taylor I, Cooke T, Nicholson R, Griffiths K (1987) Adjuvant chemotherapy for T1-2, N0, M0 estrogen receptor negative breast cancer: preliminary results of a randomized trial. In: Salmon SE (ed) Adjuvant therapy of cancer, vol 5. Grune and Stratton, Orlando, pp 233–241

Significant Survival Benefit of Node-Negative Breast Cancer Patients Treated with Adjuvant Chemotherapy: Seven-year Results

R. Jakesz, G. Reiner, M. Schemper, A. Reiner, G. Blijham, H. Rainer, D. Dittrich, J. Spona, B. Schutte, M. Reynders, C. van Assche, and T. Waldhör

Abteilung für Chirurgie, Gynäkologie, Chemotherapie und Pathologie, Universität Wien, Alser Straße 4, 1090 Wien, Austria

There is general agreement about a significant beneficial effect of adjuvant chemotherapy in premenopausal node-positive breast cancer patients. However, there is confusion about the efficacy of adjuvant treatment modalities in node-negative patients. The obvious good prognosis in this stage has led to a less rigorous and systematic investigation in this patient group compared with patients with poor prognosis. Perioperative cyclophosphamide is the only treatment so far adequately tested that has demonstrated a long-term benefit in relapse-free (RFS) and overall survival (OS) for treated patients (Nissen-Meyer et al. 1987). Results from the OSAKO trial (Senn et al. 1986) showed an increase in the OS in patients treated with chemotheraopy for up to 8 years. However, after a longer observation period, this survival benefit was not longer present. Several other trials report after a short follow-up a significant increase in the survival of node-negative patients (Bonadonna et al. 1987; Dalton et al. 1987). A major difficulty might be the fact that the pool of node-negative patients has turned out to be heterogeneous. Several prognostic risk factors among node-negative patients have been shown to influence the OS significantly. Among these factors are tumor stage, hormone receptor level, tumor grading and DNA ploidy.

In this report, we present the 7-year OS data of 128 node-negative breast cancer patients followed for 7–11 years. We randomized patients between a 3-year chemotherapy protocol and an untreated control. We found a significant improvement in survival for patients treated with chemotherapy. Furthermore, we investigated the prognostic influence of several factors and found that only the estrogen receptor (ER) content was significantly associated with OS.

Patients and Methods

All patients with operable breast cancer who had had either quadrantectomy plus axillary dissection or modified radical mastectomy performed at our institution between 1977 and 1982 and who in the final pathological report had no evidence of axillary lymph node metastases were eligible for this trial. Exclusion criteria included patients over 70; those with distant metastases, previous malignant disease, and bilateral or inflammatory breast carcinoma; patients lactating or pregnant; and those with serious emotional or additional medical problems. Patients were randomly allocated for surgical treatment in pathological T1, T2, N0 to quadrantectomy plus axillary dissection or to modified radical mastectomy. No radiotherapy was given to any patient postoperatively. Although it was intended to determine histologic tumor grade and ER and progesterone (PR) receptor levels, this was not a prerequisite for inclusion in this study. Stratification criteria were by tumor stage (T1, T2) and menopausal status. The histologic grade was determined by the method of Bloom and Richardson (1957). ER and PR were measured with the dextran-coated charcoal method, with a cut-off of 10 fmol/mg cytosol protein.

Flow cytometric determination of DNA ploidy levels were performed in nuclei isolated from paraffin-embedded tissue by a method previously described (Schutte et al. 1985). DNA content was measured by the method of Vindelov et al. (1983). A tumor with a single G1 peak was considered to be diploid, whereas evidence of an additional G1 peak indicated the presence of aneuploidy. The DNA index was calculated as the ratio of the G1 peak with the highest DNA content to the G1 peak with the lowest DNA content.

The proliferative activity was calculated by counting the number of cells between the inclination points of the descending G1 peak and the ascending G2-M peak. Histograms with coefficients of variations of less than 8% were considered to be of good quality.

Method of Randomization

Randomization was by telephone to a central office using the method of Pocock and Simon (1975). No patient once randomized was subsequently withdrawn.

Treatment

Patients were randomized in three groups:

1. Untreated surgical control
2. Chemotherapy consisting of cyclophosphamide (100 mg daily for 10 days orally), and on days 1 and 7 i.v. 5-fluorouracil (750 mg), vinblastine (5 mg), and methotrexate (25 mg). Four cycles were administered in the 1st year and two cycles in the 2nd and 3rd years
3. Chemoimmunotherapy included an additional administration of azimexon, an unspecific immunostimulant

Follow-up

All patients were regularly followed at 3-monthly intervals for the first 3 years, 6-monthly for 2 more years, and then annually. No patient was lost during follow-up. Blood chemistry included a liver function test, and a chest X-ray was performed every 6 months. Additional investigations were done if indicated by the clinical course. Recurrent disease was proven histologically whenever possible. Local recurrences were verified by local excision, other recurrences by radiologic means.

Statistical Analysis

Probabilities of survival for a given time period are described by survival functions estimated by Kaplan and Meier (1957). Calculations of the significance of observed differences were made using the log-rank test (Mantel-Cox) and the generalized Wilcoxon test (Breslow). Since survival data of patients treated with chemo- and chemoimmunotherapy showed identical behavior, we pooled these two groups and compared them with the untreated control group.

Results

Over a 4-year accrual period, 128 patients entered this trial. A total of 32 patients were treated surgically with quadrantectomy plus axillary dissection. In 96 patients, a modified radical mastectomy was performed. Table 1 demonstrates the characteristics of all accrued patients. Patient distribution with respect to ER, PR, tumor grade, and tumor ploidy shows the expected percentages of literature reports. To evaluate the relations between tumor characteristics, we performed correlations between tumor ploidy and tumor proliferation on the one hand and

Table 1. Patient characteristics of 128 node-negative breast cancer patients

	n	(%)
Control	46	36
Chemotherapy	82	63
T1	52	41
T2	76	59
Premenopausal	50	40
Postmenopausal	78	60
ER+	59	62
ER−	36	38
PR+	39	41
PR−	56	59
Grade I + II	84	76
Grade III	27	24
Diploid	38	38
Aneuploid	62	62
Slow proliferation (percentage S phase ≤ 13)	48	69
Fast proliferation (percentage S phase < 13)	22	31

Table 2. Relation between tumor ploidy, proliferation rate, and ER, PR, and tumor grading in 100 node-negative breast cancer patients

	χ^2 (P value)
Tumor ploidy	
ER status	0.56
PR status	0.13
Grading	0.03
Proliferation rate	
ER status	0.16
PR status	0.07
Grading	0.006

Table 3. Prognostic factors in node-negative breast cancer patients as derived from Kaplan-Meier plots

	P value	
	Breslow	Mantel-Cox
T1 vs T2	0.130	0.086
Pre- vs postmenopausal	0.830	0.960
ER+ vs ER−	0.0045	0.0025
PR+ vs PR−	0.077	0.070
Grade I+II vs III	0.097	0.192
Diploid vs aneuploid	0.467	0.594
Slow vs fast proliferation	0.951	0.802

ER and PR status and grading on the other. Tumor ploidy and tumor proliferation correlated significantly with tumor grading, but not with ER and PR status (Table 2).

We then evaluated the influence of several risk factors on the OS of patients derived from Kaplan-Meier plots (Table 3). We investigated tumor stage, menopausal stage, hormone receptor levels, tumor differentiation, tumor ploidy, and tumor proliferation. We found that only the ER status correlated significantly with OS ($P<0.005$). The survival rate of patients with ER-negative tumors was only 57%, compared with 93% of patients with ER-positive tumors. No other investigated factor influenced the OS significantly. Interestingly, tumor ploidy and tumor proliferation did not show any impact on OS.

Figure 1 shows the survival curves of patients treated with chemotherapy and the surgical control. Postoperative chemotherapy significantly improved the survival of patients compared with the untreated control. The survival rate of the untreated control patients at 7 years was 74%, compared with 90% of patients treated with chemotherapy ($P<0.01$; Breslow).

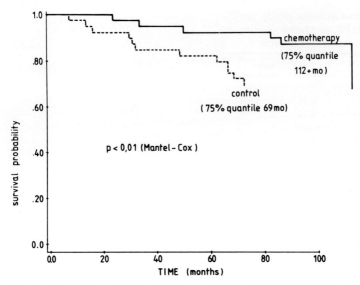

Fig. 1. Comparison of 46 surgical controls *(dashed line)* with OS of 82 node-negative patients treated with CMFV *(solid line)*

Discussion

Our 7-year results confirm earlier findings that long-term postoperative chemotherapy significantly improved the OS of node-negative patients. This result is in agreement with several reports in the literature dealing with this patient group (Bonadonna et al. 1987; Dalton et al. 1987). Although the number of accrued patients in our trial is relatively small in size, it should be especially noted that the 5-year survival rate of our control group (88%) is nearly identical with the data of the Natural History Data Base (86%) of the Arizona Group representing data from roughly 1000 patients (Dalton et al. 1987).

However, it has to be mentioned that not all node-negative breast cancer patients require some sort of postoperative chemotherapy. Roughly three out of four patients with stage I disease will remain disease free without any systemic treatment. Therefore, the definition of prognostic factors in stage I disease seems to be especially important. Our data show that the ER status of the primary tumor represents the only factor significantly influencing OS. Patients with ER-negative tumors exhibit a threefold increase in the 7-year death rate (25% vs. 7%). Especially patients with ER-negative tumors seem to respond more favorably to adjuvant chemotherapy (Jakesz et al. 1988). Interestingly, several other strong prognostic factors in stage II breast cancer patients (Reiner et al. 1987) do not show a significant influence on the OS of node-negative patients (grading, PR, ploidy).

We conclude from our trial that postoperative adjuvant chemotherapy represents an important tool in prolonging survival of node-negative patients. Furthermore, the ER status in this patient group has proved to be an important prognostic parameter. It should be recommended that only ER-negative stage I breast cancer patients should be included in adjuvant chemotherapy protocols.

References

Bloom HJG, Richardson WW (1957) Histological grading and prognosis in breast cancer. Br J Cancer 11: 359–377

Bonadonna G, Valagussa P, Zambetti M et al. (1987) Milan adjuvant trials for stage I–II breast cancer. In: Salmon SE (ed) Adjuvant therapy of cancer, vol 5. Grune and Stratton, Orlando, pp 211–221

Dalton WS, Brooks RJ, Jones SE et al. (1987) Breast cancer adjuvant therapy trials at the Arizona Cancer Center using adriamycin and cyclophosphamide. In: Salmon SE (ed) Adjuvant therapy of cancer, vol 5. Grune and Stratton, Orlando, pp 263–269

Jakesz R, Kolb R, Reiner G et al. (1988) The effect of chemo-(immuno)-therapy in breast cancer seems to be dependent on estrogen receptor status. In press

Kaplan EL, Meier P (1958) Nonparametric estimation from incomplete observation. J Am Stat Assoc 53: 457–481

Nissen-Meyer R, Host H, Kjellgren K, Mansson B, Norin T (1987) Neoadjuvant chemotherapy in breast cancer: as single perioperative treatment and with supplementary long-term chemotherapy. In: Salmon SE (ed) Adjuvant therapy of cancer, vol 5. Grune and Stratton, Orlando, pp 253–261

Pocock StJ, Simon R (1975) Sequential treatment assignment with balancing for prognostic factors in the controlled clinical trial. Biometrics 31: 103–115

Reiner A, Kolb R, Reiner G et al. (1987) Prognostic significance of steroid hormone receptors and histopathological characterization of human breast cancer. J Cancer Res Clin Oncol 113: 285–290

Schütte B, Reynders MMJ, Bosman FTG, Blijham GH (1985) Flow cytometric determination of DNA ploidy level in nuclei isolated from paraffin embedded tissue. Cytometry 6: 26–30

Senn HJ, Jungi WF, Amgwerd R et al. (1986) Swiss adjuvant trial (OSAKO 06/74) with chlorambucil, methotrexate, and 5-fluorouracil plus BCG in node-negative breast cancer patients: nine-year results. NCI Monogr 1: 129–134

Vindelov LL, Christensen IJ, Nissen NI (1983) A detergent trypsin method for the preparation of neuclei for flow cytometric DNA analysis. Cytometry 3: 323–327

Adjuvant Immunotherapy in Node-Negative Patients: Results of a Scandinavian Study

R. Nissen-Meyer, H. Høst, and K. Kjellgren

Tyribakken 10, 0280 Oslo 2, Norway

Introduction

The Scandinavian Adjuvant Chemotherapy Study group (SACS) demonstrated in its first study (initiated January 1965) a significant benefit from a short perioperative cyclophosphamide course, with clinically insignificant side effects (Nissen-Meyer et al. 1982). In our second study, a similar short perioperative course was therefore given to all patients, but the monodrug course was replaced by a multi-drug course, in accordance with the general development of cancer chemotherapy.

The second study was designed to serve two purposes:

1. To compare the single, short perioperative chemotherapy course with the same course and continued chemotherapy for 12 months (SACS-2A). Owing to the expected side effects of the long-term chemotherapy, this part of the study was restricted to node-positive patients. Preliminary reports have been published (Nissen-Meyer et al. 1987).
2. To study the effect of a local injection of *Corynebacterium parvum* (SACS-2B), the results of which are reported here.

Material and Methods

The hospitals and principal investigators participating in study 2 are listed in Table 1.

The case material comprises 1094 routine, operable primary breast cancer cases, treated in routine surgical clinics. The intake period was from March 1977 to November 1985. After a modified radical mastectomy, all patients received cyclophosphamide 500 mg, vincristine 1 mg, and 5-FU 750 mg on day 0, and cyclophosphamide 500 mg, vincristine 1 mg, and methotrexate 50 mg on day 7. These were the doses for a patient of 70 kg or more, and were adjusted in patients of lower weight. All drugs were given intravenously. After stratification into node-positive and node-negative cases, the patients were randomized by the sealed envelope method.

Recent Results in Cancer Research, Vol. 115
© Springer-Verlag Berlin · Heidelberg 1989

Table 1. Hospitals and principal investigators in SACS-2

In Norway	
Central Hospital Akershus:	T. Brøyn, N. Helsingen, F. W. Vaagenes
Central Hospital Bodø:	R. Aune, R. Capoferro, S. M. Sivertsen
Aker Hospital, Oslo:	S. Hagen, T. Harbitz, H. O. Myhre,
	R. Nissen-Meyer (coordinator)
Norwegian Radium Hospital, Oslo:	I. O. Brennhovd[a], S. Gundersen, H. Høst,
	O. G. Jørgensen, S. Kvaløy
In Sweden	
Central Hospital Borås:	S. Ahlström, C.-A. Ekman, B. Månsson[a]
Central Hospital Kalmar:	B. Pallin
Central Hospital Norrköping:	H. O. Ahnlund, K. Kjellgren, R. Peterhoff
Municipal Hospital, Västervik:	K. Wiegener

[a] Deceased.

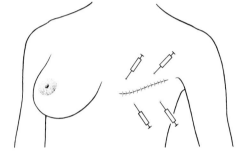

Fig. 1. The immunotherapy schedule: SACS 2 b: *Corynebacterium parvum* 70 µg subcutaneuosly in each of the 4 quadrants about 2 weeks after mastectomy

The 746 node-negative patients were randomized to immunotherapy (386 cases) or control (360 cases). The 348 node-positive patients were randomized according to a 2×2 factorial design to immunotherapy (82 cases), intravenous cyclophosphamide, methotrexate, 5-fluorouracil (CMF) for 12 months (90 cases), a combination of immunotherapy and CMF (106 cases), or control (70 cases). When preparing the sealed envelopes, the groups with CMF were deliberately made larger than the others in order to secure an earlier evaluation of the side effects of our intravenous CMF schedule.

The immunotherapy was given about 2 weeks after mastectomy with *Corynebacterium parvum* 70 µg (0.1 ml of a standard suspension diluted 10 times), injected subcutaneously in each of the four quadrants around the tumor site, as indicated in Fig. 1.

The relapse-free survival curves (RFS, or event-free) and their standard errors were constructed according to Cutler and Ederer (1958). As events, we have included local recurrences, distant metastases, new primary tumors in the opposite breast, or death from a nonrelated cause (we will differentiate among these various events in a later report, after we have achieved longer follow-up times and more events have been registered). The computer based log-rank method with a X^2 test was also used.

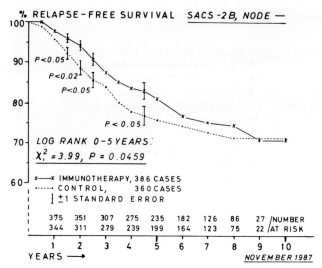

Fig. 2. Results in the node-negative patients

Results

Node-Negative Cases

We found a significant effect from the immunotherapy, with events being delayed (Fig. 2). The largest difference between the RFS curves was 6.1%, observed 4.5 years after mastectomy. Later, the differences were reduced, and after 9 years the curves overlapped. With the method of Cutler and Ederer (1958), the difference after 2 years had a P value of <0.02. The logrank test for the period from 0 to 5 years had a value of $\chi_1^2 = 3.99$, which gives a P value of <0.05.

Node-Positive Cases

Owing to the side effects from long-term chemotherapy, the clinicians soon became reluctant to enter node-positive patients in the trial. The four randomization groups are therefore small, and a separate analysis of them presently seems unreliable.

For a main effects analysis of the immunotherapy, we have combined the two groups with and the two groups without immunotherapy (Table 2). In this way, we had two groups with 188 and 160 cases respectively. Of the patients in these two groups, 56.4% and 56.3% also received long-term CMF treatment. Postoperative irradiation of the scar region and the regional lymph nodes was given to 41.0% and 35.6% respectively.

The number of events was higher in the immunotherapy groups than in the control groups (53.2% versus 46.9%), but the difference was not significant.

Table 2. Main effects analysis of immunotherapy in 348 node-positive patients

Randomization

Immunotherapy   Immunotherapy   CMF   Control
                          CMF +

	Immunotherapy CMF + / CMF	
Number of patients	188	160
Events	53.2%	46.9%
CMF 12 months	56.4%	56.3%
Local irradiation	41.0%	35.6%
CMF and/or irradiation	75.0%	73.1%

Side Effects

Side effects from the immunotherapy were not observed.

Discussion

The simple type of local immunotherapy which we tried had a delaying effect on the growth of breast cancer tissue in node-negative patients. The effect observed was modest, but statistically significant, and without side effects. The number of cases and the observation time were sufficient, and there were no obvious methodological problems in this part of the trial.

The positive results in the node-negative cases are not really contradicted by the negative results in the node-positive cases, for several reasons. The node-positive groups were small, and coincidental variations may have played a major role in the results observed. In particular, the control group of only 70 cases showed an unexpected and unrealistically good result, with few events during the observation time.

There is reason to believe that the ability of the immune system to cope with tumor cells is dependent on the tumor burden. Lymphokines are released from activated lymphocytes in response to stimulating antigens, and these may be unspecific. One of the lymphokines is interleukin-2, a growth factor for activated T cells which activates cytotoxic lymphocytes and may produce lymphokine-activated killer cells (LAK). The best clinical results in advanced metastatic cancer have been obtained by removing lymphocytes from the patient, activating them in culture with interleukin-2 (produced in large amounts by genetic engineering), and readministering them to the patient in conjunction with the administration of large doses of interleukin-2 (Durant 1987; Rosenberg et al. 1987). Large doses of interleukin-2 alone may also have some effect in advanced cancer (West et al. 1987). These procedures, however, are associated with serious complications and side effects. The hope is that an unspecific stimulation of the natural reactions leading to the production of tumor killing factors may be sufficient in cases with the smallest tumor burden, e.g., node-negative cases after removal of the primary tumor.

There are also reasons to believe that both long-term chemotherapy and irradiation of the injection sites and the regional lymph nodes will reduce the possibility that *Corynebacterium parvum* may stimulate the production of LAK (Dinarello and Mier 1987). In the immunotherapy groups of our node-positive patients, 75% had long-term CMF and/or local irradiation.

Conclusion

We find recommending our treatment schedule for routine use not reasonable now. However, our observations support the concept that immunologic factors do play a role in the growth of breast cancer metastases, and that it is possible to improve the immunologic defenses by very simple means. They suggest that immunotherapy may become clinically important in the future and should stimulate further investigations along these lines in the search for a more effective, but tolerable, immunotherapy schedule.

References

Cutler SJ, Ederer F (1958) Maximum utilization of the life table method in analyzing survival. J Chronic Dis 8: 699–712
Dinarello CA, Mier JW (1987) Lymphokines. N Engl J Med 317: 940–945
Durant JR (1987) Immunotherapy of cancer: The end of the beginning? N Engl J Med 316: 939–941
Nissen-Meyer R, Kjellgren K, Månsson B (1982) Adjuvant chemotherapy in breast cancer. In: Mathé G, Bonadonna G, Salmon S (eds) Adjuvant therapies of cancer. Springer Berlin Heidelberg New York Tokyo, pp 142–148 (Recent results in cancer research vol 80)
Nissen-Meyer R, Høst H, Kjellgren K, Månsson B, Norin T (1987) Neoadjuvant chemotherapy in breast cancer: As single perioperative treatment and with supplementary long-term chemotherapy. In: Salmon SE (ed) Adjuvant therapy of cancer, vol 5. Grune and Stratton, New York, pp 253–261
Rosenberg SA, Lotze MT, Muul LM, Chang AE, Avis FP, Leitman S, Linehan WM, Robertson CN, Lee RE, Rubin JT, Seipp CA, Simpson CG, White DE (1987) A progress report on the treatment of 157 patients with advanced cancer using lymphokine-activated killer cells and interleukin-2 or high-dose interleukin-2 alone. N Engl J Med 316: 881–897
West WH, Tauer KW, Yanelli JR, Marshall GD, Orr DW, Thurman GB, Oldham RK (1987) Constant-infusion recombinant interleukin-2 in adoptive immunotherapy of advanced cancer. N Engl J Med 316: 898–905

Breast-Conserving Surgery and the Role of Adjuvant Radiotherapy: A Review

A. Wallgren

Department of Oncology, Sahlgrenska Hospital, Gothenburg, Sweden

As a reaction against radical mastectomy, breast conservation in the treatment of breast cancer has rapidly gained popularity, both among the lay public and among members of the medical profession. Breast conservation is neither a new type of treatment nor will it abolish the psychosocial trauma of breast cancer. Still, there are many reasons to believe that it will continue to constitute an alternative to mastectomy in the treatment of this disease.

The title of this contribution – the role of radiotherapy – might imply that radiotherapy should be considered as a fixed and unchangeable treatment modality. It is obvious, however, that the amount and extent of radiotherapy, as well as the resultant effects, are variable. The same is, of course, true for surgery.

Objectives of Local Treatment

The Halstedian concept of the continuous spread of breast cancer was the rationale for extensive radical and mutilating surgery. The changing concept that early dissemination determines the outcome in breast cancer has modfied the belief in the importance of local treatment and has probably accelerated the acceptance of breast conservation. It should be recognized, however, that techniques for breast preservation in breast cancer have so far been as radical as Halstedian surgery. Radical surgery has been replaced by radical radiotherapy. The objectives of breast-conserving treatment are primarily to eradicate the malignant tumor in the breast and leave a cosmetically acceptable breast. Local treatment can cure breast cancer patients at least in the sense that death from breast cancer can be avoided if treatment is instituted early enough, a fact which studies on mammography screening have indicated (Tabar et al. 1985). This is most probably due to the local eradication of a source of future dissemination.

Can These Objectives be Achieved by Radiotherapy?

As early as 1929, Keynes reported his first 5 years of radiotherapy alone in the treatment of breast cancer. Nearly a decade later, he was able to demonstrate survival figures similar to those of breast cancer patients with the same stage of disease but treated with conventional surgery (Keynes 1937). The advantage was that with this technique the breast was preserved in most cases. Keynes implanted radium needles in the breast and in the lymph node regions of the axilla, the supraclavicular fossa, and the internal mammary area. The volume included in this treatment was thus at least as extensive as that of a surgical radical mastectomy.

There are several reports which show that even when the primary tumor is large and considered "inoperable," it is often possible to "sterilize" the tumor of the breast (Baclesse 1959; Calle 1978; Strickland 1973). Such studies have also shown that the dose of radiotherapy necessary to achieve this goal increases rapidly as the tumor increases in size. According to a retrospective study by Arriagada et al. (1985), the tumor dose was the most significant independent factor for local control, and a dose increase of 15 Gy could decrease the relative risk of local recurrence two-fold (Arriagada et al. 1985). The morbidity associated with intensive treatment of large tumors may be considerable (Strickland 1973).

The risk of late sequelae depends on the dose but also on the irradiated volume. Therefore, implantation of radioactive sources into the tumor volume may increase the dose where it is most needed and may reduce the risk of late effects in comparison with external irradiation. However, as Keynes observed in 1937, "the bulk of tissue to be irradiated did seem to be a serious obstacle," and even after high-dose radiotherapy, local regrowth is common when there is a palpable tumor.

Role of Surgery

It should be remembered that the aim of surgery in the treatment of breast cancer is the same as that of radiotherapy, i.e., the local eradication of the tumor. In addition, surgical excision of the tumor may give valuable prognostic information. Only a few patients series report breast-conserving treatment using surgery alone. Crile has reported three recurrences in 42 patients treated with a wide excision, with 3–4 cm around the primary tumor (Crile 1975). In Toronto, 154 patients were treated by excision, but without irradiation. At 5 years, the relapse rate in the breast was 24.4% in spite of the fact that in this group there was a larger proportion of patients with more "favorable disease." This is in contrast to a recurrence rate of 7.6% in the breast if it was irradiated (Clark et al. 1982). A similar frequency of recurrence in the breast has been reported in other series (e.g., Lagios et al. 1983). The most informative series of patients treated with less than mastectomy by surgery alone is the NSABP study B-06, in which one third of the patients were treated with a local excision with "tumor-free margins" and without irradiation. With this technique, approximately 70% remained free of breast tumor in the ipsilateral breast at 5 years, in contrast to about 90% of those who were also irradiated. For patients with lymph node involvement who were also given adjuvant chemotherapy, the difference was even more pronounced (64% versus 98%) (Fisher et al. 1985).

These studies, using different surgical techniques and selection of patients, indicate that many patients with limited tumors could be treated with surgery alone. There seem to be considerable differences in breast recurrence rates which can possibly be explained by differences in patients selection and surgical technique.

Role of Combined Surgery and Radiotherapy in the Conservative Treatment of Breast Cancer

Most published series on breast conservation in breast cancer concern patients who have been treated by a combination of surgery and radiotherapy. The extent of surgery ranges from excisional or incisional biopsy to extensive dissection including pectoral fascia and overlying skin. The doses of radiotherapy and the target volume also vary in these studies. As observed by Keynes (1937), the excision of the bulk of the tumor before radiotherapy increases the possibility of controlling the disease.

Bedwinek et al. (1980) found in their analyses of patients included in the radiation therapy oncology group (RTOG) a local-regional failure rate of 8.5% in 234 patients with stage I and II carcinoma of the breast and who had been followed for up to 5 years. These patients had been treated by a variety of surgical and radiologic methods in several member institutions in the USA. A clear relation between the size of tumor and failure rate was observed. Only two recurrences were found in 117 T1 tumors (tumors smaller than 2 cm). In T2 tumors (2–5 cm in diameter), such failures were more common if surgery consisted of an incisional biopsy than if an excisional biopsy of a segmental mastectomy had been performed. In the case of incisional biopsy, the frequency of relapses in the breast was related to the dose of radiation that had been delivered. If only external irradiation up to a dose of about 45–50 Gy was given, seven of 25 patients developed a breast cancer recurrence, but the rate was one in 14 if the tumor volume was further irradiated by means of an interstitial iridium implant.

In a clinical-pathologic study, Harris et al. (1983) observed that if intraductal carcinoma was found within and around the tumor and if the tumor had a high nuclear grade, the local relapse rate was considerable, especially if the irradiation dose was less than 60 Gy. This finding has not yet been confirmed by other studies. The same group also found that recurrence in the breast was more common in patients under 35 years old than in older patients (Recht et al. 1988).

Most series of patients have only reported results after a limited period of follow-up, but Kurtz and his colleagues published their results from the Cancer Institut of Marseille relating to patients who had been treated 10–20 years earlier (Kurtz et al. 1983). After limited surgery and radiotherapy, breast recurrences continued to appear during the entire period of follow-up. In T1 tumors, more than half of the recognized cancer treatment failures appeared after the first 5 years.

Is the Breast Cancer Recurrence a Second Ipsilateral Cancer or a True Recurrence?

There are obvious difficulties in determining whether the reappearance of a tumor in the breast is a true recurrence or a second primary Tumor. Most tumor reappearances seem to be recurrences, since a comparison with the contralateral breast indicated that there were 43 breast recurrences of the treated breast during 15 years in 276 treated patients in the above-mentioned series of patients in Marseille (Kurtz et al. 1983). If the number of new cancers of the other breast is considered as the maximum number of new primary tumors in the treated breast, then most of the breast events in the treated breast must be considered as "recurrences."

Sequelae of Radiotherapy

The effects of radiotherapy are related to the dose of radiation given. The target volume is also probably of importance in addition to the dosage. Harris et al. (1978) have reported a 16% incidence of minor complications such as rib fractures, pulmonary reactions, and pleural effusion and a 1% incidence of major complications. The treatment volume for these patients included not only the breast but also the regional lymph nodes and the internal mammary nodes (Harris et al. 1978). Areas of overdosage are difficult to avoid in this region. The degree of fibrosis in the breast was shown to be dose dependent (Harris et al. 1979). In a recent overview of randomized trials on radiotherapy in addition to various types of ablative surgery, excess mortality in the irradiated patients was found after 10 years of observation (Cuzick et al. 1987). An analysis of one of the series in this overview indicates that the excess mortality consisted at least in part of cardiac deaths, and the reason for this could be the dose of radiation to the heart (Høst et al. 1986).

The risk of future malignant tumors in a breast treated with doses equivalent to 50 Gy or more is not known. A new primary tumor due to radiotherapy is not discernible from a new primary tumor due to any other cause. A dose of this size is likely to reduce the volume of duct and lobular epithelium, and hence a linear extrapolation from facts derived from moderate dose irradiation probably exaggerates the risk.

The usual technique for irradiation of the breast uses two opposing tangential fields. The medial portion of the contralateral breast may be included within the tangential fields, and the remaining breast receives a small but measurable dose of radiation. It has been estimated that the mean dose of the contralateral breast may amount to 2%–3% of the target-absorbed dose, i.e., about 1.5 Gy if the target absorbed dose is 50 Gy (Landberg 1988) personal communication. Assuming a linear relationship between dose and cancer risk, this would lead to an increase of less than 1% of the spontaneous breast cancer risk (NCRP 1986). In the Milan study, after a mean follow-up of 108 months, there was a similar frequency of contralateral breast cancer whether the patient had been treated by means of radical mastectomy or quadrantectomy plus radiotherapy (Zucali et al. 1987).

Resources for Radiotherapy

The increasing number of breast cancer patients who are treated by breast-conserving surgery also increase the need for resources for radiotherapy. Our experience in Sweden is that in areas with regular mammography screening, breast-conserving treatment is administered to approximately one third of the patients with breast cancer. With a rate of approximately 500–550 cases per one million inhabitants, 0.5 treatment units per million inhabitants (CO^{60} machine of linear accelerator) will be expended on these patients.

Conclusions

Without radiotherapy, tumorectomy is complicated by a breast cancer recurrence rate of about 30% within 3 years. Radiotherapy reduces this risk of recurrence but prolongs the treatment and is associated with some morbidity. Whether careful selection of patients and a wide excision including a defined width of apparently healthy tissue outside the tumor will reduce the risk of recurrence to such an extent that radiotherapy can be avoided is the subject of ongoing trials.

References

Arriagada R, Mouriesse BS, Sarrazin D, Clark RM, Deboer G (1985) Radiotherapy alone in breast cancer. I. Analysis of tumor parameters, tumor dose and local control: The experience of the Gustave-Roussy Institute and The Princess Margaret Hospital. Int J Radiat Oncol Biol Phys 11: 1751–1757

Baclesse F (1959) Roentgenotherapy alone in the cancer of the breast. Univ Int Cancer Acta 15: 1023–1026

Bedwinek JM, Carlos AP, Kramer S, Brady L, Goodman R, Grundy G (1980) Irradiation as the primary management of Stage I and II adenocarcinoma of the breast. Cancer Clin Trials 3: 11–18

Calle R, Pilleron JP, Schlienger P, Vilcoq R (1978) Conservative management of operable breast cancer. Cancer 42: 2045–2053

Clark RM, Wilkinson RH, Lahoney LJ, Reid JG, MacDonald WD (1982) Breast cancer: A 21-year experience with conservative surgery and radiation. Int J Radiat Oncol Biol Phys 8: 967–975

Crile G (1975) Results of conservative treatment of breast cancer at ten and 15 years. Am J Surg 181: 26–30

Cuzick J, Stewart H, Peto R, Baum M, Fisher B, Host H, Lythgoe JP, Riberio G, Scheurlen H, Wallgren A (1987) Overview of randomized trials of postoperative adjuvant radiotherapy in breast cancer. Cancer Treat Rep 71: 15–29

Fisher B, Bauer M, Margolese R, Poisson R, Pilch Y, Redmond C, Risher E, Wolmark N, Deutsch M, Montague E, Saffer E, Wickerham L, Lerner H, Glass A, Shibata H, Deckers P, Ketcham A, Oishi R, Russel I (1985) Five-year results of a randomized clinical trial comparing total mastectomy and segmental mastectomy with or without radiation in the treatment of breast cancer. N Engl J Med 312: 665–673

Harris JR, Levene MB, Hellman S (1978) Results of treating stage I and II carcinoma of the breast with primary radiation therapy. Cancer Treat Rep 62: 985–991

Harris JR, Levene MB, Svensson Goran, Hellman S (1979) Analysis of cosmetic results following primary radiation therapy for stages I and II carcinoma of the breast. Int J Radiat Oncol Biol Phys 5: 257–261

Harris JR, Connolly JL, Schnitt SJ, Cohen RB, Hellman S (1983) Clinical-pathologic study of early breast cancer treated by primary radiation therapy. J Clin Oncol 1: 184–189

Høst H, Brennhovd IO, Loeb M (1986) Postoperative radiotherapy in breast cancer – long term results from the Oslo study. Int J Radiat Oncol Biol Phys 12: 727–732

Keynes G (1929) The treatment of primary carcinoma of the breast with radium. Acta Radiol 10: 393–401

Keynes G (1937) Conservative treatment of cancer of the breast. Br Med J 643–647

Kurtz JM, Spitalier J-M, Amalric R (1983) Late breast recurrence after lumpectomy and irradiation. Int J Radiat Oncol Biol Phys 9: 1191–1194

Lagios MD, Richards VE, Rose MR, Yee E (1983) Segmental mastectomy without radiotherapy. Cancer 52: 2173–2179

196   A. Wallgren

National Council on Radiation Protection (1986) Mammagraphy - A user's guide. Report on 85

Recht A, Conolly J, Schnitt SJ, Silver B, Rose MA, Love S, Harris JR (1988) The effect of young age on tumor recurrence in the treated breast after conservative surgery and radiotherapy. Radiat Oncol Biol Phys 14: 3-10

Strickland P (1973) The management of carcinoma of the breast by radical supervoltage radiation. Brit J Surg 60: 569-573

Tabar L, Gad A, Holmberg LH, Lundquist U, Fagerberg CJG, Baldetorp L, Gröntoft O, Lundström B, Månsson JC (1985) Reduction in mortality from breast cancer after mass screening with mammography. Lancet i: 829-832

Zucali R, Luini A, Del Vecchio M, Sacchini V, Sverzellati E, Stucchi C, Banfi A, Veronesi U (1987) Contralateral breast cancer after limited surgery plus radiotherapy of early mammary tumors. Eur J Surg Oncol 13: 413-417

New Trends in Breast Cancer Surgery

U. Veronesi

Istituto Nazionale per lo Studio e la Cura dei Tumori, Via Venezian 1, 20133 Milano, Italy

Introduction

There is no doubt that breast surgery had undergone a true revolution in the last 20 years and that the traditional Halsted mastectomy, which was the treatment of choice for all woman with breast cancer in the first half of this century, has been gradually replaced initially by less mutilating techniques and later by treatments designed to preserve the breast.

This evolution has been the result of different combined factors. The first is the new concepts on the natural history of breast cancer. According to the most recent views, breast cancer cells spread in the body fairly early and their growth in distant organs is conditioned by immunologic and biological factors, while the type of surgery involved in the removal of the primary carcinoma plays a limited role in the prognosis of breast cancer. The main problem in breast cancer is, therefore, the control of distant metastases.

The second factor is the change in the patient population. In fact, in recent years the characteristics of breast cancer patients have changed considerably. The introduction of mammography, improvements in the cancer education of the public, and the development of mass screening programs have greatly increased the number of patients presenting with small cancers. In most series of breast cancer cases in Western countries, the number of cases involving tumors less than 2 cm in diameter represent 30%–50% of the total, whereas only 20 years ago they accounted for only 5%–10%. Clinically occult cases and those identified only at mammography are not rare, and their number is progressively increasing, as are the noninvasive carcinomas.

A third aspect is the improved interpretation of borderline lesions: atypical hyperplasia, diffuse papillomatosis, in situ lobular carcinoma, and noninfiltrating intraductal carcinoma (all lesions that form a mixed group, requiring a treatment which must be individually designed). Moreover, infiltrating carcinoma is now better identified by the pathologist. The description of peritumoral lymphatic invasion and improved grading provide better information on the aggressiveness of the tumor. Evaluation of the presence of estrogen receptors is common, and soon the evaluation of the growth rate (labelling index and ploidy), might also become common.

Recent Results in Cancer Research, Vol. 115
© Springer-Verlag Berlin·Heidelberg 1989

Finally, an important new component is the participation of the patient in the choice of treatment. There has been an explosion on interest among women about the problem of breast cancer. This interest has generated a large number of articles in the lay press with public debates on the issues connected with breast cancer treatment. What women now ask of their surgeons is a complete description of the type of operation or radiation requested and the risks connected with conservative and ablative procedures.

The First Milan Trial

The long-term results of the first Milan trial, which started 15 years ago, have now definitely shown that the so-called QUART technique provides results equal (if not superior) to those obtained with the Halsted mastectomy.

The Milan trial was in fact the first to show that conservative treatment, if appropriate, can safely replace the Halsted mastectomy (Veronesi et al. 1981). The trial began in 1973. The new conservative treatment to be matched to the Halsted mastectomy was the QUART technique, QUART being an abbreviation of "quadrantectomy, axillary dissection, radiotherapy." The principle of the "quadrantectomy" was that, in small cancers, the "radical" removal of cancer cells from the breast can be achieved by a conservative surgical technique, which would involve excision of a good amount of normal tissue around the tumor, including the overlying skin and the underlying muscular fascia.

Radiotherapy was given to all patients treated with quadrantectomy and limited to the ipsilateral breast. The breast tissue was irradiated with a linear accelerator or with a cobalt 60 unit. The prescribed dose of 50 Gy was reached in 5 weeks. During the 6th week, a boost of 10 Gy was delivered with photons or with 10 MeV electrons.

From June 1973 to May 1980, a total of 701 patients were accrued in the trial: 349 were treated by Halsted mastectomy and 352 with QUART. From January 1976, all patients of both groups with positive nodes were treated with 12 cycles of chemotherapy with the cyclophosphamide-methotrexate-5-fluorouracil (CMF) regimen.

Fifteen years after the beginning of the trial, seven patients in the Halsted group and eight in the QUART group had had a local recurrence of the primary cancer as the first sign of failure. Moreover, in the conservative group eight more cases developed a second primary cancer in the ipsilateral breast treated with quadrantectomy and radiotherapy. The long-term results of the trial showed similar 10-year relapse-free (77.0% in the conservative treatment and 76.0% in the Halsted mastectomy group) and overall survival rates (79.0% in the first and 78.0% in the second) in the two groups of patients (Fig. 1).

Analysis of the case series according to the presence or absence of axillary node metastases showed similar 8-year survival rates in patients with negative axillary nodes (Halsted, 86%; QUART, 86%), whereas in patients with positive nodes, higher survival rates were observed in patients treated by means of QUART (82%) compared with those treated by means of Halsted mastectomy (70%) (Table 1, Fig. 2).

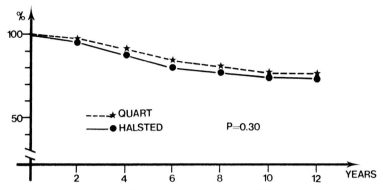

Fig. 1. Disease-free survival curves according to type of treatment, Milan Trial I

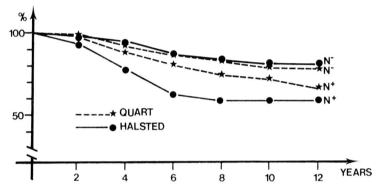

Fig. 2. Disease-free survival curves of patients treated with Halsted mastectomy and with quadrantectomy, axillary dissection, and radiotherapy (QUART) according to absence (N−) or presence (N+) of axillary node metastases. Milan Trial I

Table 1. Actuarial 8-year survival (±SE) in patients treated with Halsted or QUART

	Halsted (%)	QUART (%)
Disease-free survival	78	80
Overall survival		
All patients	83	85
Patients with negative lymph nodes	86	86
Patients with postivie lymph nodes	70	82

The conclusions drawn from the Milan trial are the following:

1. After a quadrantectomy of the breast supplemented by adequate radiotherapy, the incidence rate of local recurrence is the same as in Halsted mastectomy.
2. This vigorous local-regional conservative treatment produces survival rates equal, if not superior, to the Halsted mastectomy.
3. Radiotherapy and chemotherapy can be administered simultaneously without need of dose reduction.
4. The number of new primary carcinomas in the irradiated breast is largely inferior to the number of contralateral breast carcinomas, showing that radiotherapy has a protective action, at least in the first decade after treatment.

There are many unanswered questions in conservative treatments. The first is the size of the primary carcinoma which may be considered amenable to conservative treatment. The long-term results of the Milan trial show, without reasonable doubt, that, in patients with a tumor of less than 2 cm, conservative treatment can replace total mastectomy. Therefore, for these patients the indication for quadrantectomy (or large excision) plus axillary dissection and radiotherapy on the ipsilateral breast is a formal one, while mutilating techniques are ethically difficult to justify. For patients with carcinomas of 2–4 cm in diameter, the indications for conservative treatments are less formal. In fact, although breast excision, radiotherapy, and axillary dissection seem to produce long-term results similar to those of total mastectomy and axillary dissection, the data available are still preliminary.

A second problem concerns radiotherapy. For the time being, radiotherapy on the ipsilateral breast must be part of conservative treatment, with dosages of at least 50 Gy.

Whether the boost, either by external irradiation or by iridium implant, is needed has not been clarified as yet. Other problems to be faced by future trials are the extent of surgery (limited excision versus extensive resection, axillary dissection versus no dissection, total axillary dissection versus axillary sampling), the type of radiotherapy (immediate versus delayed, whole breast versus limited direct field, regional node irradiation versus no nodal irradiation), the comparison with other forms of surgery providing good cosmetic results (conservative treatments versus total mastectomy plus immediate reconstruction), and the pathologic patterns requiring differentiated conservative technique (lobular carcinoma in situ, intraductal noninfiltrating carcinoma, Paget's disease, and minimal carcinoma).

A second generation of trials have been designed and are being conducted at the Milan Cancer Institute in the hope of answering at least some of these questions.

The Second Milan Trial

At the Milan Cancer Institute a second randomized trial was conducted between 1985 and 1987, with the aim of comparing the classic QUART technique with a more reduced surgical intervention followed by aggressive radiotherapy treatment, consisting of 45 Gy by external high-energy source plus an implant of Ir^{192} wires, which would deliver an additional 14–17 Gy to the tumor bed. The operation consisted of a simple "tumorectomy," which removed the tumor mass with a very limited amount of peripheral normal tissue. A total of 706 cases, all with a carcinoma of less than 2.5 cm on macroscopic examination, were accrued to the trial; 360 of them were treated with QUART and the other 346 treated with TART (tumorectomy, axillary dissection, radiotherapy). Of the QUART cases 2% and of the TART cases 14% were found to have positive resection margins, but no modification of treatment was introduced in these cases.

The Third Milan Trial

In November 1987, a new trial was initiated at the Milan Cancer Institute, the aim being to compare the classic QUART with quadrantectomy and axillary dissection alone, followed by radiotherapy only in case of a local recurrence. The possible advantages of breast conservation with surgery alone are: a) that treatment is easier and cheaper, b) that a local recurrence is easier to discover, as there is no fibrosis due to radiotherapy, c) that possible late effects of radiotherapy (such as pulmonary fibrosis and cardiac damage as well as any hypothetical oncogenic risk) are avoided.

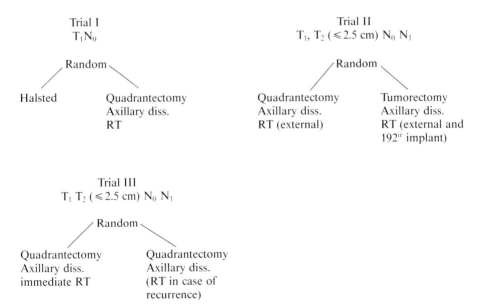

Trial I
$T_1 N_0$

Random

Halsted   Quadrantectomy
                 Axillary diss.
                 RT

Trial II
$T_1, T_2 (\leqslant 2.5 \text{ cm}) N_0 N_1$

Random

Quadrantectomy   Tumorectomy
Axillary diss.   Axillary diss.
RT (external)   RT (external and
                        192^{ir} implant)

Trial III
$T_1 T_2 (\leqslant 2.5 \text{ cm}) N_0 N_1$

Random

Quadrantectomy   Quadrantectomy
Axillary diss.   Axillary diss.
immediate RT   (RT in case of
                        recurrence)

Fig. 3. Sequence of clinical trials on conservation surgery at the National Cancer Institute of Milan (adjuvant treatments are not mentioned)

Conclusions

From the trials published, a number of conclusions can be formulated:

1. Quadrantectomy, axillary dissection, and radiotherapy for small tumors is as safe a procedure as the Halsted mastectomy in terms of local, regional, and distant recurrences and long-term survival [Milan trial (Veronesi et al. 1981, 1986), Villejuif trials (Sarrazin et al. 1983)]
2. Limited resection plus axillary dissection without radiotherapy exposes the patients to a high risk of local recurrences [NSABP trial (Fisher et al. 1985)]
3. Large resection without axillary dissection and with inadequate radiotherapy will increase the risk of axillary recurrences [Guy's Hospital trial (Hayward 1983)]. Whether the increase of local-regional recurrences will decrease the long-term survival rates (Guy's Hospital) or will not influence the survival (NSABP) must be clarified.

Future trials will deal with the extent of the surgical act, the need for radiotherapy, the type of radiotherapy, the comparison with total mastectomy plus immediate reconstruction, and the size of the primary tumor to be submitted to conservation procedures.

References

Fisher B, Bauer M, Margolese R et al. (1985) Five-year results of a randomized clinical trial comparing total mastectomy and segmental mastectomy with or without radiation in the treatment of breast cancer. N Engl J Med 312: 665–673
Hayward JL (1983) Prospective studies, the Guy's Hospital trials on breast conservation. In: Harris JR, Hellman S, Silen WJB (eds) Conservative management of breast cancer. Lippincott, Philadelphia pp 77–90
Sarrazin D, Lê MG, Fontaine MF et al. (1983) Conservative treatment versus mastectomy in T_1 or small T_2 breast cancer: A randomized trial. In: Harris JR, Hellman S, Silen W (eds) Conservative management of breast cancer. Lippincott, Philadelphia. pp 101–114
Veronesi U, Saccozzi R, Del Vecchio M et al. (1981) Comparing radical mastectomy with quadrantectomy, axillary dissection, and radiotherapy in patients with small cancers of the breast. N Engl J Med 305: 6–11
Veronesi U, Banfi A, Del Vecchio M et al. (1986) Comparison of Halsted mastectomy with quadrantectomy, axillary dissection, and radiotherapy in early breast cancer: long-term results. Eur J Cancer Clin Oncol 22: 2085–2089

Therapy of Early Breast Cancer: Preliminary Results of the German Breast Cancer Study*

R. Sauer[1], H. F. Rauschecker[2], A. Schauer[3], M. Schumacher[4], and J. Dunst[1]

[1] Strahlentherapeutische Universitätsklinik, Universitätsstraße 27, 8520 Erlangen, FRG
[2] Chirurgische Universitätsklinik, Robert-Koch-Straße 40, 3400 Göttingen, FRG
[3] Pathologisches Institut der Universität, Robert-Koch-Straße 40, 3400 Göttingen, FRG
[4] Institut für Medizinische Biometrie und Informatik, Stefan-Meier-Straße 26,
7800 Freiburg, FRG

Introduction

In 1983, the German Breast Cancer Study Group, sponsored by the Federal Ministry of Research and Technology (BMFT), started a multi-institutional prospective trial for patients with early breast cancer (pT1 pN0 M0). A total of 70 institutions, mostly community hospitals, are taking part in this study. The aims of the study are

1. To compare the incidence of local recurrences, distant metastases, and patient survival after conservative surgery plus radiotherapy and after mastectomy
2. To promote breast-preserving treatment in West-Germany
3. To improve the therapeutic standard in community hospitals, especially in the field of pathology and radiotherapy
4. To examine whether or not favorable results can be achieved by breast-preserving treatment even in a large group of participating institutes
5. To evaluate the prognostic value of certain clinical and pathohistologic factors in the case of early breast cancer
6. To investigate the "quality of life" after these different types of local treatment modalities

The planning period for this protocol lasted almost 5 years because of the conservative attitude of surgeons and gynecologists in Germany and because of many ethical and legal problems which arose in connection with the design of this protocol.

Treatment Protocol

Patients with clinically proven early breast cancer (T1 N0 M0) initially undergo tumorectomy with resection of all palpable tumor and a small amount of surrounding tissue. A lower axillary dissection (level I an II) with the removal of at least eight lymph nodes is also performed (Fig. 1).

---

* Sponsored by the Federal Ministry of Research and Technology (BMFT).

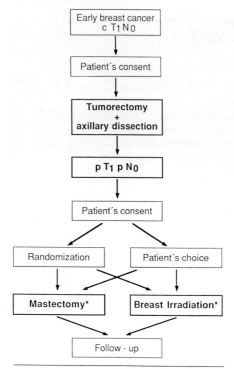

* In case of medially or centrally located tumors, the parasternal and supraclavicular region is also irradiated (in mastectomy patients as well as in patients with breast conserving treatment).

Fig. 1. The design of the BMFT breast cancer study I

Only patients who present with a pathohistologically confirmed pT1 pN0 M0 breast cancer may enter the protocol. This procedure reflects the restrictive practice in breast-preserving therapy in Germany 5–8 years ago. Multifocal and multicentric tumors are excluded from the protocol.

Following the pathohistologic staging, the patients are informed that they are participating in the clinical trial, as well as about the treatment modalities and their advantages and possible disadvantages. After informed consent, patients are randomized to one of the two treatment arms: mastectomy or breast irradiation. Patients who refuse the randomization (more than 90% of the eligible women) but are willing to be treated according to the protocol, can choose one of the two treatment modalities and are considered to be a cohort group. A prerandomization as performed in other protocols (Fisher et al. 1985; Veronesi et al. 1983) is considered inappropriate in clinical trials because of the legal situation in our country.

Irradiation Technique and Dosage

The irradiation volume includes the whole breast. The parasternal and supraclavicular area is also irradiated if the tumor has been located medially or centrally. We do not include the surgically treated axilla in the radiation volume because of the low risk of axillary recurrences in node-negative patients.

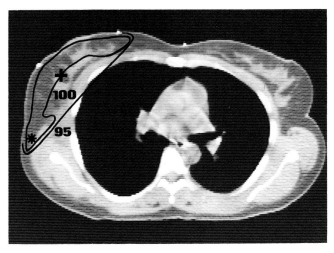

Fig. 2. Dose distribution in an irradiated breast. The 95% isodose line covers the target volume. +, reference point (100% of dose); *, maximum dose (105%)

The radiotherapeutic technique and dosage correspond with well-known protocols in Europe and the United States (Amalric et al. 1982; Calle et al. 1985; Clark et al. 1982; Fisher et al. 1985; Harris et al. 1985; Hünig et al. 1983; Veronesi et al. 1983). Radiotherapy starts within 2–6 weeks of tumorectomy and axillary dissection.

It is performed with 4–6 MV linear accelerators or cobalt-60 machines, using tangential opposing portals with wedge filters for treating the breast. The total dose to the whole breast should not exceed 50 Gy in 25 fractions over a period of 5 weeks. A boost of 12 Gy in four fractions is given to the tumor bed.

To standardize the dosage in the participating institutions, both the single dose and the total dose are calculated at a reference point in the middle of the breast at least 2 cm below the skin. The dose inhomogeneity within the target volume should be less than 10% when using a linear accelerator and less than 20% in the case of a cobalt machine (Fig. 2). The supraclavicular and parasternal lymphatics are treated by an anteroposterior portal up to total dose of 50 Gy at a depth of 3 cm. In the parasternal field, half of the dose is given by 12–15 MeV electrons.

Patient Recruitment

From November 1983 to January 1988, 762 patients were recruited. A total of 537 patients (69%) received breast-conserving therapy, 225 (31%) were treated by mastectomy (Fig. 3). As shown in Table 1, patient entry increased over the last years. Unfortunately, the randomization rate has decreased, and at the moment about 10% of the women have been randomized.

At the present time (January 31, 1988), the return of follow-up data to the data center in Freiburg is insufficient to draw final conclusions. Figure 3 also demonstrates that a remarkable number of patients entered the protocol in 1987; some of

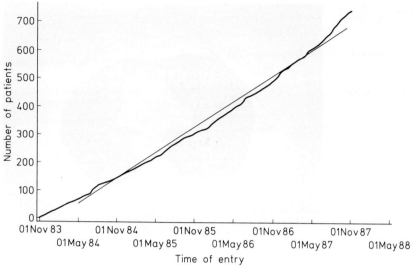

Fig. 3. The German Breast Cancer Study I: Patient recruitment (data of analysis: November 20, 1987)

Table 1. Patient recruitment from November 1983 to January 1988 with complete and incomplete follow-up and according to the treatment performed

Year of entry	Mastectomy Follow-Up		Breast-conserving treatment Follow-up	
	Complete (n)	Not complete (n)	Complete (n)	Not complete (n)
1983	6	3	10	11
1984	27	14	70	34
1985	31	13	93	27
1986	48	20	95	52
1987	48	14	110	32
1988	1	–	3	–
Σ	161	64	381	156

them have not yet completed the course of therapy. The rate of incomplete follow-up data is 29% in both treatment arms. These facts explain the relatively short median follow-up time of 15 months.

Quality of Radiation Therapy

One aim of the study was to improve the quality of radiation therapy. Therefore, in the Radiotherapeutic Reference Center, we check the dosimetric data, the treatment protocols, the localization films, and the verification portals for each patient.

Table 2. Quality criteria in radiation therapy

	Correct	Acceptable	Major deviations
Start of RT postoperatively	<6 weeks	6–8 weeks, due to postoperative complications	>8 weeks
Irradiation technique	standard	other techniques with adequate dose distribution	inadequate dose distribution
Dose deviation	<5%	5%–10%	>10%
Total treatment time	<6–7 weeks	<7–8 weeks	>8 weeks
Regional irradiation	correct	not correct	–

RT, radiation therapy.

Table 3. Quality control of radiation therapy (date of analysis: January 31, 1988)

	Breast-conserving treatment (patients)	
	(*n*)	(%)
Total	537	100
Data available	455	85
Radiotherapy correct	309	68
Radiotherapy acceptable	119	27
Protocol deviations (including refusal of treatment)	27	5
Documents not reviewed (Radiotherapy not completed, lost cases)	82	15

Radiotherapy is considered to be correct if it is performed exactly according to the protocol with dose deviations of less than 5%. Minor protocol deviations concerning the time-dose relationship or a variation in treatment technique are considered acceptable if an impact on local control or cosmesis is not to be expected (Table 2). So far, 95% of the reviewed documents of patients who have undergone radiation therapy of the breast have been correct and acceptable. In only 5% of the patients was the radiation therapy not acceptable. This means that major deviations have occurred, including delayed start of treatment, major dose deviations or refusal of radiation therapy (Table 3). Most of the protocol deviations have occurred during the first years of the protocol.

Recurrences

At present, the recurrence rate is very low; this might be explained by the short follow-up period. Table 4 summarizes the first event of recurrences only. In January 1988, there was an even distribution of local and distant relapses as well as intercurrent diseases in both treatment groups: nine vs. six local recurrences, two vs. one axillary recurrence, eight vs. two distant metastases, etc. (Table 4).

Table 4. Recurrences (first event only) in 762 patients treated with breast-conserving therapy ($n = 537$) or mastectomy ($n = 225$) (date of analysis: January 31, 1988)

	Recurrences (as of January 31, 1988) Breast-conserving therapy (n)	(First event only) Mastectomy (n)
Local recurrence	9	6
Axillary recurrence	2	1
Supraclavicular recurrence	1	
Distant metastases	8	2
Contralateral breast cancer	2	2
Other malignancy	3	
Noncancer death	1	3
Overall	26	14

Unresolved Problems

The three major problems we have observed in our group are

1. The randomization rate
2. The quality control
3. Collecting the follow-up data

The randomization of the patients to the different treatment modalities is important from a statistical point of view. In this study, it is performed by the data center in Freiburg, where a so-called "randomization telephone" is manned throughout the day. Patients are randomized immediately after having been announced by telephone call.

However, the randomization rate is very low in this study. This fact reflects the patients' and physicians' attitude towards early breast cancer treatment. The presumed equivalence of conservative treatment and mastectomy known from the recent literature has induced patients, as well as surgeons and gynecologists, to favor breast-preserving procedures. In this situation, the feasibility of further randomization seems questionable.

Adequate quality control is strongly needed in multi-institute trials to avoid institute-related differences in diagnosis or treatment. In this trial, our aim is to look for pathologic factors which may be associated with an increased incidence of local or distant failures in the treatment of early breast cancer. To assure an adequate pathohistologic work-up including immunohistology, all pathologic specimens are reviewed by a pathologic reference center.

For hormone receptor analysis, a special laboratory has been established. The radiation treatment data of all irradiated patients are reviewed by a radiotherapeutic study center. The strong regulations in this study to ensure quality not only in pathology and radiotherapy have improved the standard of breast cancer diagnosis and treatment in the participating institutions. So far, our study has had an important educational effect in the fields of pathology, radiotherapy, and surgery of early breast cancer in our country.

Collecting adequate follow-up data is a major problem. This is partly due to the fact that different disciplines (e. g., gynecologists, surgeons, radiotherapists, and general practitioners) are involved in the individual patient's follow-up. The percentage of patients with incomplete follow-up data is nearly 30%, although this figure is slowly decreasing. We are making further efforts to improve these figures and to obtain the complete data of all patients.

Summary

The German Breast Cancer Study Group has a large, homogeneous patient population with pT1 pN0 breast cancers who have undergone a detailed pathohistological work-up and uniform treatment. Seventy institutions take part in this study, mostly community hospitals. All pathologic specimens are reviewed by the Pathology Reference Center. Moreover, in order to improve the quality of radiation therapy, all dosimetric data, radiation protocols, and localization, and verification films are reviewed by the Radiotherapeutic Study Centre. By January 31, 1988, 762 patients had been recruited.

At the moment, after an admittedly short follow-up period for the majority of our patients, there is no evidence of differences between the two treatment arms concerning the incidence of local and distant recurrences, contralateral breast cancers, and other malignancies. However, the study demonstrates several unresolved problems, mainly the collection of follow-up data which can arise when many institutions especially community hospitals and general practitioners, are involved in a prospective trial.

References

Amalric R, Santamaria F, Robert F, Seigle J, Altschuler C, Kurtz JM, Spitalier JM, Brandore H, Ayme Y, Pollet JF, Burmeister R, Abed R (1982) Radiation therapy with or without primary limited surgery for operable breast cancer. A 20 year experience at the Marseilles Cancer Institute. Cancer 49: 30–34

Calle R, Vilcoq R, Pilleron JP (1985) Conservative treatment of operable breast carcinoma by irradiation with or without limited surgery – Ten year results. In: Harris J, Hellman S, Silen W (eds): Conservative management of breast cancer. Lippincott, Philadelphia, pp 3–10

Clark RM, Wilkinson RH, Mahoney LJ, Reid JG, MacDonald WD (1982) Breast cancer: A 21 year experience with conservative surgery and radiation. Int J. Radiat Oncol Biol Phys 8: 967–975

Fisher B, Bauer M, Margolese R, Poisson R, Pilch Y, Redmond C, Fisher E, Wolmark N, Deutsch M, Montague E, Saffer E, Wickersham L, Lerner H, Glass A, Shibata H, Deckers P, Ketcham A, Oishi R, Russel I (1985) Five-year results of a randomized clinical trial comparing total mastectomy and segmental mastectomy with or without radiation in the treatment of breast cancer. New Engl J Med 312: 665–673

Harris JR, Recht A, Schnitt S, Connolly J, Silver B, Come S, Henderson IC (1985) Current status of conservative surgery and radiotherapy as primary local treatment for early carcinoma of the breast. Breast Cancer Res Treat 5: 245–255

Hünig R, Walther E, Harder F, Almendral AC, Torhorst J, Roth J (1983) The Basel lumpec-
    tomy protocol: 5-year experience with a prospective study for conservative treatment of
    breast cancer. In: Harris JR, Hellman S, Silen W (eds). Conservative management of
    breast cancer. Lippincott, Philadelphia, pp 23–35
Veronesi U, DelVecchio M, Greco M (1983) Results of quadrantectomy, axillary dissection
    and radiotherapy (QUART) in T_1 N_0 patients. In: Harris JR, Hellman S, Silen W (eds.),
    Conservative management of breast cancer. Lippincott, Philadelphia pp 91–99

Methodology of Adjuvant Trials and Interpretation of Results

Methods for Assessing Treatment Efficacy in Trials for Adjuvant Therapy for Breast Cancer

R. D. Gelber and A. Goldhirsch

Division of Biostatistics and Epidemiology, Dana-Farber Cancer Institute, 44 Binney Street, Boston, MA 02115, USA

Introduction

Findings from randomized clinical trials have demonstrated an improvement in the treatment of patients with operable breast cancer. These show that systemic adjuvant therapies are effective in reducing mortality both for premenopausal and postmenopausal patients (Bonadonna et al. 1985; Nolvadex Adjuvant Trial Organisation 1985; UK-BCTSC/UICC/WHO 1984). Despite these improvements, it is predicted that almost 30% of patients with operable breast cancer will die within 5 years of the appearance of the disease. Treatments which achieve universal cure have not yet been identified. In fact, the improvements in survival are far less than the challenges which remain. This modest effect of available treatments upon mortality was the basis for a decennial controversy on defining the usefulness of adjuvant systemic therapy. The public health impact of even moderate improvement is however large because of the relatively high incidence of the disease.

Methodologies that are able to identify small real advantages in terms of meaningful end points are those which are feasible for a disease as heterogeneous as breast cancer. The development and general acceptance of adjuvant therapy for cancer have benefited perhaps more than any other treatment philosophy from the application of statistical methodologies. Especially in breast cancer, reliance on well-conducted, large-scale, randomized studies for identifying effective therapies has been the rule rather than the exception. Because the basic tenets of what constitutes reliable scientific evidence in clinical research are already well known to the reader, we will devote the majority of this chapter to a discussion of new methodologies that are useful in defining therapeutic benefit.

The Dilemma of Obtaining Statistical Evidence for Patient Care Decisions

Five features are worthy of consideration when assessing the efficacy of treatments for operable breast cancer. These are:

1. The wide variety of prognoses
2. The heterogeneity of treatments

Recent Results in Cancer Research, Vol. 115
© Springer-Verlag Berlin · Heidelberg 1989

3. The typical small treatment effect differences
4. The time lag for differences to become evident
5. The spectrum of psychosocial and quality-of-life issues

There is an obvious conflict between the desirability of defining effective therapies for specific patient groups having a homogeneous type of prognosis and the necessity of evaluating large numbers of patients (with heterogeneous prognostic characteristics) to detect the small treatment effects likely to be present.

The randomized controlled clinical trial is a particularly important methodology when prognostic factors exert a greater influence on outcome for treated patients than the effect of the treatment itself (Zelen 1974).

The requirement for randomized clinical trials has already been established in this field (Gelber and Goldhirsch 1986a). Although some controversy still exists concerning the precise cost-versus-benefit analysis of randomized trials compared with nonrandomized control studies, there is little disagreement that, all else being equal, the randomized trial will have a greater coefficient of credibility. This may or may not be warranted because a randomized design does not itself guarantee control of bias. Postrandomization case exclusions, prognostic factor imbalances, and extensive subset analyses can result in misleading conclusions. Nevertheless, despite the difficulties in execution, the randomized controlled clinical trial is the best means of evaluating treatment comparisons for operable breast cancer today. It is interesting to note that the recommendations of the NIH Concensus Development Conference on Adjuvant Therapy for Breast Cancer (1986) were based almost entirely on the results derived from such trials.

Prolonged survival is a major and, for some, a unique requirement for defining a beneficial treatment. Unless the therapeutic advantage is consistently striking, randomized trials do not therefore provide a prescription for the patient care decision. For operable breast cancer, the variety of treatments tested and the slight benefit observed rendered it necessary to explore new methodologies for focusing upon patient-oriented benefit.

Meta-Analysis for Patient Care

Meta-analysis of randomized clinical trials (or overview) is a methodology to combine the results of many separate studies and thus provide a large number of patients to answer a question of clinical interest. Table 1 describes the goals and limitations of overview procedures. The main strength of an overview is to accumulate evidence properly from many trials in order to detect treatment effects which are too small to be found in the individual studies alone. In addition, positive effects might be demonstrated earlier in an overview than if individual trials are permitted time to mature. The main weakness of an overview is the tendency to obscure the differences between studies being combined and to perform indirect comparisons between trials that ask different questions (UK-BCTSC/UICC/WHO 1984; Yusuf et al. 1985; Gelber and Goldhirsch 1986b; Cuzick et al. 1987a, 1987b; Redmond and Rockette 1987; Gelber and Goldhirsch 1987).

The current approach to overviews relies on an arithmetic construction. The principle is that comparison of two randomized groups provides an estimate of the

Table 1. Overview of randomized clinical trials of operable breast cancer: the goals and the limitations

Goals	Limitations
– Pool large number of patients in which the effect of treatment is modest.	– While a "typical" effect of treatment can be identified, the magnitude of the effect may be masked by heterogeneity of trials, patients, and treatments (arithmetic construction).
– Indirectly compare results of two overviews (e.g., endocrine therapy vs chemotherapy which were individually compared to their controls) in order to identify the best treatment by these means.	– The "typical" effect seen in each of the overviews does not necessarily apply to the same population, and this conclusion derived from such an indirect comparison may be inaccurate.
– For a more patient-oriented approach, pool results from subgroup analysis of trials with intent to find larger treatment effects for a selected subpopulation.	– Subgroup analysis is usually a retrospective one, with reporting influenced by outcome and a tendency to interpret quantitative differences as if they were qualitative.
– Design future trials with intention to study prospectively treatment effects in subpopulations and include results in overviews.	– The hyperstratification of trials complicates conduct.

effect of the experimental treatment if the two groups differ only with respect to the treatment's presence in one and its absence in the other. If the treatment has no effect, then in fact this arithmetic construction will provide a valid test for the null hypothesis. If, however, the experimental treatment has a positive effect, the magnitude of that effect is likely to depend upon a variety of factors relating to study conduct, patient population, concomitant therapies, and control group. Thus, the magnitude of treatment effect estimated from an overview must be considered as a "typical" effect rather than what might be achieved in a more focused analysis.

A future development for performing overviews designed to obtain estimates of magnitude of effects within patient subpopulations might be based upon limiting the approach to a specific question, prognostic group, or treatment modality. A danger of this analysis is the tendency to reach conclusions based upon indirect comparison of results across subgroups. If, however, interpretation were limited to explorations that were prospectively defined focusing on prognostic variables which dictate a differentiated approach to patient care (e.g., endocrine therapies based upon receptor status), these difficulties could be minimized. Specific examples of current questions that might benefit from a meta-analysis are: (a) Does chemoendocrine therapy reduce mortality compared with endocrine therapy alone for postmenopausal patients? (b) Does chemoendocrine therapy reduce mortality compared with chemotherapy alone for premenopausal patients? (c) What evidence is available to support the routine use of endocrine therapy alone (tamoxifen, oophorectomy) in premenopausal patients?

Other questions that might benefit from an overview relate to the causes of death (e.g., mortality in radiation therapy trials), incidence of specific sites of first failure in different treatment programs (e.g., local and regional recurrences in systemic adjuvant therapy trials), and long-term toxic effects of adjuvant programs.

The possibility of performing overviews reliably in subpopulations across trials might be given if each one of these groups had been defined prospectively via a stratification prior to randomization. Although hyperstratification of trials runs counter to statistical and trial logistical considerations, this would have rendered a more precise definition of magnitude of treatment effect within patient subgroups and thus provided a more patient-care-oriented approach. Very large-scale studies, however, with a high compliance for defining prognostic variables for the majority of the patients also offer some guarantee for reliable overviews of subpopulations.

Treatment Comparisons Considering Relative Patient Well-being

A second methodology, developed under the name TWiST (time without symptoms of disease and toxicity of treatment) (Gelber and Goldhirsch 1986c; Gelber et al. 1987), was designed to compare treatments considering amounts of time which are assumed to be of similar acceptable quality (i.e., without symptoms of recurrent disease or toxic effects of treatment). This approach is an extension of attempts to define patient-oriented benefit (Table 2). In general, the TWiST methodology is relevant whenever one population receives a subjectively toxic treatment for a finite period, while its control group experiences a higher rate of disease recurrence. The question for patient care decision-making is whether the delay in recurrence achieved by some patients is sufficient to justify exposure of the entire population to subjective toxic effects. In order to illustrate this new approach and to follow its evolution toward improved applicability for individual patient care, the Ludwig Trial III (Goldhirsch and Gelber, this volume

Table 2. Development of patient well-being oriented approaches for the definition of treatment benefit

Goals	Limitations
– Define the feeling of the individual patients seen by the physician (Karnofsky's index or performance status).	– (Historically, this was the first attempt to include subjective features into measurement parameters). Measures only indirectly the patients' well-being and might be biased by the observer.
– Define the feeling of the individual patient, allowing self-expression.	– Spectrum of variability is large. Methods are difficult to validate.
– Comparisons of treatment effects in terms of the amount of time spent under conditions considered to be of equivalent quality across treatment groups (e.g., side effects of drugs, symptomatic relapse); the TWiST methodology.	– The comparisons must rely upon predetermined relative values given arbitrarily to amount of time spent under different conditions. Future developments must incorporate some mechanism for individual value assignment.

Table 3. Definition of periods of time associated with differing quality of life: components of Q-TWiST

Event	Label	Time
Any subjective toxic effect reported during a month[a]	TOX	1 month
Alopecia and weight gain	TOX	3 additional months
Isolated scar recurrence or contralateral breast carcinoma	LR[b]	3 months (for recovery)
Any other relapse[c]	REL	Remaining survival time
None of the above	TWiST	

[a] Excluding hematologic toxicity only.
[b] Included in REL for analysis.
[c] Bone = when symptomatic or treated.

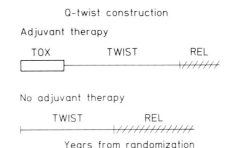

Fig. 1. Periods of TOX, TWiST, and REL for representative patients who receive adjuvant therapy or no adjuvant therapy

pp. 153–162) is considered. For the development of the TWiST end point, the first evaluation assigned zero value to the periods of time with toxicity (TOX) and the time following systemic, symptomatic relapse (REL) (Table 3, Fig. 1). Thus, TOX and REL were equated to death. Adjustments can be made to this severe construction by allowing the periods TOX and REL to be assigned utility values between 0 and 1 (u_t and u_r, respectively) to reflect their values relative to TWiST. These values represent the patients' perception of the impact of treatment toxicity and disease recurrence on their quality of life. For example, if a patient considers the toxic effects of therapy after mastectomy to be almost intolerable (based upon her bias, knowledge, and expectations) the utility value that can be set for such a patient will be near 0. The same reasoning can apply to defining the value for the utility of REL.

From a particular randomized trial, the distributions of time spent in TOX, TWiST, and REL can be calculated for each treatment, and average values for Q-TWiST (quality-adjusted analysis of TWiST) can be obtained as weighted averages of these quantities according to the equation

$$Q\text{-}TWiST = u_t \cdot TOX + TWiST + u_r \cdot REL$$

Treatment comparisons can be performed based upon values for Q-TWiST, and the range of utility values (u_t, and u_r) for which each treatment is preferred can be

Table 4. Components of Q-TWiST estimated from Ludwig Trial III[a]

	CMFp+T	p+T	Observation
TOX	9.6 (0.4)	2.0 (0.3)	0.0 (0.0)
TWiST	50.3 (2.5)	47.1 (2.7)	41.5 (2.6)
REL	7.1 (1.1)	12.9 (1.4)	20.9 (1.8)
Q-TWiST $(u_t=u_r=0.5)$	58.7 (2.2)	54.6 (2.3)	51.9 (2.2)

[a] Average months (S.E.) of TOX, TWiST, and REL accumulated within 7 years of randomization, with Q-TWiST calculated for arbitrary utility coefficients.

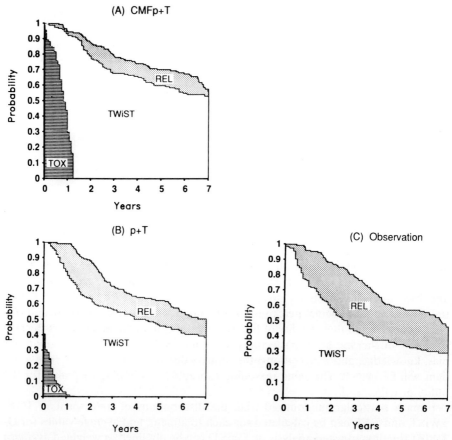

Fig. 2 A–C. Partitioned survival plots by treatment in Ludwig Trial III. Survival plots are shown for three end points, *from left to right:* time in toxicity (*TOX*), systemic disease-free survival (*SDFS*), and survival. This divides the 7 years since randomization into the three stages TOX, TWiST and REL, as indicated. The mean times (equal to the areas between the curves) are given in Table 4. The 7-year overall survival and SDFS percentages are: 57% and 53% for CMFp+T, 51% and 39% for p+T, and 47% and 31% for observation

determined. Individual patient decisions can then be made according to the presumed values the patient or physician might assign to the utility coefficients.

Specifically, for Ludwig III, the average months of TOX, TWiST, and REL accumulated within 7 years from mastectomy with a calculated Q-TWiST for arbitrary utility coefficients of $u_t = 0.50$, $u_r = 0.50$ are described in Table 4.

In order to visualize the different contributions of events for the three treatments, Fig. 2 represents the TOX, TWiST, and REL components of overall survival time for each group. Average TOX is the area under the curve defining the amount of time spent with subjective side effects of treatment. TWiST is the time to systemic relapse (systemic disease-free survival; SDFS) but not including TOX. Average REL is the area between the overall survival time distribution (top curve) and the SDFS curve. As reported elsewhere in this volume (Goldhirsch and Gelber, this volume pp. 153–162), disease recurrence was significantly delayed for postmenopausal patients treated with cyclophosphamide-methotrexate-5-fluorouracil-prednisone + tamoxifen (CMFp + T), as compared with either p + T alone or observation. This superior control of disease had a significant influence on overall survival compared with observation first appearing only after 6 years of follow-up. The difference in overall survival between CMFp + T and p + T was not statistically significant. The choice of therapy for an individual patient will, however, depend upon the relative weights assigned to the three regions, TOX, TWiST, and REL. The evolution of benefit in terms of TWiST or its adjustment (the Q-TWiST) indicates that, by 7 years' median follow-up, the more toxic treatment, the CMFp + T, is also the most advantageous for the patient for a wide range of utility coefficients (Goldhirsch et al. 1989).

Methodologies for New Adjuvant Approaches

Conventionally, a treatment is considered to be a legitimate option for an adjuvant trial if it has demonstrated efficacy in advanced disease and if some long-term observation for potential toxicities is available. Clinical trials methodology is also available to aid in the recruitment of new therapies into the adjuvant setting. Despite the advances achieved for the adjuvant treatment of early breast cancer, substantial additional progress is required for developing and evaluating new therapeutic strategies for this disease. The administration of systemic treatments preoperatively represents an approach that has a biological and theoretical rationale for anticipated additonal benefit. The use of such "neoadjuvant" therapies in clinical trials requires the development of new methodologies for their conduct and evaluation (Gelber 1985; Gelber and Goldhirsch 1986d). One issue, for example, is understaging and the possible modification of prognostic variables if systemic therapy is given preoperatively. Preoperative treatment will also have an effect on the status of the primary tumor that might influence cosmetic results and patient well-being. Prospective planning to evaluate such end points is required.

Because patients with operable breast cancer continue to relapse and die many years after the initial diagnosis, the opportunity exists to observe either therapeutic benefit and/or adverse treatment effects after a long-term follow-up. The overall survival advantage for chemoendocrine therapy for postmenopausal patients in

Ludwig III was observed at a median follow-up of 6 years. In other trials, the advantages for single-agent cyclophosphamide administered immediately postoperatively (Nissen-Meyer et al. 1978), and for oophorectomy plus continuous, low-dose prednisone (Meakin et al. 1983) were also seen only after extended follow-up of the study cohorts. In a recent overview (Cuzick et al. 1987a), the increased mortality observed for the patients who received postoperative irradiation became apparent in analyses restricted to events occurring beyond 10 years from diagnosis. Investigations are underway to elaborate possible reasons for this increased mortality.

The requirement of waiting for the appearance of late advantages or disadvantages frustrates the desire to provide the best treatment for patients diagnosed today. It is vital to consider the results of individual trials, and overviews of them, within the time frame for which the detected differences are reliable and meaningful (Zelen and Gelman 1986).

New treatment modalities, new methodologies for evaluating benefits from adjuvant therapies, and pooling all available results to detect moderate treatment effects are all needed for reasonable progress in this field.

Acknowledgement. We thank Drs. R. J. Simes, P. Glasziou, and A. S. Coates for significant contributions to the development of the Q-TWiST methodology.

References

Bonadonna G, Valagussa P, Rossi A, et al. (1985) Ten-year experience with CMF-based adjuvant chemotherapy in resectable breast cancer. Breast Cancer Res Treat 5: 95–115

Cuzick J, Stewart H, Peto R, et al. (1987a) Overview of randomized trials of postoperative adjuvant radiotherapy in breast cancer. Cancer Treat Rep 71: 15–29

Cuzick J, Stewart H, Peto R, et al. (1987b) Overview of randomized trials comparing radical mastectomy without radiotherapy against simple mastectomy with radiotherapy in breast cancer. Cancer Treat Rep 71: 7–14

Gelber RD (1985) Methodological and statistical aspects in perioperative chemotherapy trials. In: Metzger U, Largiader F, Senn H-J (eds) Perioperative chemotherapy. Springer, Berlin Heidelberg New York Tokyo, pp 53–63 (Recent results in cancer research, vol 98)

Gelber RD, Goldhirsch A (1986a) The requirement for clinical trials in breast cancer. In: Forbes JF (ed). Breast disease. Churchill Livingstone, Edinburgh, pp 106–122 (Clinical surgery international, vol 10)

Gelber RD, Goldhirsch A (1986b) The concept of an overview of cancer clinical trials with special emphasis on early breast cancer. J Clin Oncol 4: 1696–1703

Gelber RD, Goldhirsch A for the Ludwig Breast Cancer Study Group (1986c) A new endpoint for the assessment of adjuvant therapy in postmenopausal women with operable breast cancer. J Clin Oncol 4: 1772–1779

Gelber RD, Goldhirsch A (1986d) Methodological issues in neoadjuvant chemotherapy trials. In: Jacquillat C, Weil M, Khayat D (eds) Neoadjuvant chemotherapy: first international congress. Libbey, London, pp 799–809 (Colloque INSERM, vol 137)

Gelber RD, Goldhirsch A (1987) Interpretation of results from subset analyses within overviews of randomized clinical trials. Stat Med 6: 371–378

Gelber RD, Goldhirsch A, Castiglione M, et al. for the Ludwig Breast Cancer Study Group (1987) Time without symptoms and toxicity (TWiST): A quality-of-life-oriented endpoint to evaluate adjuvant therapy. In: Salmon SE (ed) Adjuvant therapy of cancer V. Grune and Stratton, Orlando, pp 455–465

Goldhirsch A, Gelber RD, Simes RJ, et al. for the Ludwig Breast Cancer Study Group (1989) Costs and benefits of adjuvant therapy in breast cancer: a quality adjusted survival analysis. J Clin Oncol 7: 36–44

Meakin JW, Allt WEC, Beale FA, et al. (1983) Ovarian irradiation and prednisone following surgery and radiotherapy for carcinoma of the breast. Breast Cancer Res Treat 3 [Suppl]: 45–48

Nissen-Meyer R, Kjellgren K, Malmio K, et al. (1978) Surgical adjuvant chemotherapy: results with one short course of cyclophosphamide after mastectomy for breast cancer. Cancer 41: 2088–2098

Nolvadex Adjuvant Trial Organisation (1985) Controlled trial of tamoxifen as single agent in management of early breast cancer: analysis at 6 years. Lancet i: 836–839

Proceedings of the NIH Consensus Development Conference on Adjuvant Chemotherapy and Endocrine Therapy for Breast Cancer (1986) NCI Monogr 1: 1–159

Redmond CK, Rockette HE (1987) Meta-analysis: considerations of its worth and its limitations. In: Salmon SE (ed) Adjuvant therapy of cancer. Grune and Stratton, Orlando, pp 467–475

UK-BCTSC/UICC/WHO (1984) Review of mortality results in randomized trials in early breast cancer. Lancet ii: 1205

Yusuf S, Peto R, Lewis J, et al. (1985) Beta-blockade during and after myocardial infarction: an overview of the randomized trials. Prog Cardiovasc Dis 27: 335–371

Zelen M (1974) The randomization and stratification of patients to clinical trials. J Chronic Dis 27: 365–375

Zelen M, Gelman R (1986) Assessment of adjuvant trials in breast cancer. NCI Monogr 1: 11–17

Overview of Adjuvant Radiotherapy for Breast Cancer

J. Cuzick

Imperial Cancer Research Fund, P.O. Box 123, Lincoln's Inn Fields, London, WC2A 3PX, Great Britain

Two papers (Cuzick et al. (1987a, 1987b)) have recently been published, in which mortality results from all available mature randomized trials of adjuvant radiotherapy were updated and analyzed collectively. These overviews were based on individual patient data for over 10000 patients, of whom more than 6000 had died. Brief details of the individual trials are shown in Table 1. As shown in Figs. 1 and 2, no effect of radiotherapy could be found in the first 10 years of follow-up in the two types of pure radiotherapy trials – radical mastectomy with or without radiotherapy and simple mastectomy with or without radiotherapy. There was no indication of heterogeneity between different trials. In trials of simple mastectomy with radiotherapy vs. radical mastectomy without radiotherapy, a slightly worse prognosis ($P = 0.05$) was observed in the irradiated patients (Fig. 3). This was due to poor survival in one trial (Southeast Scotland) in the first 5 years of follow-up and appears to be a chance finding.

However, the data suggested rather strongly ($P < 0.001$) that at least some forms of radiotherapy had a deleterious effect on long-term survival as measured by subsequent survival in those patients who survived at least 10 years. This result was based primarily on the earliest generation of trials in which radiotherapy was a randomised option after all patients had received a radical mastectomy (Fig. 4), but was also supported by the Kings/CRC trial of simple mastectomy with or without radiotherapy (hazard ratio after 10 years = 1.50, 95% confidence interval 1.08, 2.09, $P < 0.05$). The other trials of simple mastectomy with or without radiotherapy were not sufficiently mature to yield very much information about survival after 10 years. However, from the information available, there was no suggestion of heterogeneity between trials. Overall the death rate after 10 years in 10-year survivors was estimated to be 35% higher (95% confidence interval 15%–58%) in those who had been randomised to receive radiotherapy.

These results have prompted further questions which were not addressed in the original study. These are of two types: (a) limitations in the data base and (b) limitations in the analysis. These are briefly addressed below.

Recent Results in Cancer Research, Vol. 115
© Springer-Verlag Berlin·Heidelberg 1989

Table 1. Details of radiotherapy regimens in trials under review

Trial	Year of onset	Type of therapy	Dose (Gy)	Fractions (n)	Duration (days)	Biologic dose (rets)
Radical mastectomy ± XRT						
Manchester Q	1949	250 kV	35.0–40.0	15	21	1438–1693
Manchester P	1952	250 kV	32.5–42.5	15	21	1335–1746
Oslo I	1964	200 kV	18.0–36.0	20	28	681–1362
Oslo II	1968	^{60}Co	50.0	20	28	1689
Heidelberg	1969	^{60}Co	54.0	30	42	1905
Stockholm	1971	Nodal, ^{60}Co	45.0	25	35	1406[a]
Simple mastectomy ± XRT						
Manchester Regional	1970	300 kV or	37.0	15	21	1493
		Nodal, 4 meV	40.0	15	21	1464 (1211[b])
			30.0	15	21	
CRC	1970	Ortho or	32.5–46		21–42	1335–1483
		meV	35.7–50.6		21–42	1306–1453
NSABP-B04	1971	meV	40–50	25	35	1224–1530
Edinburgh I	1974	4 meV	42.5	10	28	1661
Simple mastectomy + XRT vs. Radical Mastectomy − XRT						
Copenhagen	1951	Nodal, 400 kV	42.0	18	21	1592 (1652[c])
Southeast Scotland	1964	2 meV	42.5	10	28	1695
Manchester Regional	1970	300 kV or	37.0	15	21	1493
		Nodal, 4 meV	40.0	15	21	1464 (1211[b])
			30.0	15	21	
NSABP-B04	1971	meV (node-negative)	40–50	25	35	1224–1530
		meV (node-positive)	50–60	25	35	1531–1837

XRT, X-ray therapy.

[a] Chest wall, 10–15 meV; [b] Chest wall, 300 kV; [c] Chest wall, 250 kV.

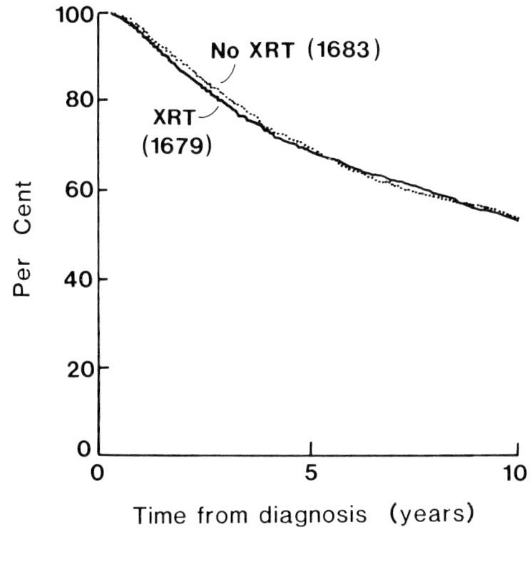

Fig. 1. Combined 10-year survival according to allocated treatment for trials employing a simple mastectomy. *Curves* do not include material from NSABP-B04 trial. *Numbers in parentheses* are total patients at risk in each arm (excluding NSABP)

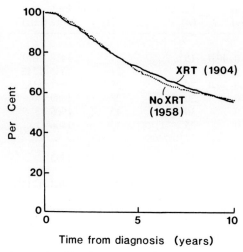

Fig. 2. Combined 10-year survival according to allocated treatment for all trials employing a radical mastectomy. Numbers in parentheses are total patients at risk in each arm

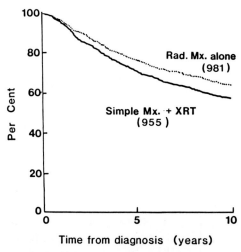

Fig. 3. Combined 10-year survival curves in trials comparing radical mastectomy alone vs. simple mastectomy with radiotherapy. Survival was marginally better in the nonirradiated arm ($P=0.05$). Numbers in parentheses are total patients at risk in that arm (excluding NSABP). Curves do not include data from NSABP-B04 trial, although all calculations do

Limitations in the Data Base

Because of the large amount of effort necessary to extract data from very old trials, the data collected were kept to a minimum. We were interested in long-term mortality, so it was essential to record the vital status and date of death of each individual patient. The essential core data collected on all patients consisted of (a)

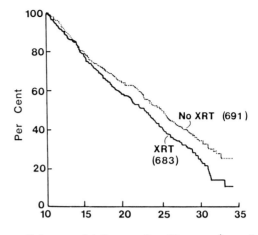

Fig. 4. Subsequent survival in patients surviving 10 years who where in a trial employing radical mastectomy. There is a significant difference favouring patients treated by radical mastectomy alone ($P=0.002$). Numbers in parentheses are total patients at risk in each arm

randomised treatment option, (b) age at diagnosis and (c) clinical nodal status. The results of the overview have prompted a number of further questions, including:

1. Which specific cause(s) of mortality are elevated? In particular are leukaemia, other cancers, or heart disease mortality elevated?
2. The relation of excess mortality to type of radiotherapy given. The scattering profile and organ doses vary considerably according to whether orthovoltage or megavoltage machinery is used and also depend on the particular fields irradiated and doses given.
3. The laterality of the primary tumour. This will affect doses to other tissues, especially the heart, and an examination of heart disease mortality in relation to which breast was irradiated may be informative.
4. The actual treatment given, not just allocated treatment. Few patients did not receive to allocated initial treatment, but many had radiotherapy for local recurrence and some of these will have survived more than 10 years.

In order to answer these questions, we plan to collect the following additional information on each individual patient who survived 10 years or more:

1. Whether breast cancer was present at death
2. Cause of death with special attention to the following major groups: (a) breast cancer; (b) other cancer; (c) cardiac; (d) other vascular
3. Type of radiotherapy given, especially kilovoltage vs. megavoltage X-rays
4. Actual radiotherapy given to primary site (dose and fields both at presentation and for relapses in the first 10 years)
5. Laterality of original primary tumour
6. Radiotherapy given for contralateral disease

We hope this more detailed overview will help to answer questions about the long-term effects of radiotherapy, which are particularly revelant now because of a shift in primary treatment towards breast conservation with its associated increase in the use of radiotherapy.

Methodological and Statistical Issues

Two points have arisen regarding the methods of analysis used: (a) the emphasis on subsequent mortality in patients surviving more than 10 years, and (b) the need to accommodate treatment variability in the analysis.

The Subgroup of 10-Year Survivors

The majority of deaths in the first 5–10 years are due to occult distant micro-metastases which would be unaffected by radiotherapy to the chest wall or axilla. Thus, by focussing on long-term survivors, we are avoiding the great mass of deaths which are likely to contribute more to the variance of any treatment difference than to any mean difference. However, the subgroup of 10-year survivors is necessarily a post-randomisation selected group and, potentially, could be biased. This could happen if radiotherapy affected survival in the first 10 years in a way such as to unbalance the future survival prospects of those who achieved 10-year survival. For example, if the effect of radiotherapy was only to delay deaths in the 9th year until the 10th year, then the poorer survival after 10 years would be the result of better survival in the first 10 years. However, the survival curves in the first 10 years do not support such a possibility, but because of the far larger number of deaths at early follow-up times such an effect could be masked. This possibility seems sufficiently unlikely on a priori grounds in this particular instance, and most likely it can be discounted.

Treatment Heterogeneity

Although the precise treatment may vary among centres, doctors, or even on an individual patient basis, this fact is usually ignored in clinical trials, except for occasionally stratifying by centre. The question arises more naturally when attempting an overview since differences in treatment are usually apparent in the separate trial protocols.

The question of a specific treatment difference has already arisen in discussion of the radiotherapy trials. In attempting to explain the differences in long-term survival, one possible explanation is a delayed effect of scattered irradiation on heart disease rate. This could be quite different for kilovoltage vs. megavoltage treatment. By collecting more information this specific question can be addressed, but there also remain other differences in the treatments, and it would be unreasonable to suspect that they do not have at least a small effect on survival. A test for heterogeneity between trials can give some idea of the magnitude of this variability, but problems still remain in the interpretation of a single summary treatment effect obtained from an overview.

Interpretation will depend to some extent on the degree of heterogeneity, as measured for example by a χ^2 test. When this is sufficiently large that treatment effects differ by more than their estimated standard error, an attempt should be made to discover which specific treatments were superior, and further trials should be undertaken to confirm this. When differences in treatment effects are small compared with their estimated standard errors, as in the case for the radiotherapy trials, then it is probably more fruitful to think in terms of some average treatment effect and accept that treatment itself has some measurable variability in addition to that due to the unpredictable nature of the patient's response. This variability can be modelled in various ways, but the most important component will be its variance. Empirical Bayes arguments can then be invoked to estimate the variance and to determine its effect on confidence limits for the mean treatment effect. Generally, the variance and confidence intervals will only be increased if the χ^2 test for heterogeneity exceeds its expected value, and then by an amount related to the magnitude of this difference. Often, these considerations have little effect on the resulting estimates, but they are important in principle and need to be considered in each specific overview.

References

Cuzick J, Stewart H, Peto R, Baum B, Fisher B, Host H, Lythgoe JP, Ribeiro G, Scheurlen H, Wallgren A (1987a). Overview of randomized trials of postoperative adjuvant radiotherapy in breast cancer. Cancer Treat Rep 71: 15–29

Cuzick J, Stewart H, Peto R, Fisher B, Kaae S, Johansen H, Lythgoe JP, Prescott RJ (1987b). Overview of randomized trials comparing radical mastectomy without radiotherapy against simple mastectomy with radiotherapy in breast cancer. Cancer Treat Rep 71: 7–14

Randomized Multicenter 2 × 2-Factorial Design Study of Chemo/Endocrine Therapy in Operable, Node-Positive Breast Cancer (Protocol 2)*

H. Scheurlen

Institut für Medizinische Biometrie und Informatik, Universität Heidelberg,
Im Neuenheimer Feld 325, 6900 Heidelberg, FRG

Introduction

In 1984, the West German Breast Cancer Study Group (see Appendix A) set up a controlled clinical trial on adjuvant therapy in "early" breast cancer to answer the following question: Is it possible to reduce six cycles of cyclophosphamide, methotrexate, and 5-fluorouracil (CMF), to be given within 6 months starting perioperatively, to half the dose within half the time without decreasing the patient's chance of survival? At that time, we started out from the following assumptions:

1. Polychemotherapy is superior to monotherapy (Fisher et al. 1981).
2. No other drug combination has so far been proved superior to the modified Bonadonna scheme (Bonadonna et al. 1981).
3. Twelve cycles of CMF can safely be reduced to six cycles (Bonadonna et al. 1981).
4. Early onset of adjuvant systemic chemotherapy is important: "Small is sensitive" (Nissen-Meyer 1982; Shackney et al. 1978).
5. Prolonged chemotherapy might be for the benefit of a small group of patients only, and therefore costs and benefits of cytotoxic chemotherapy in terms of side effects and gains in survival time should be taken into account.

As a physician might feel tempted to compensate the lower-dose regimen by adding endocrine therapy, the use of tamoxifen should be regulated by protocol in order to avoid confounded effects. We did not know, however, whether to recommend combined chemo- and endocrine therapy, and therefore we decided that patients should again be randomized to receive either tamoxifen (tam) for 2 years or no endocrine therapy during that time, irrespective of the patient's hormone receptor and menopausal state. Such a four-armed or 2 × 2-factorial setting would also enable us to investigate components of the combined therapy.

Owing to legal regulations in the FRG, we have to inform patients of possible treatment alternatives and uncertainties in choosing the optimal therapy, in addi-

* Supported by Bundesministerium für Forschung und Technologie (BMFT), Contract 01ZPO43.

tion to details of random allocation if the patient asks for this information (Eber-bach 1988). In an attempt to clarify selection mechanisms arising from the patient's consent or refusal, we have decided to include all clinically eligible patients, whether randomized or not. We call this concept Comprehensive Cohort Study (Scheurlen et al. 1984; Olschewski and Scheurlen 1985; Schumacher and Davis 1988).

Patients and Methods

Figure 1 explains the Comprehensive Cohort Study (CCS) concept. We may suppose for the sake of simplicity that only two treatment alternatives A and B are provided by the protocol instead of the four in our protocol 2. X may be any other treatment not provided by the protocol. Decision tree notation has been used merely to demonstrate that nothing is left to be decided by the clinician. If the clinician were a negligible quantity in decision-making, the number of those patients per hospital who consent to randomization or prefer one of the treatments should be highly correlated. This assumption corresponds poorly to reality, as we shall see later.

The treatment schedules are depicted in Fig. 2. It should be noticed that, exept for a 3-month overlap in the "CMF+tam" arm, the chemotherapy and the endo-crine therapy follow each other sequentially in time in the two combined therapy arms. Preferably, patients should be randomized after initial therapy (three cycles of CMF) has been completed. Many patients, however, want to plan ahead soon and therefore ask their doctor at an earlier stage of therapy to inform them of the whole procedure they will have to go through. As a consequence, we are not able to avoid randomization taking place somewhere during initial therapy (as symbolized by the hatched triangle in Fig. 2). This, however, will certainly raise the risk of protocol violations. Furthermore, this is why we have to consider a node-positive

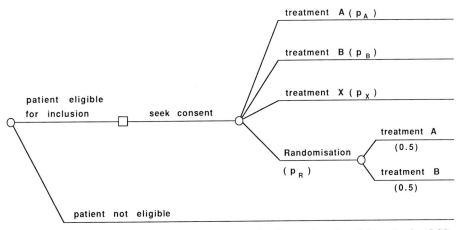

Fig. 1. Decision analysis under informed consent: the Comprehensive Cohort Study (CCS) concept

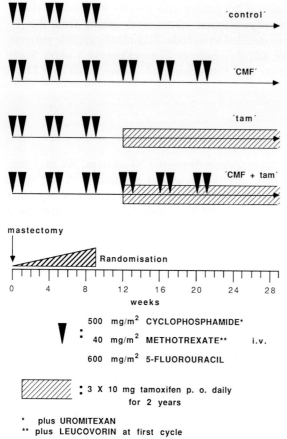

Fig. 2. Protocol 2: randomization and treatment schedules

patient for the cohort study as soon as her initial CMF therapy has started periop-eratively.

The most characteristic selection criteria are outlined in Table 1. Table 2 shows the main prognostic factors to be considered in the trial.

Results

The trial has been running since June 1984 and will be closed in 1989. After two-thirds of the running time, we should raise the question of to what extent the medical profession in the FRG has responded to the trial and how well the doctors and the patients participating in the trial have complied with the protocol.

Out of a total of 549 institutions in the FRG which initially expressed some interest in a cooperative trial (Scheurlen and Schumacher 1982) no more than 39, or 7%, finally took part in this trial. These institutions are among the smaller ones, covering less than 5% of the total breast cancer incidence in a country where medical care of breast cancer patients appears to be rather decentralized as compared with other European countries (Fig. 3).

Table 1. Patient selection

Eligibility criteria	Comprehensive Cohort Study	
	Controlled trial	Observational study
Surgery		
Breast	Mastectomy (Patey)	
Axilla	En bloc dissection with at least 6 lymph nodes to be identified in the specimen	
Primary tumor	T_{1a-3a}	
Axillary lymph nodes (Histologic status)	Positive	
Initial CMF therapy (Perioperative onset)	3 Cycles completed or presumably to be completed	At least first course completed
Random allocation of treatment alternatives	Accepted	Not accepted or patient unsuitable for randomization

Table 2. Pretreatment laboratory investigation: prognostic factors

Variable	Investigator
Tumor size	Regional pathologist
Number of metastatic lymph nodes	Regional pathologist
Histologic classification	Reference pathologist
Grading (Bloom, Richardson)	Reference pathologist
Hormone receptor status	Regional laboratory, quality control by reference laboratory

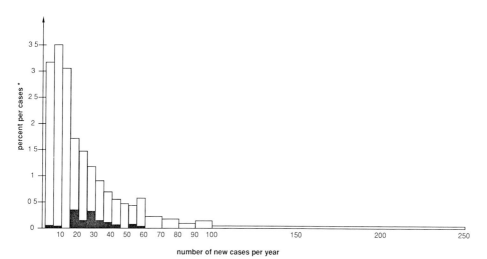

Fig. 3. Distribution of hospitals by new breast cancer patients per year in the FRG in 1979 ($N = 549$ hospitals reporting 15 786 cases). *Black columns,* participating hospitals. * The percentage of hospitals reporting an incidence as indicated on the abscissa is equal to the area, not the height of a rectangle, e.g. $3.5 \times 5 = 17,5\%$ hospitals reported 5 to 10, $0.0034 \times 150 = 5\%$ hospitals reported 100 to 250 new cases in 1979

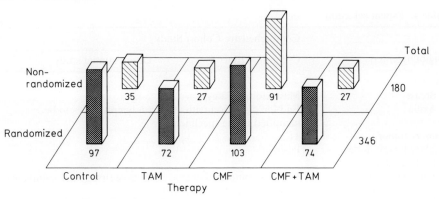

Fig. 4. Distribution of patients by treatment group and randomization state (January 31, 1988)

During the previous 3-4 years, 526 patients have been admitted to the trial, and of these 346 have been randomized (Fig. 4). However, a total of 1500-2000 randomized patients would be required to answer the questions posed, assuming only a weak synergistic interaction, if any, between CMF and tamoxifen, and taking into account that preference will be given to the least aggressive regimen should the trial fail to yield any significant difference. Thus, at the closure of patient entry we will have reached only one third to one quarter of the required sample size. Note also that an imbalance occurs in Fig. 4 between the two tamoxifen arms and the two control arms. This is due to the fact that in December 1986 we discontinued tamoxifen therapy in premenopausal women.

To see how well the physicians were able to manage the requirement of informed consent, the numbers of randomized and nonrandomized patients entered so far per hospital should be compared. The respective pairs of numbers are presented in Fig. 5 as a scatter diagram. The nonrandomized patients are further subdivided by the numbers of CMF cycles intended to be given. The respective numbers of (nonrandomized) patients per hospital can be seen in Fig. 6. It appears that not even a weak correlation can be discerned in either figure, indicating that a patient's willingness for giving consent to randomization and her preference for a particular therapy depend largely on the caring hospital, or, to put it more clearly, that ultimately it is the doctor who has the say and not the patient.

An assessment of side effects and early recurrences during initial treatment is clearly beyond the scope of a randomized trial that preferably randomizes patients towards the end of this part of therapy. The distribution of discontinuations, indicating intolerability, among both the randomized and the nonrandomized patients is given in Table 3. There are still some hidden reserves of treatment failures according to the preliminary figures in the last row of Table 3.

Table 4 and Fig. 7 supply information about the compliance of CMF therapy subsequent to initial therapy in terms of mean actual doses in percent of target doses according to random allocation. It should be noted that this and Table 5 are confined to the randomized patients. There was a rather stable gradient of about 75% to be noticed between the two groups treated for six cycles and the two groups treated for three cycles throughout the previous life time of the trial.

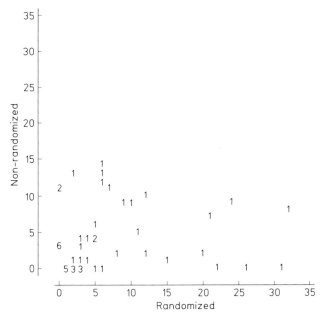

Fig. 5. Numbers of randomized and nonrandomized patients by hospitals (January 31, 1988)

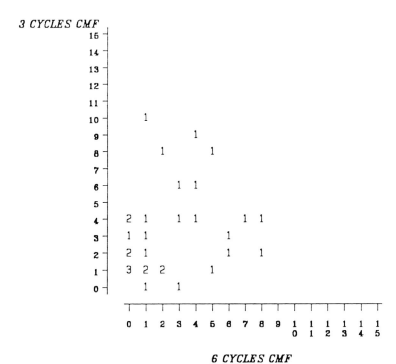

Fig. 6. CMF (3 vs. 6 cycles) in nonrandomized patients: numbers entered into the trial by hospitals (January 31, 1988)

Table 3. Tolerability of initial CMF therapy - distribution of patients by discontinuation and randomization state (January 31, 1988)

Allocation of therapy (acceptance into CCS)	Initial CMF therapy			
	Completed (*n*)	Discontinued (*n*)	State unknown (*n*)	Total (*n*)
Random (accepted)	325	3	18	346
Nonrandom (accepted)	178	2	0	180
Nonrandom (not accepted)[a]	87	11	unknown	un-known

[a] Results of an ad hoc survey.

Table 4. CMF compliance in randomized patients - mean actual in percent of target doses by components and treatment groups (January 31, 1988)

Treatment group	C	M	F	CMF	*N*
Control	100.9	101.0	100.2	100.7	92
CMF	92.7	92.4	91.3	92.1	94
tam	97.8	98.2	96.8	97.6	70
CMF+tam	91.0	90.8	89.3	90.3	71

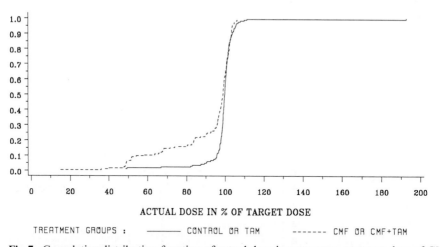

ACTUAL DOSE IN % OF TARGET DOSE

TREATMENT GROUPS :   ——— CONTROL OR TAM   ------- CMF OR CMF+TAM

Fig. 7. Cumulative distribution function of actual dose in percentage to target dose of CMF

At present, we know little about tamoxifen usage during the 2nd year of therapy. Table 5 shows compliance during the 1st year, and we compare the patients randomized to receive tamoxifen plus three further CMF cycles with those to receive tamoxifen only, after completion of initial CMF therapy. Apparently, there is no essential difference between the two arms, and there are few refusers, as should be the case.

Table 5. Tamoxifen compliance in randomized patients – distribution of patients by completeness of therapy during the 1st year and by treatment groups (tam *vs* CMF + tam)

Treatment group	Tamoxifen supposed to be taken in accordance with the protocol			
	Yes (n)	No (n)	Unknown (n)	Total[a] (n)
tam	47	2	12	61
CMF + tam	48	5	12	65
Total	95	7	24	126

[a] Patients who have been under observation for less than 1 year not included.

Discussion

In summary, the trial is running fairly well and seems to address an important question, despite a rather complicated infrastructure comprising so many hospitals scattered all over the country and limited entry rates. However, the everlasting conflict between scientific honesty, the right to patients' determination of treatment and an irrational expectation of an all-knowing physician still raises problems. Nevertheless, the success of our efforts is still questioned as the total numbers of patients realistically expected to be entered in the trial by the year 1990 will fall considerably short of the numbers required to give valid answers to the questions posed. This latter point is mainly due to a regrettable unwillingness of the larger institutions in the FRG to cooperate with the smaller ones. In the second place, the effects of several announcements in the press in 1985 are hard to overcome (Fisher et al. 1985; Consensus Conference 1985). Since then, many clinicians feel pressed to perform limited surgery even in node-positive cases, or to avoid tamoxifen in premenopausal, or not to avoid tamoxifen in postmenopausal receptor-positive women, or the like. In order not to lose more of these potential participants, we have already had to agree to some minor alterations in the protocol.

In conclusion, we only can invite all those who are already involved in or who want to contribute to the dose problem in ajduvant chemotherapy of breast cancer to cooperate with us or even to join the trial.

Appendix A
West German Breast Cancer Study Group

Participants in the study include:
Prof. G. Bastert (chairman), Universitäts-Frauenklinik Heidelberg; Dr. H. Scheurlen (chairman, advisory board), Heidelberg; Prof. K. Hübner (reference pathologist), Frankfurt; Prof. H. Bojar (reference laboratory for hormone receptor assays), Düsseldorf; Prof. H. Schumacher, Mr. M. Olschewski, Mrs. D. Leibbrand, Mr. W. Sauerbrei (methodological center), Freiburg; Dr. R. Neumann, Marienhospital Essen; Prof. H.J. Peiper, Dr. H. Rauschecker, Chirurgische Universitäts-Klinik Göttingen (advisory board); Dr. W. Lenz, Dr. G. Ott, St. Jo-

sef-Hospital Oberhausen; Prof. P. Kopecky, Knappschafts-Krankenhaus Würselen; Dr. J. Pulheim, St. Katharinen-Hospital Frechen; Prof. W. Schmidt, Universitäts-Frauenklinik Homburg; Dr. A. Wilhelm, Dr. M. Hall, Städtisches Krankenhaus München-Neuperlach; Prof. K. v. Maillot, Mrs. R. Kirst, Frauenklinik Aalen; Dr. W. Haisken, Dr. B. Huth, St. Josef-Krankenhaus Essen-Kupferdreh; Prof. H. Mickan, Dr. A. Warecka-Speichermann, Dr. J. Maier, Städtische Krankenanstalten Eßlingen, Dr. H. Bruch, Dr. G. Neuser, Kreiskrankenhaus Groß-Umstadt; Dr. D. Wagner-Kolb, Dr. W. Czopnik, Evangelisches Amalie-Sieveking-Krankenhaus Hamburg; Prof. D. Tenhaeff, Dr. G. Job, Dr. R. Bentler, Kreiskrankenhaus Herford; Prof. G. Rotthoff, Dr. G. Hopf, Städtische Kliniken Kassel; Prof. E. Marx, Dr. J. Uy, St. Antonius-Hospital Kleve; Dr. C. Beyerle (advisory board); Dr. J. Bühler, Kreiskrankenhaus Kronach; Dr. W. Liedtke, Mrs. J. Kroke, Borromäus-Hospital Leer; Dr. O. Brandt, Dr. P. Lehmann, Kreiskrankenhaus Lichtenfels; Dr. F. Peters, Dr. H. Ruppert, St. Hildegardis-Krankenhaus Mainz; Dr. H. Mittelbach, Dr. H. J. Steinbrei, Städtisches Krankenhaus Pirmasens; Dr. H. Wolfart, Dr. B. Stahl, DRK-Krankenhaus Saarlouis; Prof. W. Seidel, Dr. P. Rebsam, Städtisches Krankenhaus Sindelfingen; Prof. Dr. K. Meinen, Dr. D. Mankarella, Dr. A. Fritz, St. Lukas-Klinik Solingen-Ohligs; Prof. V. Zahn, Dr. S. Stahl-Kuschel, Elisabeth-Krankenhaus Straubing; Dr. V. Schwanitz, Dr. B. Heien-Conrads, St. Josef-Krankenhaus Wuppertal; Prof. J. Jaeger, Dr. G. Füchsel, Evangelisches Krankenhaus Mülheim; Dr. K. Decker, Dr. P. Hofmann, Paracelsus-Krankenhaus Ostfildern; Dr. J. Ferstl, Dr. L. Kronpaß, Kreis-Krankenhaus Rotthalmünster; Prof. W. Wiest, Dr. H. Zander, St. Vincenz-Hospital Mainz; Dr. U. Prasser, Dr. A. Köppl (advisory board), St. Josef-Krankenhaus Regensburg; Dr. K. Hördemann, Dr. St. Bartos, St. Martinus-Krankenhaus Langenfeld; Dr. J. W. Holze, Dr. E. Horsch, Verbandskrankenhaus Schwelm; Prof. J. Schnell, Mrs. J. Heinze, St. Franziskus-Hospital Bielefeld; Dr. D. Langnickel, Dr. H. Franz, Zentralkrankenhaus Bremen; Dr. G. Opitz, Dr. W. Gallenmüller, Klinik Dr. Opitz Regensburg; Dr. N. Schöndorf, St. Elisabeth-Krankenhaus Saarlouis; Prof. H. Hennekeuser, Dr. B. Orth, Krankenhaus der Barmherzigen Brüder Trier

References

Bonadonna G, Valagussa P, Rossi A, Tancini G, Brambilla C, Marchini S, Veronesi U (1981) Multimodal therapy with CMF in resectable breast cancer with positive axillary nodes. The Milan Institute expericence. In: Salmon SE, Jones SE (eds) Adjuvant therapy of cancer, vol 3. Grune and Stratton, New York, pp 435–444

Consensus Conference (1985) Adjuvant chemotherapy for breast cancer. JAMA 254: 3461–3463

Eberbach WH (1988) Individual cases and the scientific method – a conflict? In: Scheurlen H, Kay R, Baum M (eds) Cancer clinical trials: a critical appraisal. Springer, Berlin Heidelberg New York Tokyo, pp 185–190 (Recent results in cancer research, vol 111)

Fisher B, Redmond C, Wolmark N, Wieland HS (1981) Disease-free survival at intervals during and following completion of adjuvant chemotherapy: The NSABP experience from three breast cancer protocols. Cancer 48: 1273–1280

Fisher B, Bauer M, Margolese R, Poisson R, Pilch Y, Redmond C, Fisher E, Wolmark N, Deutsch M, Montague E, Saffer E, Wickerham L, Lerner H, Glass A, Shibata H, Deckers P, Ketcham A, Oishi R, Russel I (1985) Five-year results of a randomized clinical trial comparing total mastectomy and segmental mastectomy with or without radiation in the treatment of breast cancer. N Engl J Med 312: 665–673

Nissen-Meyer R (1982) The Scandinavian clinical trials. In: Baum M, Kay R, Scheurlen H (eds) Clinical trials in early breast cancer. Birkhäuser, Basel pp 571–579

Olschewski M, Scheurlen H (1985) Comprehensive cohort study: An alternative to randomized consent design in a breast preservation trial. Methods Inf Med 24: 131–134

Scheurlen H, Schumacher M (1982) Planning breast cancer trials in the Federal Republic of Germany. Statistical Software Newsletter 2: 47–53

Scheurlen H, Olschewski M, Leibbrand D (1984) Zur Methodologie kontrollierter klinischer Studien über die Primärbehandlung des operablen Mammakarzinoms. Strahlentherapie 160: 459–468

Schumacher M, Davis K (1988) Combining randomized and nonrandomized patients in the statistical analysis of a clinical trial. In: Scheurlen H, Kay R, Baum M (eds) Cancer clinical trials: a critical appraisal. Springer, Berlin Heidelberg New York Tokyo, pp 130–137 (Recent results in cancer research, vol 111)

Shackney SE, McCormack GW, Cuchural GJ (1978) Growth rate patterns of solid tumors and their relation to responsiveness to therapy. Ann Intern Med 89: 107–121

Critical Review: Methodology of Adjuvant Trials and Interpretation of Results

R. D. Gelber

Harvard Medical School, Harvard School of Public Health, and Dana-Farber Cancer Institute, Boston, MA, USA

The development of new methodologies is essential in order to obtain reliable information about treatment effects based upon results from clinical investigations. Substantial progress has been made with the acceptance of the large, multicenter, randomized clinical trial as the "gold standard" for establishing comparative treatment efficacy. This is because effects of treatments available today are modest and the course of breast cancer (small yearly risk for relapse, which continues for long periods of follow-up) provides only a small fraction of patients who might benefit. Further advances are required if more rapid progress is to be made for improving the care of patients with breast cancer.

Evaluating a large number of patients is required in order to detect modest treatment effect differences. The results of several trials have been combined here in meta-analyses or overviews to answer questions relating to the impact of post-operative irradiation of the breast on survival, and the reduction in mortality associated with the use of adjuvant systemic therapy (tamoxifen or chemotherapy) (Early Breast Cancer Trialists' Collaborative Group 1988). Meta-analysis has been used in the social sciences for a number of years. Statistical methods for combining the results of several independent investigations have been well developed since the 1950s and relate primarily to issues of the appropriate weights to apply to each of the independent contributions. The methods are those used for a stratified analysis in which the studies themselves are considered as the separate strata. The term "overview" has been recently introduced to distinguish a methodology for combining results which also establishes principles designed to reduce systematic bias as well as random variability. Overviews include only randomized trials, seek to include all relevant trials, consider all subjects as randomized, and accumulate evidence on the basis of comparisons of "like with like." Specifically, relevant trials are all those in which the only difference between two randomized treatment options is the presence of the experimental (or test) therapy in one arm and the absence of this therapy in the other. Treatment effect estimates are based on an "arithmetic construct" which first calculates treatment differences within each trial separately and then accumulates these differences across all trials. By applying these principles, the resulting treatment effect estimates are more precise (based upon large patient numbers) without introducing systematic bias.

Recent Results in Cancer Research, Vol. 115
© Springer-Verlag Berlin · Heidelberg 1989

The most important practical positive contribution of meta-analysis is to focus attention on questions of clinical relevance by putting all available data in front of the clinical investigator. Separate evaluation of individual studies may be misleading by creating the impression of no effect owing to low statistical power, or a positive effect owing to selective reporting of promising results. The lure of large number, however, must not supercede our responsibility to evaluate critically the individual trials which contribute to an overview in order to improve patient care.

The overview presented by Cuzick suggests that patients who received postoperative breast irradiation had a diminished survival exclusively beyond 10 years from randomization. Many of the trials contributing to the overview were conducted several decades ago, raising the question of whether long-term results of therapies which are subject to changing technologies (such as radiation therapy) are applicable to current patient care decisions. The poorer survival is suggested only for patients who were treated 10–30 years ago.

The results described by Peto on the overviews of tamoxifen and chemotherapy are very important in establishing a basis for adjuvant-treated control groups within trials. The initial objective was to test the null hypothesis (no treatment effect) for adjuvant tamoxifen and for adjuvant chemotherapy on overall mortality. The concrete findings are: a) the effects of the therapies are real, but modest, b) the tamoxifen advantage is largest for older women, and c) the chemotherapy advantage is largest for younger women.

The interpretation of results of overviews requires an appreciation of the characteristics of the individual trials that are combined. Features of patient eligibility criteria, nature of the experimental and control therapies, dates of active accrual and follow-up time, and study quality are important. The combination of studies that differ in these aspects may confuse rather than clarify, even if the mathematical criteria of the "arithmetic construct" are satisfied. The overview of studies to evaluate the effect of perioperative chemotherapy (PeCT) provides an example (see Table 1).

Table 1. Perioperative chemotherapy overview: Risk ratio (RR) for first event

Trial	RR	P value
Scandinavian[a]	0.78	0.001
PeCT vs. nil		
CRC[a]	0.83	0.04
PeCT vs. nil		
PeCT + TAM vs. TAM		
Ludwig V (node-positive)[b]	1.06	0.61
PeCT + ConCT vs. ConCT		

PeCT, perioperative chemotherapy; TAM, tamoxifen; ConCT, conventionally timed chemotherapy.

[a] Houghton, data presented at 3rd international conference on adjuvant therapy of primary breast cancer, St. Gallen 1988.

[b] The Ludwig Breast Cancer Study Group 1988.

Each of the three trials satisfies the arithmetic condition requiring PeCT to be the only difference between two randomized treatment groups. The interpretation of the overview value for the magnitude of the effect of PeCT is problematic because the trials are substantially different. Although the PeCT for the first two trials was the same (6 days of cyclophosphamide), the estimate derived from the CRC trial is based on a much shorter follow-up than the Scandinavian trial, which suggests that the estimated risk ratio (RR) might change (showing greater treatment effect) with additional follow-up. Study follow-up time may influence effect size estimates. The Ludwig V trial results presented in Table 1 are for node-positive patients only, all of whom received 6 months of conventionally timed chemotherapy (ConCT) with or without an initial cycle of combination chemotherapy (days 1 and 8, CMF) initiated within 36 h after mastectomy (PeCT). The Ludwig V trial for node-positive patients does not evaluate the effect of PeCT alone versus no adjuvant treatment, but rather investigates the role of very early commencement of adjuvant chemotherapy. Owing to the interaction of treatment effects, it does not make medical sense to include these results in the PeCT overview even if it makes arithmetic sense.

Another new methodological area which was applied to aid the interpretation of data from adjuvant trials involves the aspect of quality of life. While methods for objectively defining the well-being status or impact of various therapies are ongoing, some thoughts about the statistical comparison of periods of time considered by the patient to be of similar quality of life were presented. Certainly these methodologies will develop to incorporate findings from prospective collection of patient self-assessments to balance the burden of symptoms of disease against the subjective toxicity of treatment.

The report by Scheuerlen introduced a vivid reminder of the practical difficulties of conducting clinical research on human subjects where the scientific goals of randomization and focused investigation conflict with the realities of personal prejudice and patient management. It is our obligation to remind the community that advances in clinical cancer research, especially in the field of breast cancer, would have been achieved more rapidly and more precisely had the acceptance of conducting clinical trials been greater. To date, the acceptance of clinical trials is almost exclusively limited to the enthusiasm of receiving the results, while little scientific effort and moral acceptance resulting in a broad-based participation in clinical trials can be observed. Increased participation required to speed progress might be achieved if a clinical trial were considered to be the treatment of choice for the majority of patients with breast cancer.

References

Early Breast Cancer Trialists' Collaborative Group (1988) Effects of adjuvant tamoxifen and of cytotoxic therapy on mortality in early breast cancer: an overview of 61 randomized trials among 28,896 women. N Engl J Med 319: 1681–1692

The Ludwig Breast Cancer Study Group (1988) Combination adjuvant chemotherapy for node-positive breast cancer: inadequacy of a single perioperative cycle. N Engl J Med 319: 677–683

Quality of Life: Psychological Aspects of Adjuvant Therapy of Breast Cancer

Adjuvant Therapies in Breast Cancer and Quality of Life: A Critical Review of the TWiST Concept

K. W. Brunner

Institut für Medizinische Onkologie, Inselspital, Universität Bern, 3010 Bern, Switzerland

The conventional end points of any curative cancer treatment are disease- and re-currence-free survival and overall long-term survival. It is customary to assume that any increase in the number of cured patients at 5 or 10 years justifies and compensates for all early and late side effects of treatment, not only for the cured but also for the unsuccessfully treated patients. Quality of life assessments rarely influence the evaluation of truly curative therapies.

The conventional end points for the assessment of adjuvant chemotherapy are essentially the same as for curative treatment because the final aim of adjuvant therapy is an increase in cure rates. However, more than 15 years of clinical re-search in this area have demonstrated that the truly curative effects of adjuvant chemotherapy in breast cancer are marginal and possibly limited to small sub-groups. The main effect is on disease-free survival and much less, if at all, on over-all survival and definitive cure rates.

If adjuvant chemotherapy preponderantly increases life spent without recurrent and symptomatic disease but not the cure rate, then such treatment approaches palliative chemotherapy, and considerations which are relevant in palliative chemotherapy and relate to the quality of life become important. The main ques-tion in palliative chemotherapy is whether palliation of disease symptoms and time without tumor progression outweighs the toxic side effects of treatment and to what extent (Brunner 1987). Analogously, in adjuvant chemotherapy of breast cancer with a very limited curative potential the question arises of whether the prolongation of the time spent without symptoms of recurrent disease for a limited number of patients compensates for the toxic side effects of all treated patients, in-cluding those who are unsuccessfully and those who are unnecessarily treated.

The assessment of toxicity and cost-benefit ratios which are quality-of-life oriented become less and less important, the higher the curative potential of a can-cer treatment is. Short-term toxic side effects are then of little concern, and only long-term sequelae of treatment have to be considered. On the other hand, the less effective a cancer treatment is, the more important are the short-term toxic side ef-fects and the question of their acceptability in relation to the treatment result. Late toxic events such as second neoplasias and infertility can be largely neglected. These relations are demonstrated in Fig. 1.

Recent Results in Cancer Research, Vol. 115
© Springer-Verlag Berlin·Heidelberg 1989

Intent of treatment	Intensity of treatment	Acceptable short-term treatment toxicity	Acceptable long-term treatment toxicity	Quality of life considerations during treatment
1. Curative CT	+ + +			Of secondary importance
2. Curative adjuvant CT	+ + +			Dependant upon additional numbers of cures or DFS
3. Palliative CT with prolongation of life	+ +			Of primary importance
4. Limited palliative effects of CT	+			The only important consideration

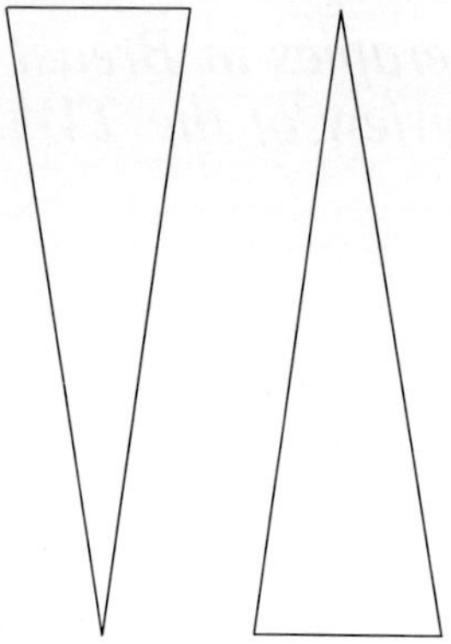

Fig. 1. Acceptable early and late treatment toxicities in relation to intent of treatment. *CT*, chemotherapy; *DFS*, disease-free survival

The problems of assessments of adjuvant chemotherapy which are quality-of-life oriented are demonstrated more specifically in Fig. 2. Assuming that in a randomized study with 200 patients, 48 of 100 treated and 60 of 100 untreated patients have a recurrence at 5 years, then the recurrence rate is decreased by 20%. The number of patients who are disease free at 5 years is increased by 30% due to the additional 12 treated patients who did not have a recurrence. If we try to evaluate the real cost-benefit ratio of such a result, which is close to reality in the adjuvant chemotherapy of breast cancer, two assessments have to be made. Firts, we have to assess whether the longer life span without symptoms of recurrent disease for the 12 successfully treated patients compensates for their loss in quality of life during the 6–12 months of toxic adjuvant chemotherapy. The second assessment is more difficult: Does the gain for the 12 successfully treated patients outweigh the loss in quality of life in the 48 unsuccessfully and in the 40 unnecessarily treated patients?

This leads us immediately to the basic problems involved in the assessment of quality of life. Firstly, we have no absolute or direct way of measuring and comparing the quality of life of different groups of patients. Secondly, even in relative terms it is impossible to weigh the gain in quality of life of one group (the 12 successfully treated patients) against the loss of another group (the 88 unsuccessfully and unnecessarily treated patients). Any attempt to make such a comparison on a statistical basis seems artificial and questionable because it cannot replace the subjective and ethical judgment which is involved in such a comparison. It may be possible to compare the losses in terms of toxic side effects with the gains in terms of additional time without symptoms of disease in the same group of patients, but comparing the losses of one group with the gains in another group is an entirely different matter.

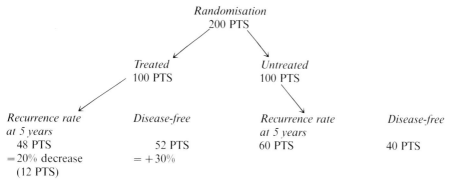

1st assessment: coast-benefit ratio for the 12 successfully treated patients
2nd assessment: coast-benefit ratio of 48 unsuccessfully and 40 unnecessarily treated patients versus the 12 successfully treated patients

Fig. 2. Problems of quality-of-life oriented assessment of adjuvant chemotherapy

Thirdly, comparative assessment of quality of life is in itself a difficult and methodologically unsolved problem. It involves quantification of an essentially qualitative attribute (Coates et al. 1983; Spitzer et al. 1981). It can only be done by measuring and comparing factors which are normally, but not necessarily always correlated with quality of life. Such indirect factors are tumor regression or time spent without tumor progression and without symptoms of disease and time spent without toxic side effects of treatment (TWiST – time without symptoms and toxicity). From these factors, evaluated by the physician or by the patient, it is possible to construct a disease- and therapy-related index, which may be correlated to the quality of life for this group (Brunner 1987; Coates et al. 1987).

Gelber and Goldhirsch (1986) have proposed a different model for an assessment of adjuvant chemotherapy in breast cancer which is quality-of-life oriented. They correct the projected individual and collective survival times by time deductions for subjective toxic side effects during adjuvant treatment, for local recurrence or contralateral breast cancer and for the life span with recurrent metastatic disease (TWiST). Each month with subjective toxicity of any form or intensity is subtracted from projected survival. For local recurrence or contralateral breast cancer, a uniform 3-month period is deducted, with the assumption that 3 months are needed to re-establish a normal life after local treatment. For distant metastases, originally all time spent with metastatic disease was deducted from projected survival. More recently, the authors have corrected this projection and calculate their model under the assumption, that patients with distant metastases are statistically not counted as not living but as 50% alive. The cumulative distribution of TWiST is calculated according to the Kaplan-Meier method, based on the amount of TWiST that each patient in the treated or untreated group accumulates after mastectomy. The comparison of cumulative TWiST in both groups demonstrates, that with the assumptions described above, early losses in "valuable" life span due to toxicity in the treated group are more than compensated for later on (after 3–4 years) by a longer life span without symptomatic metastatic disease. Furthermore, the model demonstrates that, under the assumptions made, the gain in the treated group is much more impressive than the difference in crude overall survival would suggest.

The model of TWiST is a unique and interesting attempt at defining a new end point for the evaluation of adjuvant chemotherapy. But it is doubtful whether the model reflects a more realistic or truly quality-of-life oriented assessment of adjuvant therapies or whether it has any advantage over objective evaluation based on differences in disease-free and overall survival alone. The reasons are the following:

1. Time deductions from survival in the TWiST model are arbitrary, uniform, and not really quality-of-life oriented.
2. Total or even 50% deduction of survival time spent with metastatic disease is also arbitrary and is not based on any data on the quantity or quality of symptoms during metastatic disease.
3. The model is a construction, designed in such a way that it automatically determines a certain outcome. It is an interesting computer model which demonstrates how certain assumptions statistically modify conventional survival curves.
4. The model obscures rather than clarifies the basic problem of how gains in valuable life for a small group of patients can be weighed against toxicity-related losses in the quality of life of unsuccessfully or unnecessarily treated patients. This basic problem cannot be solved by statistical manipulations. It probably remains a matter of more or less well-informed subjective judgment.

The next obvious question is: Can we improve the TWiST model or find a better quality-of-life-based assessment of the limited effects of adjuvant chemotherapy in breast cancer?

The model could certainly be improved by more realistic and individually adapted time deductions for different degrees of toxic side effects and for disease symptoms during the life span with distant metastases. This would enable the model to compare not only no treatment, hormonal treatment, and chemotherapy, but also different chemotherapies, a comparison which is not possible with arbitrary assumptions. In fact, it seems more important to be able to differentiate between the effects of various intensities and durations of chemotherapy than between a treated and an untreated group. The TWiST model is too coarse a tool for such assessments.

A truly quality-of-life-oriented assessment of adjuvant chemotherapy would also have to include linear analogue self-assessments of the patients concerning their physical well-being, mood, subjective toxicity of adjuvant treatment, and disease symptoms during local recurrence or metastatic disease. A move in this direction has been made in the International Breast Cancer Trials VI and VII. These studies are accompanied by quality-of-life questionnaires to be filled out by the patients within 4 weeks of surgery and every 3 months there-after. The information gained from these studies may put us in a better position to truly assess the impact of adjuvant chemotherapy on the patients quality of life.

References

Brunner KW (1987) Evaluation criteria in comparative clinical trials in advanced breast cancer: a proposal for improvement. In: Cavalli F (ed) Endocrine therapy of breast cancer II. Springer, Berlin Heidelberg New York Tokyo, p 45

Coates AS for the Australian-New Zealand Breast Cancer Trials Group (1987) Improving the quality of life during chemotherapy for advanced breast cancer. N Engl J Med 317: 1490–1495

Coates AS, Fischer Dillenbeck C, McNeil DR, et al. (1983) On the receiving end. II. Linear analogue self-assessment (LASA) in evaluation of aspects of the quality of life of cancer patients receiving therapy. Eur J Cancer Clin Oncol 19: 1633–1637

Gelber RD, Goldhirsch A (1986) A new endpoint for the assessment of adjuvant therapy in postmenopausal women with operable breast cancer. J Clin Oncol 4: 1722–1779

Spitzer WO, Dobson AJ, Hall J, et al. (1981) Measuring the quality of life of cancer patients: a concise QL-index for use by physicians. J Chronic Dis 34: 585–597

Rehabilitation of Patients with Primary Breast Cancer: Assessing the Impact of Adjuvant Therapy*

P. A. Ganz, M. L. Polinsky, C. A. C. Schag, and R. L. Heinrich

Departments of Medicine and Psychiatry, UCLA-San Fernando Valley Program, VAMC, Sepulveda, CA 91343, USA
and the Division of Cancer Control, Jonsson Comprehensive Cancer Center, UCLA, Los Angeles, CA 90024, USA

Introduction

During the past decade, the primary treatment of breast cancer has become increasingly complex owing to the use of radiation therapy as an alternative to mastectomy (Fisher et al. 1985; Veronesi et al. 1981) and the more extensive use of adjuvant chemotherapy and adjuvant hormonal therapy (Bonadonna and Valagussa 1987; Lippman 1986, Report from the Breast Cancer Trials Committee 1987). With these changes in primary therapy has come increased participation of the patient in treatment decisions, frequently intensifying the psychologic difficulties she must face (Holland and Rowland 1987; Sinsheimer and Holland 1987). Primary therapy is often protracted and no longer ends with the initial surgery, but continues for an additional 2–3 months if breast conservation therapy is used, with further extension of the period of initial treatment from months to years if adjuvant therapy is used. In addition, adjuvant therapy is now being extended to a larger segment of the population with breast cancer (e.g., treatment of node-negative patients) (Report from the Breast Cancer Trials Committee 1987; Bonadonna et al. 1986). Breast cancer patients currently face a wide range of physical, psychosocial, and economic problems as a consequence of these events.

The 1985 NIH Consensus Conference on Adjuvant Therapy of Breast Cancer made a number of specific recommendations about the adjuvant treatment of breast cancer (Lippman 1986). In addition, the conference participants suggested that there be systematic evaluation of the psychological, social, and economic consequences of adjuvant therapy (Lippman 1986). In spite of the widespread utilization of adjuvant chemotherapy in this common disease, very few studies have examined the nonmedical problems which patients experience as a result of this treatment (Meyerowitz et al. 1979, 1983; Knobf 1986; Cassileth et al. 1986; Taylor et al. 1985; Maguire et al. 1980).

Most of these studies have been cross-sectional and retrospective, but nevertheless they begin to examine the impact of adjuvant therapy on women's lives.

* Supported by grant no. CA 43461 from the National Institues of Health/National Cancer Institute.

Knowledge of the range and frequency of problems which patients experience is crucial for successful patient education, as well as for the development of interventions to modify the negative sequelae of adjuvant therapy. This is becoming particularly important, as the population of patients receiving adjuvant therapy is expanding (Report from the Breast Cancer Trials Committee 1987; Bonadonna et al. 1986).

During the past 4 years, we have been prospectively evaluating the rehabilitation needs of newly diagnosed breast cancer patients during the 1st year after primary treatment. This has been accomplished using a combination of structured interviews as well as expert and patient-rated standardized instruments (Ganz et al. 1986, 1988). In a previous paper, we explored potential differences in rehabilitation needs in relation to the type of surgical procedure used (Ganz et al. 1988). For a wide range of physical and psychologic problems, we did not find any major differences between patients undergoing mastectomy and patients receiving segmental resection and radiation therapy. However, the mastectomy patients experienced more difficulty with clothing and body image, and the patients receiving primary radiation had more disruption of their social and recreational activities as a result of the protracted course of primary treatment. Our data suggest that there is a broad spectrum of rehabilitation needs common to all breast cancer patients independent of the primary surgical treatment modality.

In order to extend these observations, we now examine the impact of adjuvant therapy in our current sample of patients with breast cancer. We have found that patients receiving adjuvant therapy report a frequency and range of physical and constitutional problems similar to those who are not receiving adjuvant therapy. However, the adjuvant group reports more frequent psychologic concerns, treatment-related problems, problems interacting with the health care setting, and vocational and economic concerns. These findings suggest that adjuvant therapy has an impact the rehabilitation and recovery process of newly diagnosed breast cancer patients which is independent of the experience of the cancer diagnosis and primary surgical treatment.

Materials and Methods

Subjects

This report describes our findings in 50 patients who were evaluated between May 20, 1987, and January 7, 1988. Study entry criteria included the following: all patients were English speaking, had stage I or II breast cancer at diagnosis, did not have a history of major psychiatric illness, did not have other disabling noncancer illnesses, and lived within the geographic area (Los Angeles County, California). Patients were selected from the surgical practices of the full-time and voluntary faculty of the UCLA School of Medicine as well as from a number of community physicians and health maintenance organizations. Permission to approach the patient was obtained from the physician, and then the research study was explained to the patient. Consenting patients agreed to participate in four interviews during the year following diagnosis. This paper describes information obtained from the first interview.

Procedures and Instruments

Initial interviews with all subjects were conducted between 3 and 5 weeks after their primary cancer surgery. The interviews were comprehensive, structured, and reviewed a broad range of rehabilitation needs. The details of the interview procedure are described fully elsewhere (Ganz et al. 1986, 1988). At the end of each interview, a specific problem list was coded for each subject using an existing comprehensive list of rehabilitation problems. A severity rating was determined for each problem using a four-point scale with 1 representing "a little" and 4 representing "very much." The severity rating was a combination of the patient's self-report and the clinical judgment of the interviewers.

Each subject also completed several standardized instruments including the Profile of Mood States (POMS) (McNair et al. 1971), a 65-item, Likert scale measure of affective states which has been widely used with cancer patients (Cassileth et al. 1985); the Functional Living Index-Cancer (FLIC) (Schipper et al. 1984), a 22-item visual-analogue scale with Likert format; and a single visual-analogue scale rating the quality of life before cancer and currently (Gough et al. 1983). The clinicians conducting the interview rated the Karnofsky Performance Status (KPS) (Karnofsky and Burchenal 1949), which is an established measure of functional performance used in oncologic practice, and the Global Adjustment to Illness Scale (GAIS) (Morrow et al. 1981), which is a single global rating scale designed to record the judgment of a trained clinical observer concerning the psychosocial adjustment of patients to a medical illness.

Data Analysis

Descriptive statistics were used to evaluate the medical and demographic characteristics of the study sample. The coded interview problem lists served as the main source of data for this paper. The severity code of each problem was not utilized in these analyses. Rather, the codes were dichotomized to indicate the presence or absence of a problem. As a first step, the number of subjects with each problem was calculated for the entire group of subjects. Then the most frequently occurring problems (where greater than 40% of the sample reported the problem) were examined according to whether or not adjuvant therapy was being received. A two-sided T-test was used to test for differences in the age distribution of the adjuvant and nonadjuvant therapy groups. Other statistical tests of significance were not performed because of the small sample size and exploratory nature of the study.

Results

Medical and Demographic Characteristics of the Sample

The medical characteristics of the study sample are shown in Table 1. Slightly more than two-thirds of the sample had undergone modified radical mastectomy, and these subjects were equally distributed between the nonadjuvant and adjuvant

Table 1. Medical characteristics

	No treatment (n=30)		Adjuvant therapy (n=20)	
	(n)	*(%)*	*(n)*	*(%)*
Type of Surgery				
MRM	19	63.3	14	70
SM	11	37.7	6	30
Nodal Status				
+nodes	1	3	13	65
−nodes	29	96.7	7	35
Type of therapy				
Chemotherapy	0		11	55
Tamoxifen	0		11	55
Radiation	4	13.3	5	25

MRM, modified radical mastectomy; SM, segmental mastectomy with axillary dissection.

therapy groups. As would be predicted, almost all of the subjects in the nonadjuvant therapy group had negative nodes, while 65% of the adjuvant group had positive nodes. The interviews were conducted an average of 32 days after primary surgery (range, 23–43 days), and at the time of interview only half of the subjects receiving a segmental mastectomy had begun their planned primary radiation therapy. All subjects had undergone axillary node dissection as part of the primary surgical treatment. Of the adjuvant therapy group 55% were receiving chemotherapy and 55% were receiving tamoxifen. Cyclophosphamide-methotrexate-5-fluorouracil (CMF) was the adjuvant chemotherapy regimen used in the vast majority of subjects, with only a few individuals receiving a regimen containing doxorubicin.

The age range for the two groups of subjects was similar, but the mean age of the adjuvant therapy group was nearly a decade younger ($P=0.017$). Other demographic characteristics, including marital status, educational background, family income, and employment status at the time of cancer diagnosis, were similar (Table 2). The sample was largely white (87.5%) with a similar distribution of religious affiliation between the two groups.

Rehabilitation Problems Identified in the Interview

As in our previous study (Ganz et al. 1988), physical and psychologic problems were the most frequently reported rehabilitation concerns described by these subjects (Fig. 1). There was little difference between the two groups of subjects in the area of physical and constitutional problems, and they reported a range and frequency of problems which are similar to our previous sample (Ganz et al. 1988).

In contrast, for psychologic problems the adjuvant group reported more frequent difficulty than the nonadjuvant group, including more frequent reports of

Table 2. Demographic characteristics

	No treatment (n=30)		Adjuvant therapy (n=20)	
Mean age (range) in years	59 (37–77)		51 (33–73)	
	(n)	(%)	*(n)*	(%)
Marital Status				
Single	3	10	1	5
Married	19	63.3	13	65
Divorced/separated	2	6.7	2	10
Widowed	6	20	4	20
Education				
Doctorate	2	6.7	0	
Masters	4	13.3	1	5
College degree	8	26.6	7	35
Partial college	7	23.4	8	40
High school or less	9	30	4	20
Income[a]				
$ 0–$ 15 000	3	10	4	20
$ 15 001–$ 30 000	6	20	2	10
$ 30 001–$ 45 000	6	20	4	20
$ 45 001–$ 60 000	2	6.7	2	20
Over $ 60 000	11	36.7	6	30
Employment status[b]				
Working	17	56.7	13	65
Volunteer	4	13.3	5	25
Retired	4	13.3	0	
Homemaker	3	10	2	10
Unemployed	2	6.7	0	

[a] Two subjects in each group did not wish to report income.
[b] Before cancer diagnosis.

worry about recurrence, anxiety, depression, anger, and being overwhelmed by emotions regarding the cancer (Fig. 2).

As might be anticipated, the adjuvant therapy group also reported a wide range of treatment-related problems which were infrequently reported by the nonadjuvant therapy group (Fig. 3). Of the adjuvant therapy group 55% reported nausea and vomiting associated with treatments, while none of the nonadjuvant group did so. Nausea and vomiting were universal findings for the subgroup of the adjuvant sample who were receiving chemotherapy as their adjuvant treatment. Of the adjuvant therapy group, 80% worried about whether their treatment(s) would be successful (treatments included surgery, radiation, and adjuvant therapy), in contrast to only 37% of the nonadjuvant group. Also, a slightly higher incidence of difficulty in interactions in the health care setting was reported by the adjuvant therapy group than the nonadjuvant group (Fig. 4), including more anxiety while waiting for the results of diagnostic tests, more difficulty communicating with doctors and nurses, and more anxiety while having diagnostic tests performed. In spite of very similar socioeconomic backgrounds (except age), the subjects receiving adju-

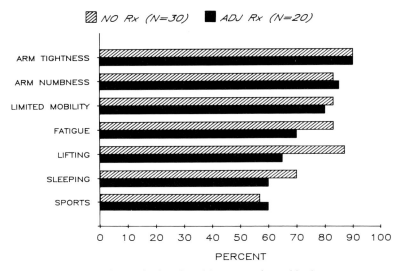

Fig. 1. Most frequent physical and constitutional problems experienced by breast cancer patients 1 month after primary surgery. There is little difference between the nonadjuvant and adjuvant therapy groups

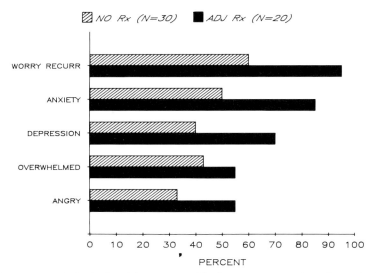

Fig. 2. Most frequent psychological problems reported by breast cancer patients 1 month after primary surgery. The adjuvant therapy group reports more frequent difficulty with all of these problems

vant therapy more frequently reported concern about the financial impact of the cancer diagnosis and had less information about their health insurance benefits than the nonadjuvant therapy group (Fig. 5). Both groups frequently expressed concern about their job performance and ability to work, with about one-fifth of each group reporting difficulty communicating with their boss and coworkers about the disease and its treatment.

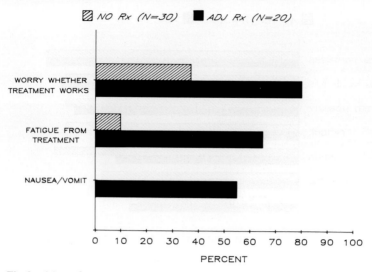

Fig. 3. Most frequent treatment-related problems reported by breast cancer patients 1 month after primary surgery. The adjuvant therapy group reports more frequent difficulty with all of these problems. None of the nonadjuvant therapy group experienced nausea or vomiting

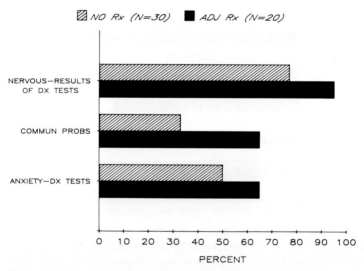

Fig. 4. Most frequent problems related to interacting with the health care setting reported by breast cancer patients 1 month after primary surgery. The adjuvant therapy group reported more frequent difficulties with all problems, especially with communication with doctors and nurses

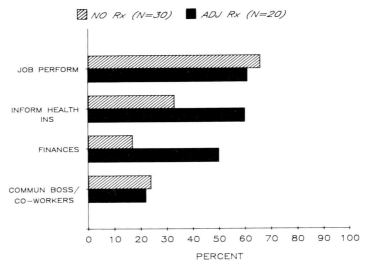

Fig. 5. Most frequent vocational and economic concerns reported by breast cancer patients 1 month after primary surgery. Both groups are frequently concerned about their job performance and ability to work, as well as communication with boss and coworkers. More of the adjuvant therapy group report lack of information about health insurance benefits and concern about the financial impact of their cancer treatment

Evaluation Using Independent Measures

The clinician-rated instruments (KPS and GAIS) detected little difference between the two treatment groups. The mean KPS for the no treatment group was 87 and for the adjuvant group was 84.5, suggesting that both groups had a relatively high performance status even at only 1 month after surgery and although they had begun postoperative treatment with radiation and adjuvant therapy. Likewise, the GAIS scores showed on average a fairly high level of adjustment for both groups with a mean score of 84.8 for the no-treatment group (range, 70-95) and a mean score of 80.6 for the adjuvant therapy group (range, 55-95). The samples are too small at this juncture to assess whether these differences are significant.

The average total mood disturbance score on the POMS for the no-treatment group was quite low (Table 3) in contrast to the score for the adjuvant therapy group. All of the subscales of the POMS were higher (showing more distress) for the adjuvant therapy group, except for the vigor scale in which a higher score reflects less disturbance. The vigor score for the adjuvant group was lower than the no-therapy group. The sample size is small, with a large standard deviation which prevents us from making a statement about statistical significance.

Both groups reported a similar quality of life before cancer on the linear analogue scale (78.3 for no treatment and 79.4 for adjuvant treatment), but their assessment of quality of life after cancer differed, with the no-treatment group reporting a mean score of 72.4 versus 67.2 for the adjuvant group. Total score on the FLIC was higher on average (indicating a better quality of life) for the no-treatment group than for the adjuvant group (120.6 versus 114.1). Examination of the

Table 3. Profile of mood states (POMS) mean scores

	No treatment (n=30)	Adjuvant therapy (n=19)
Total mood disturbance (Standard Deviation)	10.87 (31.16)	21.89 (35.06)
Tension	7.77	10.32
Depression	5.37	8.21
Fatigue	7.40	7.42
Anger	3.67	5.00
Vigor	18.73	16.16
Confusion	5.40	7.11

individual FLIC items revealed minimal differences in response except on three items: maintenance of usual recreation and leisure activities, nausea affecting daily functioning, and nausea during the past 2 weeks. These response differences might have been more striking if the adjuvant sample had included only those receiving chemotherapy.

Discussion

Our findings in this exploratory study are consistent with the reports of other authors and emphasize the differential impact of adjuvant therapy in comparison with a concurrent sample of breast cancer patients who were not receiving any adjuvant therapy. The descriptive findings from our interview problem lists and the scores from the POMS suggest increased psychological distress in the adjuvant therapy group. In addition to the increased psychologic difficulties, patients receiving adjuvant therapy also reported increased difficulty with treatment-related problems, interacting with the health care setting, vocational and economic concerns. These findings are consistent with results reported by others (Meyerowitz et al. 1979, 1983; Knobf 1986; Cassileth et al. 1986; Taylor et al. 1985; Maguire et al. 1980), but in addition explore some issues not previously investigated.

The small size of the adjuvant sample (n=20) at this time prohibits evaluation of the contribution of the physical toxicity from chemotherapy to the increased psychologic distress which these patients reported, since only roughly half of the adjuvant group was receiving chemotherapy. The adjuvant group may be experiencing more psychologic distress as a result of the knowledge of their more guarded prognosis. This could be potentiated by increased contact with physicians and visits to an oncologist's office where patients with more advanced cancer are being treated. Another possible explanation for our observation of increased psychologic distress in the adjuvant group is that on average, the patients who were receiving adjuvant therapy were younger. We and others have previously shown that elderly subjects frequently exhibit less psychologic distress than younger subjects with cancer (Ganz et al. 1985; Cassileth et al. 1984). We intend to explore the contribution of the type of adjuvant therapy and the impact of age on psychologic distress in much greater detail when we reach our target study sample of

350–400 patients who will be followed prospectively during the year following breast cancer diagnosis.

Our preliminary findings suggest that adjuvant therapy has a negative impact on quality of life as early as 1 month after primary surgery, as measured by the FLIC and the simple visual analogue scale. It is premature to determine how significant and long-lasting the impact may be; however, both Meyerowitz (1983) and Knobf (1986) found residual problems in their samples of subjects who were evaluated many months after the cessation of adjuvant chemotherapy. Certainly, the acute or long-term problems associated with adjuvant therapy may be worthwhile enduring if there is prolonged disease-free and overall survival, as suggested by Gelber and Goldhirsch (1986). Therefore, it is important that the physical, psychosocial, and economic problems associated with adjuvant therapy of breast cancer be identified and potentially modified in an attempt to diminish the negative impact on the quality of life for these cancer survivors.

In conclusion, we have found that patients undergoing primary treatment for breast cancer frequently experience a variety of physical and constitutional problems in relation to their initial surgery, irrespective of whether or not adjuvant therapy is given. However, patients receiving adjuvant therapy report more psychologic distress and mood disturbance, as well as more treatment-related, vocational, and economic problems. Two self-report measures of quality of life suggest that, as early as 1 month after breast cancer surgery, patients who receive adjuvant therapy have a poorer quality of life than those who do not. The increased psychologic distress which the adjuvant therapy group exhibits suggests that they are a high-risk subset of patients for whom early intervention is appropriate. These findings must be taken into account when designing interventions for patients receiving primary treatment for breast cancer.

*Acknowledgements.*The authors wish to achnowledge the contribution of the following individuals to this research effort: Helen Cheng, Carol Fred, Christy Harman, and Barbara Kahn. Without them, this work would not have been completed. In addition, we are grateful to the following physicians who have allowed and encouraged their patients to participate in this research study: Drs. George Bisharat, Frederick Eilber, Marjorie Fine, Armando Giuliano, Gracia Goade, Douglass Harwood, Jonathan Hiatt, James Huth, Stephen Kuchenbecker, Donald Morton, Bernhard Penner, Norman Rubaum, Lawrence Schecter, Ivan Shulman, and David Sievers.

References

Bonadonna G, Valagussa P (1987) Current status of adjuvant therapy for breast cancer. Semin Oncol 14: 8–22

Bonadonna G, Zambetti M, Valagussa P, et al. (1986) Adjuvant CMF in node negative breast cancer. Proc Am Soc Clin Onc 5: 74

Cassileth BR, Lusk EJ, Strouse TB, et al. (1984) Psychosocial status in chronic illness: A comparative analysis of six diagnostic groups. N Engl J Med 311: 506–511

Cassileth BR, Lusk EJ, Brown LL et al. (1985) Psychosocial status of cancer patients and next of kin: Normative data from the profile of mood states. J Psychosocial Oncol 3: 99–105

Cassileth BR, Knuiman MW, Abeloff MD et al. (1986) Anxiety levels in patients random-ized to adjuvant therapy versus observation for early breast cancer. J Clin Oncol 4: 972–974

Fisher B, Bauer M, Margolese M, et al. (1985) Five years of a randomized trial comparing total mastectomy and segmental mastectomy with or without radiation in the treatment of breast cancer. N Engl J Med 312: 665–673

Ganz PA, Schag CC, Heinrich RL (1985) The psychosocial impact of cancer on the elderly: A comparison with younger patients. J Am Geriatr Soc 33: 429–435

Ganz PA, Rofessart J, Polinsky ML, et al. (1986) A comprehensive approach to the assess-ment of cancer patients' rehabilitation needs. J Psychosocial Oncol 4: 27–42

Ganz PA, Schag CC, Polinsky ML, et al. (1988) Rehabilitation needs and breast cancer: The first month after primary therapy. Breast Cancer Res Treat 10: 243–253

Gelber RD, Goldhirsch A (1986) A new endpoint for the assessment of adjuvant therapy in postmenopausal women with operable breast cancer. J Clin Oncol 4: 1772–1779

Gough IR, Furnival CM, Schilder L, et al. (1983) Assessment of the quality of life of pa-tients with advanced cancer. Eur J Cancer Clin Oncol 19: 1161–1165

Holland JC, Rowland JH (1987) Psychological reactions to breast cancer and its treatment. In: Harris JR, Hellman S, Henderson IC, Kinne DW (eds) Breast diseases. Lippincott, Philadelphia, pp 632–647

Karnofsky DA, Burchenal JH (1949) The evaluation of chemotherapy agents in cancer. In: MacCleod CM (ed) Evaluation of chemotherapeutic agents. Columbia University Press, New York, pp 199–205

Knobf MT (1986) Physical and psychological distress associated with adjuvant chemothera-py in women with breast cancer. J Clin Oncol 4: 678–684

Lippman ME (1986) National Institutes of Health Consensus development conference on adjuvant chemotherapy and endocrine therapy for breast cancer. NIH publication no. 86–2860, Department of Health and Human Services, U.S. Government Printing Office, Washington, DC

Maguire GP, Tait A, Brooke M, et al. (1980) Psychiatric morbidity and physical toxicity as-sociated with adjuvant chemotherapy after mastectomy. Br Med J 281: 1179–80

McNair DM, Lorr M, Droppleman LF (1971) EITS manual for the profile of mood states. Educational and Industrial Testing Service, San Diego

Meyerowitz BE, Sparks FC, Spears IK (1979) Adjuvant chemotherapy for breast carcino-ma: psychosocial implications. Cancer 43: 1613–1618

Meyerowitz BE, Watkins IK, Sparks FC (1983) Psychosocial implications of adjuvant chemotherapy: a two-year follow-up study. Cancer 52: 1541–1545

Morrow GR, Feldstein M, et al. (1981) Development of brief measures of psychosocial ad-justment to medical illness applied to cancer patients. Gen Hosp Psychiatry 3: 79–88

Report from the Breast Cancer Trials Committee, Scottish Cancer Trials Office (MRC), Ed-inburgh (1987) Adjuvant tamoxifen in the management of operable breast cancer: the Scottish trial. Lacet ii: 171–175

Schipper H, Clinch J, McMurray A, et al. (1984) Measuring the quality of life of cancer pa-tients: the functional living index-cancer: development and validation. J Clin Oncol 2: 472–483

Sinsheimer L, Holland JC (1987) Psychological issues in breast cancer. Semin Oncol 14: 75–82

Taylor SE, Lichtman RR, Wood JV, et al. (1985) Illness-related and treatment-related factors in psychological adjustment to breast cancer. Cancer 55: 2506–2513

Veronesi U, Saccozzi R, Del Vecchio M, et al. (1981) Comparing radical mastectomy with quandrantectomy, axillary dissection, and radiotherapy in patients with small cancers of the breast. N Engl J Med 305: 6–11

Coping and Survival in Patients with Primary Breast Cancer: A Critical Analysis of Current Research Strategies and Proposal of a New Approach Integrating Biomedical, Psychological, and Social Variables

C. Hürny[1] and J. Bernhard[2]

[1] Medizinische Abteilung Lory, Inselspital, 3010 Bern, Switzerland
[2] Schweizerische Arbeitsgruppe für klinische Krebsforschung SAKK, Seidenweg 63, 3012 Bern, Switzerland

Introduction

From a theoretical point of view, it is relatively unlikely that the prognosis of breast cancer is defined exclusively by biomedical factors. Although breast cancer is usually a slow-growing neoplasia, outcome in individual patients may vary considerably. The disease-free survival time (DFS) after primary treatment ranges from several months to over 30 years. Not all of the variance can be explained by well-documented biological prognostic factors such as the size of the primary tumor, nodal status, and menopausal status, nor by less well-established factors such as estrogen and progesterone receptor status, histologic grading, locally metastatic intraductal tumors, oncogene amplifiers, aneuploidy or tumor growth rate as assessed by DNA flow cytometry (McGuire, this volume; Harris, this volume).

Interaction Between Environment and Psychological and Biological Systems

In the last 20 years, a variety of interaction and feedback mechanisms between environmental events, psychological reactions, emotional states, and the central nervous, immune, and endocrine systems have been detected (Fig. 1, p. 263). It is well documented that illness or loss of partner, divorce, marital problems, umemployment, and the stress of taking examinations is followed by the impairment of cell-mediated immune functions, sometimes of considerable duration (Kiecolt-Glaser et al. 1987a, 1987b; Irwin and Risch 1987; Arnetz et al. 1987; Schleifer et al. 1983; Locke et al. 1984). It has also been shown in animal models that immunosuppression can be elicited as a conditioned response (Ader and Cohen 1975). Lymphocytes are known to have receptors for different hormones and neuropeptides (Lippman et al. 1973; Lesniak et al. 1973; Krug et al. 1972; Bourne et al. 1974; Hadden et al. 1970). The effects of hormone levels on mood are well known, such as in premenstrual or menopausal syndromes, in steroid-induced depression or psychosis, or in anxiety states in hyperthyroidism. The growth of some breast cancers is hormone dependent, as we know mainly from antiestrogen treatment. There is also some evidence of interaction between biological vulnerability to disease and social environment. Almost every disease is more frequent in the lower socioeconomic groups (Jenkins et al. 1983). In virtually every primary cancer, survival is significantly better in patients with high as compared with low socioeconomic status (Vågerö and Persson 1987; Berg et al. 1977; Linden 1969; Lipworth et al. 1970). Therefore, breast cancer must be considered a biopsychosocial problem. As of today, the biomedical aspects of the disease have been studied extensively and with only moderate success in terms of changing the natural history of the disease for the better. In recent years, psychological and social aspects of the disease have been of growing scientific interest.

The Coping Process and Its Assessment

The diagnosis of breast cancer is one of the most stressful events a women can experience. The treatment modalities she may have to undergo, be it mutilating surgery, radiation, and/or chemotherapy, are a considerable burden she will have to bear. For her ultimate psychosocial adaptation, the importance of the way she reacts to and copes with the disease is evident. Coping is a process, not a single event. Coping strategies may change over time. Different authors have defined different periods of the illness in relation to the coping process. The most subtle one was proposed by Schain (1976), of which an apdated version is summarized below:

1. Previous biographically defined fears about breast cancer
2. Detection of irregularities and/or a lump in the breast
3. Medical work-up
4. Biopsy/diagnosis
5. Actual modified radical mastectomy, lumpectomy, or other primary treatment
6. Early postmastectomy at the hospital
7. Convalescence after hospital discharge, rehabilitation
8. Adjuvant treatments
9. Social reintegration
10. Reconstructive breast surgery
11. Relapse, local and/or distant metastases
12. Cytotoxic/radiation therapy
13. Treatment success/failure
14. Dying and death

The diversity of situations occurring during a long and usually slowly evolving disease process most likely elicits a whole range of different coping reactions depending on the patient's previous experience and personality. Only recently has a differentiated approach to the understanding and assessment of coping in breast cancer patients evolved. In their longitudinal study of 58 women with breast cancer, Heim et al. (1988) have defined the most frequently used coping strategies and have been able to show changing patterns over time. According to Herschbach and Henrich (1987), the coping process is defined by the actual problems the patient faces, the intensity of the strain the patient experiences in confronting each problem, the types of coping strategies she uses, as well as whether they are implemented in a rigid or flexible way to solve the problem or to obtain relief. In a

Table 1. Herschbach coping inventory (modified). Self-rating by the patient on three levels

---

1. *Seven problem areas*
- Information about the disease
- Treatment sequelae
- Pain
- Anxiety/emotional tension
- Capacity/efficiency
- Social behavior
- Partner/family
2. *Burden/stress for each area*
3. *Fifteen coping strategies for each area*
- Analyzing the problem and looking for counteractions
- "Stiff upper lip"
- Talking to someone
- Accepting the problem as it is
- Keeping busy to be distracted
- "Other people are far worse off"
- Crying and becoming desperate
- Feeling and expressing anger
- Consulting an expert in the field
- Self-criticism
- Taking tranquilizers or alcohol
- "There will be better times"
- Waiting for spontaneous change
- Trying to avoid the problem
- Seeing the positive side of the problem

---

cross-sectional study of over 300 breast cancer and other cancer patients, they defined seven problem areas and 15 coping strategies which are used more or less frequently (Table 1). Currently, no generally accepted methodology of coping assessment in breast cancer patients is available. This is made clear by the variety of assessment instruments used in currently available studies, most of which are not directly concerned with the coping process.

The result of the coping process is usually considered in terms of the patient's level of adaptation to the disease and its treatment. The level of adaptation is a main determinant of the patient's physical, psychological, and social well-being, or quality of life. However, most studies focussing on psychosocial reactions to primary breast cancer consider survival time as the main outcome measure, neglecting psychosocial well-being and adaptation as dependent variables and often ignoring biological factors such as axillary lymph node status at study entry as possible confounding variables (Table 2). Only a few studies have psychosocial adaptation as the outcome measure (Funch and Mettlin 1982). Similarly, in studies evaluating the effect of surgical, cytotoxic or radiation treatments the biomedical variable "survival time" [overall survival (OS) and DFS] is considered almost exclusively as hard evidence in the assessment of outcome. Psychosocial factors, such as patient coping and emotional well-being, are considered soft data and are mostly ignored. To the best of our knowledge no study integrating the coping process and its resulting psychosocial adaptation into the evaluation of medical treatments has been published.

Table 2. Overview of studies investigating the impact of the coping process on survival in patients with primary and metastatic breast cancer

Authors	Sample	Follow-up time design	Control for confounding variables	"Coping" factor	Association with outcome (+, better; –, worse; 0, none)	Assessment instruments
Derogatis et al. 1979	Thirty-five patients (metastatic, receiving chemotherapy): 13 short-term survivors, 22 long-term survivors	One year, retrospective	– Age – Disease-free interval – Menopausal status – Distribution of metastases – Karnofsky performance status – Initial response to treatment → Not controlled: duration of previous chemotherapy	Hostility, guilt Negative affect Good adjustment Positive attitude towards treatment and physician	OS + + – –	SCL – 90 (Symptom Check List) ABS (Affect Balance Scale) GAIS (Global Adjustment to Illness Scale) Structured interview
Greer et al. 1979	Fifty-seven patients stage I and II out of a sample o 69	Five years, 10 years, prospective	– Age, social class – Tumor size – Histological grading – Delay in seeking medical advice – Menopausal status – Clinical stage – Radiation therapy – Type of surgery – Habitual reaction to stressful events – Expression of anger – Loss/depression 5 years prior to study entry – social adjustment including sexual adjustment, interpersonal relationships, and work records	Denial Fighting spirit Stoic acceptance Hopelessness/helplessness Alone/poor marital relationship	OS/DFS + + – – –	*Interviews at 3 months of diagnosis* Categorial rating of interview content
1985				Depression Hostility Neuroticism Extroversion	0 0 0 0	*Preoperative psychological testing* HDS (Hamilton Depression Scale) HDHQ (Hostility and Direction of Hostility Questionnaire) EPI (Eysenck Personality Inventory)

Study	Sample	Design	Controlled variables	Psychosocial variable	Effect	Measure
			→Not controlled: histological axillary nodal status at study entry	Verbal intelligence	0	Mill Hill Vocabulary Scale
Funch and Marshall 1983	Two hundred and eight patients stage I and II out of initial 352 patients	Twenty years, retrospective	– Disease stage – Menopausal status – Past health status – Socioeconomic status →Not controlled: treatment regimens	Social involvement	OS +	*Interview at diagnosis 1958–1960 on the previous 5 years* Marital status, number of relatives and friends, organizational involvement
				"Objective stress"	–	Illness, death, or unemployment of someone in the family
				"Subjective stress"	–	Number of months the subject felt tired, upset, or perceived family income inadequate
Morgenstern et al. 1984	Thirty-four patients (all stages) participating in support group, 86 matched controls	One to ten years retrospective	– Age at diagnosis – Stage of disease – Treatments (surgery chemotherapy, radiation, hormone therapy) – Histologic type – Lag time to entry in support group – Number of sessions attended	Social support	OS/DSF +(trends)	Participation in support group of 8–12 cancer patients and invited family and friends, ECaP (Exceptional Cancer Patients); no formal assessment of effect
Cassileth et al. 1985 a	One hundred and fifty-five patients: 93 stage II breast cancer, 62 stage I melanome (high or intermediate risk) – 41 relapsers	Until relapse: median DFS 12.3 months, prospective	– Specific diagnosis (±) – Adjuvant chemotherapy (±) – Stage of disease – Socioeconomic status – Sex – Age →Not controlled: menopausal status	Marital history	DSF 0	*Self-report questionnaire within 2–8 weeks of diagnosis* Two questions about marital status
				Social ties	0	Six items of Berkman and Syme scale
				Job satisfaction	0	Six occupational questions
				Psychotropic drug use	0	One question about use of medication for anxiety and depression
				General life evaluation/satisfaction	0	Eight questions regarding life satisfaction

Table 2 *(continued)*

Authors	Sample	Follow-up time design	Control for confounding variables	"Coping" factor	Association with outcome (+, better; −, worse; 0, none)	Assessment instruments
1987	Fifty-nine relapsers	– DFS 3 years or more, prospective		Subjective view of adult health	0	One question about health before illness
				Hopelessness/helplessness	0	Beck's hopelessness scale
				"Adjustment" to illness	0	One item of PACIS (Personal Adjustment to Chronic Illness Scale)
Holland et al. 1986	Three hundred and forty-six patients stage II out of 945	Until relapse, prospective	– ER – Stage – Adjuvant treatment → Otherwise no information (abstract)	Somatization,	0	SCL-90 prior to start od adjuvant chemotherapy
				Obsessive-compulsive	0	
				Interpersonal sensitivity	0	
	CALGB 8082: 106 relapsers, 240 nonrelapsers			Depression	0	
				Anxiety	0	
				Hostility	0	
				Phobic anxiety	0	
				Paranoid ideation	0	
				Psychoticism	0	
				Three summary scales	0	
Hislop et al. 1987	One hundred and thirty-three patients all stages out of 168 under age of 55, mainly premenopausal	Four years, 26 deaths (OS), 38 relapsers (DFS), prospective	– Age – Stage – Axillary nodal status – Histologic grading – ER → Not controlled: – Treatment regimens	Expressive activities		*Self-administered questionnaire within + 3 months of diagnosis*
				– at home	+ +OS + DFS	
				– away from home	+ +OS + DFS	
				Instrumental activities		Expressive and Instrumental Activity Measure (Waxler)
				– at home	0	
				– away from home	0	

Study	Sample	Not controlled	Variable (result)	Measure/Instrument
			Extroversion ++OS	EPI
			Neuroticism 0	
			Self-esteem 0	Rosenberg Self-Esteem Scale
			Locus of control +DFS	Rotter IE-Scale
			Recent life events 0	Social Adjustment Rating Scale (Rahe)
			Coping behavior 0	Weisman and Worden Project Omega
			Anxiety 0	Psychologic Status (Illfeld)
			Anger low ++OS+DFS	
			Depression 0	
			Cognitive disturbance low +DFS	
Jensen 1987	Twenty-seven disease-free patients 3.5 year after initial diagnosis (mean time to recurrence: 911 days), 25 patients with recurrence 3.3 years after diagnosis of recurrence (mean time to recurrence: 1310 days), 34 healthy controls. Mean 624 days, retrospective (in part prospective), highly selected groups	– Age at diagnosis – Disease stage at diagnosis – Total length of disease course – Recurrence-free period – Medical status at study onset – Family history of cancer – Number of children – Socioeconomic status → Not controlled: treatments, time from diagnosis to study onset	Repressive personality Style – Reduced expression of negative affect – Comforting day-dreaming Helplessness/hopelessness – Chronic stress –	*Self-reporting measures at study onset* Crowne Marlowe Social Desirability Scale Bendig/Taylor Manifest Anxiety Scale, Sackheim-Gur Self and Other Deception Scale Imaginal Process Inventory (Huba, Aneshensel, Singer) MBHI (Millon Behavioral Health Inventory) MBHI
Jamison et al. 1987	Forty-nine patients with metastatic disease: 25 short-term. Until death, retrospective	– Age – People at home – Education level – No. of chemotherapy treatments	Well-being 0 Subjective valuation of health 0 Self-esteem 0	*Self-reporting questionnaires* General Well-Being Scale Health Value Rating Questionnaire Self-Esteem Inventory

Table 2 *(continued)*

Authors	Sample	Follow-up time design	Control for confounding variables	"Coping" factor	Association with outcome (+, better; −, worse; 0, none)	Assessment instruments
	survivors (10.8 months) 24 long-term survivors (30.4 months)		ments – No. of other illnesses – Family members with cancer, friends with cancer – No. of nodes – No. of metastases – Menopausal status – ER status – Karnofsky status → Not controlled: site of metastases, treatment regimens	Hostility Depression Anxiety Belief of health control – Internal – Chance – Powerful – Others	0 0 0 { 0 0 0 0 NKA (−, diminished; 0, not affected)	Hostility Scale of Multiple Affect Adjective Check List Zung Depression Scale Spielberger Trait Anxiety Inventory, Situation-Response Scale of General Trait Anxiousness Multidimensional Health Locus of Control Scales *Structured and audiotaped interview within 5–7 days of surgery and an 3 months* Scored interview ratings
Levy et al. 1987	Seventy-five patients stage I and II from NCI Protocol 79-C-11	Three months, prospective	– Treatments: modified radical mastectomy, wide excision plus radical radiotherapy plus axillary dissection, if positive chemotherapy with Adriamycin + Endoxan or methotrexate + 5 FU → No other information	Delay in seeking medical advice Listless apathetic pattern of response Other attitudes Little social support "Adjustment" (low distress) Fatigue Other POMS scales	0? (not stated) – (trend) 0? (not stated) – – – 0? (not stated)	Patient's delay in seeking diagnosis Patient's attitudes towards the disease and its treatment Patient's perception of interpersonal support GATS (Global Adjustment to Illness Scale; observer rated) POMS (Profile of Mood States; self-report)

DFS, disease-free suvival; OS, overall survival; ER, estrogen receptor; NKA, natural killer activity.

Coping and Survival

If survival is considered as the outcome measure of coping, the question of possible interactions between the coping process and the biological course of the disease must be clarified. Basically, there are three possibilities:

1. The coping process can have an impact on the patient's compliance with treatment and indirectly influence the disease process.
2. The coping process is mainly determined by the biological disease process.
3. The coping process directly influences the biological disease process through psycho-neuro-endocrino-immunological mechanisms (Fig. 1).

These three interactions are probably inextricably mingled, with one factor outweighing the others in a particular situation.

Considering the possible impact of the coping process on survival implies the question of whether there are good copers, who use adaptive coping strategies, as opposed to bad copers, who use maladaptive coping strategies. In his review of the literature, Heim attempts to categorize the psychosocial factors studied in the different investigations according to his own coping strategies and preliminarily defines adequate versus inadequate coping mostly by considering survival as the outcome measure (Heim 1988). However, he does not take into account possible bias due to inadequate biological sampling. To show methodological pitfalls possibly invalidating the results of a given investigation instead of comprehensively reviewing the literature, we will analyze the two most frequently cited studies in the

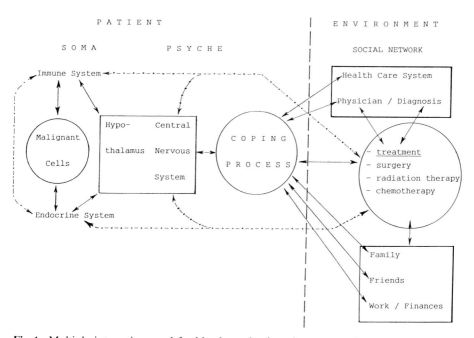

Fig. 1. Multiple interactions and feed-back mechanisms between environment and patient possibly influencing tumor growth

field with contradictory findings. An overview of recent studies in breast cancer is presented in Table 2. More comprehensive reviews are available (Hürny and Adler 1985).

Critical Analysis of Two Representative Studies

Greer and his group at King's College Hospital in London initiated the first psychosocial long-term follow-up study of stage I and II breast cancer patients (Greer et al. 1979; Pettingale et al. 1985). A total of 69 consecutively admitted patients were assessed preoperatively with a structured interview and psychological testing including a variety of psychosocial variables (see Table 2). At 3 months after surgery, 57 patients were interviewed more openly regarding their psychological response to the disease. The responses were grouped by two independent raters into four mutually exclusive categories: denial, fighting spirit, stoic acceptance, and feelings of helplessness/hopelessness. After 5 years, 28 patients were alive with no evidence of disease, 13 were alive with metastases, and 16 had died. Comparing recurrence-free survival ($n=28$) with metastatic disease alive or dead ($n=29$), there was a significant association between initial psychological response and outcome (chi-square $=9.0$, df $=3$, P <0.03). A favorable outcome was more frequent in patients with active denial or fighting spirit (15/20, 75%) than in patients who showed either stoic acceptance or helplessness/hopelessness (13/37, 35%). Of the women who subsequently died, 88% (14/16) initially reacted with stoic acceptance or helplessness/hopelessness, whereas only 46% (13/28) of the women who remained alive and well had demonstrated these reactions (chi-square $=9.35$, df $=1$, P <0.25). Apart from a tendency for patients who were living alone or who reported poor marital relationships at the time of diagnosis to have a less favorable outcome (chi-square $=6.53$, P <0.09; and chi-square $=7.00$, P <0.08 respectively), there were no significant associations between 5-year outcome and all the other psychosocial variables, including psychological testing.

At 10-years' follow-up (19 patients alive with no recurrence, two alive with metastases, and 36 dead), these results were confirmed. In a multivariate regression analysis with eight prognostic factors, psychological response was the most significant individual factor for death from any cause (P <0.003), death from breast cancer (P <0.003), and first recurrence of disease (P <0.008).

Cassileth and her coworkers at the University of Pennsylvania Cancer Center assessed 155 consecutive patients (93 with stage II breast cancer, 62 with stage I melanoma, high or intermediate high risk) with a self-report questionnaire within 2-8 weeks of diagnosis. This questionnaire assessed seven psychosocial factors found to be predictive of outcome in previous studies with cancer patients: (a) social ties, (b) job satisfaction, (c) psychotropic drug use, (d) life satisfaction, (e) subjective view of adult health, (f) hopelessness and (g) perceived adjustment to chronic illness (Cassileth et al. 1985 a, 1987). Each of the seven factors was used as a subscale for purposes of data analysis. A total psychosocial profile score was constructed for each patient by adding the subscale scores for that patient. A second group of 204 patients with advanced cancer of different sites also included in the study does not pertain to this analysis. With the exception of the well-validated

Table 3. Methodological criteria in the evaluation of studies investigating the impact of psychosocial factors on the disease course in breast cancer patients

Overview		
Hypothesis	Defined a priori	Not defined
Design	Retrospective	Prospective
Assessments	Cross-sectional	Serial/longitudinal
Instruments	Psychometrics	Interviews
Patient samples	Small	Large
	Nonrepresentative	Representative
Statistical analysis	Inappropriate	Appropriate
Characterization of patient samples		
Number of patients	Small	Large
	Non-representative	Representative
Sociodemographic characteristics		
Age	Noncomparable	Comparable
Marital status		
Life situation		
Profession		
Occupational position		
Education		
Income level		
Biological characteristics		
Menopausal status	Noncomparable	Comparable
Tumor site		
Histologic grading		
Hormone receptors		
Disease stage		
Treatments		

Beck hopelessness scale, factor items were assessed by factual criteria or simple indexes rather than by scales or instruments. At a median time to recurrence of 12.3 months, 41 of the 155 patients had relapsed. In three different types of analyses (Kaplan-Meier life table survival analyses, Mantel-Cox model, and analysis of variance), neither individual subscale scores nor total scores had any influence on length of DFS. At 3 years or more after diagnosis (84 patients disease free, 59 relapsed), these results were confirmed. Positive attitudes and hopefulness were found with equal frequency among patients who later remained in remission and those who relapsed.

The criteria used for evaluation of the two studies are summarized in Table 3. The Cassileth study (Cassileth et al. 1985a), and the Greer study (Greer et al. 1979) are clearly prospective. Many investigators claim that their studies are prospective, which in fact they are not. Funch and Marshall (1983), for instance have retrospectively analyzed data which were gathered 20 years ago for another purpose (Snell and Graham 1971). Jensen (1987) obtains highly selected groups by investigating his patients at arbitrarily chosen points in time after diagnosis and not controlling for time from diagnosis to study onset. His study is only "half" prospective. In a truly prospective study, the hypotheses must be defined beforehand, and the patient sample must be assessed at well-defined points in terms of disease development.

In the English study, the follow-up time of 10 years is considerably longer than the follow-up time of 3 or more years in the American study. Since breast cancer is a slow-growing tumor, significant benefits of adjuvant treatments usually emerge only late in the disease course, several years from diagnosis. Similarly, it is conceivable that early coping factors have only late effects. However, this is only a weak argument in favor of Greer et al. (1979).

A crucial point is the timing of assessment(s) and the choice of assessment instruments. Since coping probably changes over time, serial assessments are necessary. In both studies, the presumable predictive variables were only assessed once, within 2–8 weeks of diagnosis in Cassileth et al. (1985 a) and within 3 months of diagnosis in Greer (1979). At 3 months, according to clinical experience, the initial inner turmoil caused by the cancer diagnosis has calmed down. Cassileth et al. (1987) has made a second assessment at 3 years, which is still too early for the evaluation of survival prediction.

As discussed earlier, so far no generally accepted instruments to assess coping in breast cancer are available. Instruments developed for psychiatric patients or the general population are usually not sensitive enough for the specific problems of breast cancer patients. As shown in Table 2 in the majority of the studies, psychological tests, questionnaires and structured interviews were used. Some of them have proved to be valid, reliable, and specific in cancer patients, others have not been tested. In fact, Greer et al. (1979) is the only study using a more open-ended interview as well as structured interviews and psychological testing to assess the patients reactions to cancer.

In our opinion, there is a fundamental difference between interview data resulting from the interaction of an experienced, psychologically trained physician with a patient and data from psychological tests or questionnaires. Objective tests are usually less sensitive and more superficial than the in-depth assessment in an interview. On the other hand, considerable interviewer bias may flaw this kind of data. Greer et al. (1979) state that "in a pilot survey independent ratings (of the response categories) by two observers produced a high level of agreement." Subsequently, the four categories are well defined, but there is no clear-cut information about interrater reliability. Nevertheless, the authors were able to group their patients into four categories predictive for outcome.

In Cassileth et al. (1985 a), a self-report questionnaire of 32 questions attempting to assess seven complex psychosocial constructs is used. It is questionable whether this kind of instument is sensitive to relevant aspects of the coping process. With the exception of Beck's hopelessness scale, the questionnaire has not been formally validated.

In quite a few studies, the biological and psychosocial characterization of the patient sample is deficient and control for possible confounding variables is lacking. In both studies, sociodemographic characteristics were roughly assessed and statistically controlled for. In Cassileth et al. (1985 a) this was done in response to a letter from Funch (1985; Cassileth et al. 1985 b). In Greer et al. (1979) the assessment of "social class" is not specifically described. Since socioeconomic status is likely to have a prognostic impact on survival (Vågerö and Persson 1987), it should be assessed in greater detail.

In both studies, a variety of possible confounding biological and medical factors were considered. In Cassileth et al.(1985a), the combined analysis of two patient groups comparable for stage but with completely different primary tumors is questionable, although statistically the site of the primary tumor did not influence the psychosocial scores. This possibly shows the lack of specificity and sensitivity of the instruments. The fact that here breast cancer but not melanoma patients receive adjuvant chemotherapy may also be of importance. Since age had no confounding effect, menopausal status is unlikely to have had substantial influence. In Greer et al.(1979), a great number of possibly confounding biomedical variables were tested. However, one of the most significant predictors of outcome in early breast cancer – histologic axillary lymph node involvement – could not be assessed as a control variable, since at the time of the investigation axillary dissection was not done at that hospital. Even if axillary lymph node involvement is claimed not to be of great importance in 10-year survival (Pettingale et al.1985; Fentiman et al.1984), we cannot be sure that the differences of survival are not due to unequal distribution of lymph node-positive patients within the four categories of responses.

The number of patients is relatively small in both studies, but larger in Cassileth et al.(1985a), thus providing more statistical power. The analyses in Greer et al.(1979) comprised over 20 variables including control and dependent variables. By multiple testing in a sample of 57 patients, the possibility of obtaining statistical significance by chance cannot be neglected. However, it would be unlikely to obtain all accidental significances from the same instrument, namely the open interview. This instrument may be promising for future research. One problem is that it is burdensome and costly to have well-trained professionals repeatedly interviewing large numbers of patients.

In conclusion, weighing all the pros and cons of the different investigations, there is no conclusive evidence that coping has or does not have an impact on survival in breast cancer. Further carefully designed prospective studies are needed to elucidate this question and distinguish underlying factors.

Research Strategies in the International Breast Cancer Studies IBCS VI and VII

As stated above, no published study integrates the coping process and its resulting psychosocial adaptation into the evaluation of medical treatments. In the IBCS VI and VII, we have had the opportunity of attempting to do so in a large sample of stage II breast cancer patients. The objectives of the trial are the following:

1. To evaluate the efficacy of adding reinduction chemotherapy to an initial course of adjuvant combination chemotherapy after a treatment interval, as compared with administering an initial course of adjuvant treatment alone in pre- and perimenopausal patients (Trial VI)
2. To determine whether three cycles of initial adjuvant chemotherapy are as effective as six cycles in pre- and perimenopausal patients (Trial VI)

3. To evaluate the efficacy of adding early combination chemotherapy and late reinduction chemotherapy to adjuvant tamoxifen, as compared with administering tamoxifen alone in postmenopausal patients (Trial VII)

To answer these three questions, the patient's subjective experience is of foremost importance because (a) longer treatments are compared with treatments of shorter duration, (b) the expected differences of the regimens in terms of DFS and OS are not very large, and (c) it is the explicit goal of the trial to assess eventual improvement of the quantity and the quality of survival by integration of conventional and new end points.

It will be necessary to include over 2000 patients in the trial in order to obtain enough statistical power to give an adequate answer to the questions. In a large international trial, only simple and short, relatively superficial assessments of indicators of quality of life are feasible. This is outweighed to a great extent by the large number of biomedically and sociodemographically well-defined patient groups. To understand further the meaning and clinical significance of the short measures, a subgroup of 150 Swiss patients is being investigated in greater depth regarding their coping. As shown in Fig. 2, in all patients of the IBCS VI and VII, a global assessment of coping with the Perceived Adjustment to Chronic Illness Scale (PACIS) (Hürny et al. 1989) of well-being with a modified version of the Befindlichkeits-Skala (Bf-S) (von Zerssen 1976), and of appetite, physical well-being, and mood with Linear Analogue Self-Assessment Scales (LASA) (Coates et al. 1983) is made within 4 weeks of diagnosis and every 3 months thereafter for up to 2 years. This design enables study in a well-controlled way of the impact of the subjective-

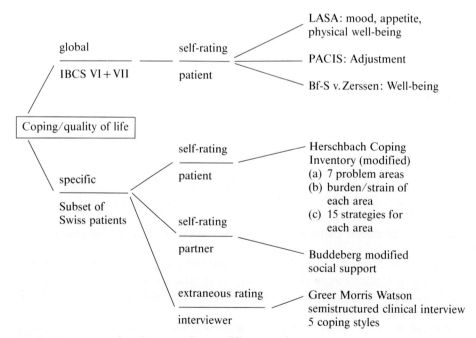

Fig. 2. Assessment of coping according to different scales

ly perceived initial crisis on biological and psychological outcome. In addition, the relatively inexact patient-rated measures will be used together with physician-rated toxicity and disease symptoms to evaluate the different treatments comprehensively.

In the Swiss subgroup, the coping process is being studied specifically and in more depth. At 3 months after diagnosis and 2 years later, simultaneously with the global measures of the IBCS, a semistructured interview according to the guidelines of Morris et al.(1985) is recorded on audiotapes for rating by independent observers (including the five response categories active denial, fighting spirit, stoic acceptance, helplessness/hopelessness, and anxious preoccupation). Additionally, the patients fill out at months 3, 6, 12, and 24 the Herschbach coping inventory, and their partners are assessed with regard to social support (Buddeberg 1985, modified). One aim of this approach is to identify patients at risk for poor psychosocial adaptation.

With the addition of the Swiss subgroup study, we will be able to replicate Greer et al.(1979) and at least partially Cassileth et al.(1985a) in a biomedically well-controlled sample. Furthermore, we will obtain more information about the clinical significance of our global measures and have the opportunity of emphasizing psychosocial outcome measures in cancer clinical trials. We hope to shed some more light on the complex virtual interactions of coping and the disease process.

References

Ader R, Cohen N (1975) Behaviorally conditioned immunosuppression. Psychosom Med 37: 333–340
Arnetz BB, Wasserman J, Petrini B, et al (1987) Immune function in unemployed women. Psychosom Med 49: 3–12
Berg JW, Ross R, Latourette HB (1977) Economic status and survival of cancer patients. Cancer 39: 467–477
Bourne HR, Lichtenstein LM, Melmon KL (1974) Modulation of inflammation and immunity by cyclic AMP. Science 184: 19–28
Buddeberg K (1985) Ehen krebskranker Frauen. Urban und Schwarzenberg, Munich
Cassileth BR, Lusk EJ, Miller DS, et al (1985a) Psychological correlates of survival in advanced malignant disease? N Engl J Med 312: 1551–1555
Cassileth BR, Lusk EJ, Miller DS, et al (1985b) Reply to letters to the editor. N Engl J Med 313: 1356
Cassileth BR, Lusk EJ, Walsh H, et al (1987) Psychosocial correlates of unusually good medical outcome 3 years or more after cancer diagnosis. ASCO Proc 6: 253
Coates A, Fisher Dillenbeck C, McNeil DR, et al (1983) On the receiving end-II. Linear analogue self-assessment (LASA) in evaluation of aspects of the quality of life of cancer patients receiving chemotherapy. Eur J Cancer Clin Oncol 19: 1633–1637
Derogatis LR, Abeloff MD Melisaratos N (1979) Psychological coping mechanisms and survival time in metastatic breast cancer. JAMA 242: 1504–1508
Fentiman IS, Cuzick J, Millis RR, et al (1984) Which patients are cured of breast cancer? Br Med J 289: 1108–1111
Funch DP (1985) Psychosocial variables and the course of cancer. N Engl J Med 313: 1354
Funch DP, Mettlin C (1982) The role of support in relation to recovery from breast cancer. Soc Sci Med 16: 91–98
Funch DP, Marshall J (1983) The role of stress, social support and age in survival from breast cancer. J Psychosom Res 27: 77–83

Greer S, Morris T, Pettingale KW (1979) Psychological response to breast cancer: effect on outcome. Lancet ii (8146): 785-787

Hadden JW, Hadden EM, Middleton E jr (1970) Lymphocyte blast transformation I. Demonstration of adrenergic receptors in human peripheral lymphocytes. J Cell Immunol 1: 583-595

Heim E (1988) Coping and Adaptivität: gibt es geeignetes oder ungeeignetes Coping? Psychother Med Psychol 38: 8-18

Heim E, Augustini KF, Blaser A, et al (1987) Coping with breast cancer - a longitudinal prospective Study. Psychoth Psychosom 48: 44-59

Herschbach P, Henrich G (1987) Probleme und Problembewältigung von Tumorpatienten in der stationären Nachsorge. Psychother Med Psychol 37: 185-192

Hislop TG, Waxler NE, Coldman AJ (1987) The prognostic significance of psychosocial factors in women with breast cancer. J Chronic Dis 40: 729-735

Holland JC, Korzun AH, Tross S (1986) Psychosocial factors and disease free survival in stage II breast carcinoma. ASCO Proc 5: 237

Hürny C, Adler R (1985) Psychoonkologische Forschung. In: Meerwein F (ed) Einführung in die Psycho-Onkologie, 3rd edn. Huber, Bern, pp 15-57

Hürny Ch, Bernhard J, Schatzmann E, Cassileth BR (1989) Assessment of adjustment to cancer in clinical trials: evaluation of the personal adjustment to chronic illness scale PACIS. J Psychosoc Oncol (accepted for publication)

Irwin MR, Risch SC (1987) Plasma cortisol and immune function in bereavement. Psychosom Med 49: 210

Jamison RN, Burish TG, Wallston KA (1987) Psychogenic factors in predicting survival of breast cancer patients. J Clin Oncol 5: 768-772

Jensen MR (1987) Psychobiological factors predicting the course of breast cancer. J Pers 55: 317-342

Jenkins CD (1983) Social environment and cancer mortality in men. N Engl J Med 308: 395-398

Kiecolt-Glaser JK, Fisher LD, Ogrocki P, et al (1987a) Marital quality, marital disruption and immune function. Psychosom Med 49: 13-34

Kiecolt-Glaser JK, Glaser R, Shuttleworth EC (1987b) Chronic stress and immunity in family care givers of Alzheimer's disease victims. Psychosom Med 49: 523-535

Krug H, Krug F, Cuatrecasas F (1972) Emergence of insulin-receptors on human lymphocytes during in vitro transformation. Proc Natl Acad Sci USA 69: 2604-2608

Lesniak MA, Roth J, Gordon P, Gavin R (1973) Human growth hormone radioreceptor assay using cultured human lymphocytes. Nature 241: 20-22

Levy S, Herberman R, Lippman M, et al (1987) Correlation of stress factors with sustained depression of natural killer cell activity and predicted prognosis in patients with breast cancer. J Clin Oncol 5: 348-353

Linden G (1969) The influence of social class in the survival of cancer patients. Am J Public Health 59: 267-274

Lippman M, Haltermann R, Perry S, et al (1973) Glucocorticoid binding proteins in human leukaemic lymphoblasts. Nature 242: 157-158

Lipworth L, Abelin T, Connelly RR (1970) Socioeconomic factors in the prognosis of cancer patients. J Chronic Dis 23: 105-116

Locke SE, Kraus L, Leserman J, et al (1984) Life change, stress, psychiatric symptoms and natural killer cell activity. Psychosom Med 46: 441-453

Morgenstern H, Gellert GA, Walter SD, et al (1984) The impact of a social support program on survival with breast cancer: the importance of selection bias in program evaluation. J Chron Dis 37: 273-282

Morris T, Blake S, Buckley M (1985) Development of a method for rating cognitive responses to a diagnosis of cancer. Soc Sci Med 20: 795-802

Pettingale KW, Morris T, Greer S, et al (1985) Mental attitudes to cancer: an additional prognostic factor. Lancet i 8431: 750

Schain W (1976) Psychological impact of the diagnosis of breast cancer on the patient. Front Radiat Ther Oncol 11: 68–89

Schleifer SJ, Keller SE, Camerino M, et al (1983) Suppression of lymphocyte stimulation following bereavement. JAMA 250: 374–377

Snell L, Graham S (1971) Social trauma as related to cancer of the breast. Br J Cancer 25: 721–734

Vågerö D, Persson G (1987) Cancer survival and social class in Sweden. J Epidemiol Community Health 41: 204–209

von Zerssen D (1976) Klinische Selbstbeurteilungsskalen (KSb-S) aus dem Münchener Psychiatrischen Informationssystem (PSYCHIS München). Die Befindlichkeitsskala-Parallelformen Bf-S und Bf-S' Manual. Beltz, Weinheim

Behavioral Side Effects of Adjuvant Chemotherapy

W. H. Redd, P. B. Jacobsen, and M. A. Andrykowski

Memorial Sloan-Kettering Cancer Center, New York, NY, USA

During the protracted course of adjuvant chemotherapy following surgery for breast cancer, a significant proportion of patients experience side effects. The most unpleasant are the nausea and vomiting, which can begin as the patient anticipates treatment and continue for up to 48 h following each infusion. In our prospective, longitudinal study of 77 women receiving outpatient chemotherapy for breast cancer, 71% of patients experienced nausea and vomiting following treatment infusions (Jacobsen et al. 1988). And, by the sixth treatment infusion, 57% of patients experienced anticipatory side effects (i.e., they felt nauseous and/or vomited as they approached the treatment clinic) (Andrykowski et al., submitted for publication). The purpose of the present discussion is to review our research on the role of psychological and behavioral factors in the development of such side effects. Results from our most recent studies of post-treatment nausea and vomiting are presented first. Discussion of our findings for pretreatment side effects follows. The last issue is the development of cost-effective behavioral interventions to control these aversive side effects.

Post-treatment Side Effects

Although the emetic properties of chemotherapy protocols can be specified and patients are routinely informed as to what aversive side effects to expect, there is considerable variability in the severity of gastrointestinal distress that patients experience from regimens with similar emetic potential. Indeed, even among patients receiving the same agents at equivalent doses, markedly different levels of post-treatment nausea and vomiting have been reported (Gralla et al. 1981). To understand these individual differences, researchers have examined whether age (Zook and Yasko 1983; Nerenz et al. 1986), sex (Zook and Yasko 1983), extent of disease (Cohen et al. 1986), susceptibility to motion sickness (Morrow 1985), and patterns of sleep and food intake prior to chemotherapy (Scogna and Smalley 1979) are related to post-treatment gastrointestinal distress. Psychological factors, such as expectations of treatment side effects (Scogna and Smalley 1979), anxiety, and psychosocial adjustment (Zook and Yasko 1983; Cassileth et al. 1985; Rhodes

Recent Results in Cancer Research, Vol. 115
© Springer-Verlag Berlin · Heidelberg 1989

et al. 1986) have also been investigated. Unfortunately, this research has generally yielded mixed results.

These confusing results are surprising since both experimental and clinical studies provide a rationale for hypothesizing that certain nonpharmacologic variables are associated with post-treatment gastrointestinal distress. Laboratory research by Epstein and Clarke (1970) indicated that expectations about an aversive event establish self-fulfilling prophecies for subjects' subsequent reactions. From these results, it has been hypothesized that patients who expect chemotherapy to make them nauseated are more likely to experience post-treatment side effects. A second variable is anxiety; the rationale for a hypothesized association with post-treatment nausea and vomiting stems from both clinical observations of individuals under stress and research on anticipatory nausea and vomiting in chemotherapy patients. Healthy individuals anticipating a stressful event often report sensations of nausea, and competitive athletes have been observed to vomit before an important race or game (Scogna and Smalley 1979).

In our research, we followed breast cancer patients scheduled to receive weekly adjuvant chemotherapy for five 6-week cycles (up to 1 year). The following drugs were administered via i.v. injection: methotrexate, fluorouracil, and vincristine. Patients also received oral cyclophosphamide. Twenty-two percent of patients used oral prochlorperazine as an antiemetic. Each patient was interviewed before and after all infusions and completed nausea and side effect questionnaires. Before their initial chemotherapy infusion, each patient was administered a battery of personality and anxiety scales.

Patients' susceptibility to gastrointestinal distress, their expectations that chemotherapy would make them nauseous, and the degree of anxiety they experienced during infusions predicted individual differences in post-treatment nausea and vomiting. Although other nonpharmacologic factors were related to post-treatment gastrointestinal distress, the factors listed above emerged most frequently as significant predictors of the frequency, severity, and duration of post-treatment nausea.

Patients with a history of motion sickness experienced post-treatment nausea for longer durations. This result corroborates a finding previously reported by Morrow (1985). Our study also demonstrated that post-treatment nausea was more likely to develop in patients who had a history of becoming nauseous when feeling anxious. Furthermore, post-treatment nausea was likely to occur more frequently in those individuals who reported nausea after eating certain foods. These results suggest that patients who have histories of susceptibility to nausea experience progressively worse nausea over the course of repeated infusions. These findings also raise the possibility that there are constitutional differences in patients' susceptibility to gastrointestinal distress: Certain individuals may have lower physiological thresholds for becoming nauseous in response to a variety of stressors, including chemotherapy.

Patients who expected that chemotherapy would make them nauseous were more likely to develop post-treatment nausea and to experience it at higher intensity and for longer durations. Two explanations can be provided. One possibility is that the relationships between expectations and post-treatment nausea reflect the patient's ability to appraise correctly how her body will react to chemotherapy. It follows from this argument that expectations of developing nausea would be based, in part, on the patient's recognition of her own past history of nausea and vomiting. However, this hypothesis was not supported by the data: No relationships were evident between patients' expectations and their self-reported past histories of gastrointestinal distress. A second explanation remains: Patient expectations establish self-fulfilling prophecies which contribute to the intensity of the side effects experienced. Unfortunately, the present study does not indicate whether self-fulfilling prophecies operate through a process in which expectations lead patients to imagine symptoms of nausea or whether, because of their expectations, patients carefully monitor themselves and thereby notice sensations of nausea which they would otherwise ignore.

Patients who reported greater anxiety during infusions were more likely to develop post-treatment nausea, to experience it more frequently, and to report it at higher levels of intensity. Several explanations can be offered for these relationships. One possibility is that the obtained relationships do not represent associations between anxiety and post-treatment nausea. They may reflect associations between pre- and post-treatment anxiety. According to this explanation, patients remain anxious after the administration of chemotherapy and mislabel their post-treatment anxiety as post-treatment nausea. This mislabelling may occur both because patients have just received emetic chemotherapy and are "set" to report post-treatment nausea and/or because of the similarities between sensations of anxiety and nausea. A second possibility is that heightened anxiety is present during infusions only because patients were anticipating the aversive sensations of post-treatment nausea. According to this explanation, anxiety during infusions does not contribute to post-treatment nausea; it merely reflects the patient's dread of the subsequent gastrointestinal distress.

In summary, our results offer strong support for the view that nonpharmacologic factors contribute to individual differences in gastrointestinal distress associated with chemotherapy. Identification of these factors was possible because of the use of a research design in which pharmacologic factors (i.e., the agents administered and the time between administrations) were held relatively constant. Under these conditions, nonpharmacologic factors were found to be even more important than the chemotherapy drug dosage in predicting gastrointesitnal distress.

Pretreatment Side Effects

In addition to post-treatment side effects, many patients experience nausea in anticipation of treatment (i.e., *before* the drugs are actually injected). Most patients begin chemotherapy treatment with considerable apprehension, most having heard stories about the horrors of "chemo." Some clinicians maintain that many patients are "primed" for problems, starting the first course of treatment with the clear expectation that treatment is going to be tough. Interestingly, most patients find the first infusion much easier than they had expected. But, as the course of treatment continues with repeated infusions, patients begin to notice side effects. Unfortunately, with subsequent infusions these side effects generally become more severe. For 57% of the patients we studied, clinic stimuli that were repeatedly associated with post-treatment side effects became elicitors of anticipatory reactions. The likelihood that a particular stimulus acquired nausea-eliciting properties depended on how closely it was associated with treatment. The most potent stimulus for adjuvant chemotherapy patients was the smell of the rubbing alcohol used to clean the skin in preparation for an infusion. After four or five infusions, the nurse's perfume, the handsoap the doctor uses, and the odor of coffee elicited it. For some of the patients visual and auditory stimuli (e.g., the sight of clinic staff, the name of the hospital printed on a road sign, the sound of the nurse's voice, and the music played in the waiting room) became powerful cues eliciting anticipatory reactions. Cognitively generated images and thoughts of treatment came to elicit nausea and vomiting in a subset of patients. For example, during patient interviews conducted by a research assistant who is not directly associated with treatment, it is not uncommon for a patient to ask that the conversation be terminated because talking about treatment brings on nausea. In many cases, the mere mention of chemotherapy, cancer, or hospitalization elecited significant nausea.

In terms of the Pavlovian, classical conditioning conceptualization of the development of anticipatory side effects, an association was formed between the nausea and vomiting (unconditioned response) experienced after drug infusion (unconditioned stimulus) and various stimuli associated with the environment in which chemotherapy is administered (conditioned stimulus). Visual, auditory, olfactory, or taste cues associated with chemotherapy administration can also function as conditioned stimuli. As a result of such classical conditioning, in vivo exposure to these stimuli trigger nausea and/or vomiting.

Severity of post-treatment nausea and vomiting, as well as patients' expectations for experiencing nausea, were predictive of the development of anticipatory nausea. Two distinct patterns of anticipatory nausea were identified: that which developed early in the course of treatment and that appearing later. Patients who developed early-onset anticipatory nausea were characterized by histories of nausea and vomiting under a variety of situations and by having received larger doses of i.v. chemotherapeutic agents during the initial infusion. On the other hand, late-onset anticipatory nausea was associated with heightened anxiety and post-treatment side effects during the treatment infusion immediately prior to the first occurrence of anticipatory nausea. For both patterns of anticipatory nausea, the severity of anticipatory nausea was mild and stable. Moreover, anticipatory nausea was intermittent (i.e., anticipatory nausea did not occur with all infusions following its initial occurrence).

Several lines of evidence point to the critical role of classical conditioning in the development of anticipatory nausea. First, the occurrence of post-treatment nausea and vomiting is necessary for the development of anticipatory nausea. In no case did one of our study patients experience anticipatory nausea without having experienced post-treatment nausea and vomiting with prior chemotherapy treatment. Second, all of the factors which reliably predicted the development of anticipatory nausea are either directly or indirectly linked to the magnitude of post-treatment nausea and vomiting. Chemotherapy drug dose and the duration and severity of post-treatment side effects predicted the development of anticipatory nausea. The strength of our data has led researchers in the area to accept the classical conditioning hypothesis of anticipatory side effects.

Clinical Interventions

In response to the failure of sedative and antiemetic drugs to control anticipatory nausea and vomiting, researchers have investigated the application of behavioral methods of symptom control. Five procedures have been studied: passive relaxation training combined with guided imagery (Burish et al. 1987; Redd et al. 1982), progressive muscle relaxation training with imagery (Lyles et al. 1982), electromyographic (EMG) feedback with relaxation training and imagery (Burish et al. 1981), systematic desensitization (Morrow and Morrell 1981), and attentional/cognitive distraction (with children) (Redd et al. 1987). All of these methods incorporate various relaxation training procedures (i.e., hynotic/passive induction and/or muscle tension/release induction) and oral descriptions of tranquil scenes. The goal is to relax the patients and to distract their attention from treatment. Results have been quite impressive: Clinically significant reductions in anticipatory nausea and vomiting have been achieved in independent studies with different patient populations (Burish et al. 1981, 1987; Lyles et al. 1982; Morrow and Morrell 1982). In those studies which included physiologic measures, the relaxation/imagery interventions resulted in the reduction of both pulse rate and blood pressure. The studies are summarized in Table 1.

Behavioral researchers in this area have speculated on the mechanisms that may underlie behavioral symptom control (Redd et al. 1982, 1985). However, researchers have not yet identified them empirically. In all of the published studies on behavioral symptom control in adults, distraction and relaxation have been confounded. Although Redd et al. (1987) have demonstrated that cognitive distraction alone is sufficient to block conditioned behavioral reactions in children, the specific effect of relaxation on symptom control has not been determined. While this issue may not be critically important to clinical care, it is relevant to the general theoretical understanding of cognitive-behavioral methods of symptom relief.

Unfortunately, almost all of the research to date has dealt with anticipatory side effects only. No one has systematically studied the use of behavioral methods to

Table 1. Behavioral control of anticipatory nausea and vomiting of cancer chemotherapy

Study	Behavioral method	Patient sample	Outcome
Burish et al. (1982)	Progressive relaxation with guided imagery	Adults	Reduction in nausea Reduction in anxiety
Burish et al. (1981)	EMG Biofeedback with relaxation and guided imagery	Adults	Reduction in nausea
Redd et al. (1982)	Passive relaxation (hypnosis) with guided imagery	Adults	Reduction in nausea Elimination of anticipatory vomiting
Morrow and Morrell (1982)	Systematic desensitization	Adults	Reduction in nausea Reduction in vomiting
Redd et al. (1987)	Attentional/cognitive distraction via video games	Children	Reduction in nausea

reduce post-treatment reactions. Although researchers have found that patients report milder post-treatment side effects when they use behavioral relaxation/distraction to control anticipatory reactions, most researchers "believe" that post-treatment nausea and vomiting is less amenable to behavioral intervention. Researchers argue that chemically based post-treatment nausea cannot be blocked as easily as psychologically based conditioned (pretreatment) nausea. Our clinical observations are consistent with such speculations; however, we have treated patients who are able to use behavioral methods to reduce post-treatment nausea. Indeed, it is our clinical experience that at least 10% of patients can literally "turn off" post-treatment nausea by focussing on deep breathing, relaxation, and tranquil images. But effective control requires considerable practice, and such skill is unusual. It is clear that this topic must be addressed more fully by behavioral researchers.

Conclusions

The results discussed here indicate the role of psychological/behavioral factors in patients' reactions to adjuvant chemotherapy. This research may help clinicians devise effective interventions as well as enable patients to understand a reaction which to them may appear bizarre. Indeed, these conditioned reactions to chemotherapy treatment reflect normal responses to "abnormal" circumstances. It is important that both clinicians and patients understand this fact and are aware of how to treat the resultant problems.

References

Andrykowski MA, Jacobsen PB, Marks E, Gorfinkle K, Hakes TB, Kaufman RJ, Currie VE, Holland JC, Redd WH (1988) Prevalence predictors and course of anticipatory nausea in women receiving adjuvant chemotherapy for breast cancer. Cancer 62: 2607–2613

Burish TG, Shartner CD, Lyles JN (1981) Effectiveness of multiple-site EMG biofeedback and relaxation in reducing the aversiveness of cancer chemotherapy. Biofeedback Self Regul 6: 523–535

Burish TG, Carey MP, Krozely MG, Greco FA (1987) Conditioned side effects induced by cancer chemotherapy: prevention through behavioral treatment. J Consult Clin Psychol 55: 42–48

Cassileth BR, Lusk EJ, Bodenheimer BR, et al.(1985) Chemotherapeutic toxicity - the relationship between patients' pretreatment expectations and posttreatment results. Am J Clin Oncol 8: 419–425

Cohen RE, Blanchard EB, Ruckdeschel JC, Smolen RC (1986) Prevalence and correlates of posttreatment and anticipatory nausea and vomiting in cancer chemotherapy. J Psychosom Res 30: 643–654

Epstein S, Clark S (1970) Heart rate and skin conductance during experimentally induced anxiety: Effects of anticipated intensity of noxious stimulation and experience. J Exp Psychol [Hum Percept] 84: 105–112

Gralla RJ, Itri LM, Pisko SE, et al.(1981) Antiemetic efficacy of high-dose metoclopramide: Randomized trials with placebo and prochlorperazine in patients with chemotherapy-induced nausea and vomiting. N Engl J Med 305: 905–909

Jacobsen PB, Andrykowski MA, Redd WH, Die-Trill M, Hakes TB, Kaufman RJ, Currie VE, Holland JC (1988) Nonpharmacologic factors in the development of posttreatment nausea with adjuvant chemotherapy for breast cancer. Cancer 61: 379–385

Lyles JN, Burish TG, Krozely MG, Oldham RK (1982) Efficacy of relaxation training and guided imagery in reducing the aversiveness of cancer chemotherapy. J Consult Clin Psychol 50: 509–524

Morrow GR (1985) The effect of a susceptibility to motion sickness on the side effects of cancer chemotherapy. Cancer 55: 2766–2770

Morrow GR, Morrell BS (1982) Behavioral treatment for the anticipatory nausea and vomiting induced by cancer chemotherapy. N Engl J Med 207: 1476–1480

Nerenz DR, Leventhal H, Easterling DV, Love RR (1986) Anxiety and drug taste as predictors of anticipatory nausea in cancer chemotherapy. J Clin Oncol 4: 224–233

Redd WH, Andrykowski MA (1982) Behavioral intervention in cancer treatment: Controlling aversion reactions to chemotherapy. J Consult Clin Psychol 50: 1018–1029

Redd WH, Andresen GV, Minagawa RY (1982) Hypnotic control of anticipatory emesis in patients receiving cancer chemotherapy. J Consult Clin Psychol 50: 14–19

Redd WH, Burish TG, Andrykowski MA (1985) Aversive conditioning during the course of cancer chemotherapy. In: Burish TG, Levy SM, Meyerowitz BE (eds) Cancer, nutrition and eating behavior. Hillsdale, New Jersey: Lawrence Earlbaum Associates, pp 117–134

Redd WH, Jacobsen PB, Die-Trill M, Dumatis H, McEvoy M, Holland JC (1987) Cognitive/attentional distraction in the control of conditioned nausea in pediatric cancer patients receiving chemotherapy. J Consult Clin Psychol 55: 391–395

Rhodes VA, Watson PM, Johnson MH (1986) Association of chemotherapy-related nausea and vomiting with pretreatment and posttreatment anxiety. Oncol Nurs Forum 13: 41–47

Scogna DM, Smalley RV (1979) Chemotherapy-induced nausea and vomiting. Am J Nurs 79: 1562–1564

Zook DJ, Yasko JM (1983) Psychologic factors: their effect on nausea and vomiting experienced by clients receiving chemotherapy. Oncol Nurs Forum 10: 76–81

Critical Review of Quality of Life: Psychosocial Aspects of Adjuvant Therapy in Breast Cancer

C. Hürny

Medizinische Abteilung Lory, Inselspital, 3010 Bern, Switzerland

Adjuvant treatment of breast cancer is considered primarily a medical problem. At first glance, the psychosocial sciences have little to contribute. Treatment evaluation focusses on the biological and clinical behavior of the tumor. The conventional end points of adjuvant trials are disease-free survival (DFS) and overall survival (OS). In the early days of chemotherapy, Karnofsky and Burchenal (1949) proposed "mood" and "the general feeling of well-being" as subjective criteria of improvement in addition to the physical performance status. In the following years, while new developments made chemotherapy more effective, these criteria of subjective improvement were lost. In recent years, the psychological and social implications of primary breast cancer treatments have been of growing scientific interest. Initial attempts have been made to integrate the subjective experience of the patient into treatment evaluation (Fig. 1).

In Part 11, four areas of intense biopsychosocial research in primary breast cancer are represented:

1. *Treatment evaluation:* integration of the subjective experience of the patient into treatment evaluation
2. *Coping process and adaptation:* physical and psychosocial adaptation to the disease and its treatments (rehabilitation needs and compliance with treatment)
3. *Psychosocial factors as prognostic indicators:* interactions between psychological and social reactions to the disease and its outcome
4. *Treatment side effects:* psychosocial implications of treatment side effects and possible psychosocial interventions

Treatment Evaluation

Brunner's critical analysis (this volume) of the concept of time without symptoms of disease and subjective toxicity of treatment (TWiST) for treatment evaluation reflects the currently ongoing discussion on appropriate study end points in the adjuvant setting. Gelber and Goldhirsch (1986) were the first to take into account the patient's burden of toxic side effects and disease symptoms in treatment evalu-

Recent Results in Cancer Research, Vol. 115
© Springer-Verlag Berlin · Heidelberg 1989

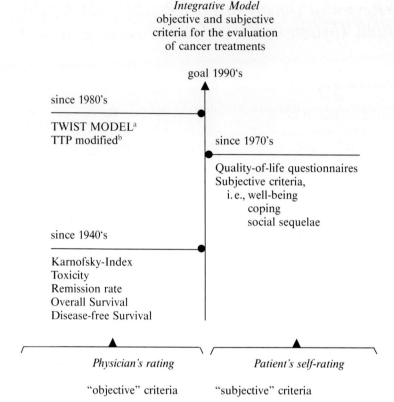

Integrative Model
objective and subjective
criteria for the evaluation
of cancer treatments

goal 1990's

since 1980's

TWIST MODEL[a]
TTP modified[b]

since 1970's

Quality-of-life questionnaires
Subjective criteria,
  i.e., well-being
    coping
      social sequelae

since 1940's

Karnofsky-Index
Toxicity
Remission rate
Overall Survival
Disease-free Survival

Physician's rating   *Patient's self-rating*

"objective" criteria   "subjective" criteria

Fig. 1. Development of treatment evaluation in oncology
[a] Gelber and Goldhirsch (1986)
[b] Brunner (1987)

ation. By simply and arbitrarily transforming toxicity, local recurrence, and occurrence of distant metastases into loss of time they defined TWiST as a new, in their opinion more appropriate, quality-of-life-oriented end point in the adjuvant setting, especially in the early phase of trials, before differences in OS begin to emerge or when OS differences are lacking. They were able to show that early losses of quality of life by toxicity are more than compensated for later on, as the majority of patients remain diseasefree for a longer period of time. Brunner claims that the TWiST concept is a theoretical construct far removed from the subjective reality of the patient and therefore of questionable value as a study end point. To extrapolate the potential benefit for an individual patient from results of studies comparing groups of patients is always a problem. TWiST in its current version (total loss of time with subjective toxicity and recurrent disease) is actually a crude reflection of the patient's subjective experience, but at least it is an attempt (and the first one since Karnofsky!) to integrate some patient-relevant aspects other than survival into treatment evaluation. And since time penalties for toxicity and recurrent disease are so severe, there is no bias in favor of treatment. TWiST has to be refined and it will be. In the International Breast Cancer Studies VI and VII, we are periodically assessing patients' coping and well-being (Hürny and Bernhard, this volume). This will allow for a more differentiated definition of TWiST.

Coping Process and Adaptation

In her prospective study of the rehabilitation needs of 50 patients treated for primary breast cancer, Ganz and coworkers found a wide range of physical and psychosocial problems 1 month after surgery. During the following year, the majority of physical problems were resolved; however, over 50% of subjects still experienced anxiety, worry about recurrence, and increased fatigue 13 months after initial surgery. Patients undergoing adjuvant treatment reported a higher frequency of anxiety, depression, and worry about recurrence.

This study shows that the process of adaptation is not completed with physical healing and that adjuvant treatment can temporarily jeopardize the patient's well-being to a considerable degree. An important issue not addressed in this study is the possible influence of the patient's coping on compliance with treatment.

Interestingly, Ganz and coworkers found only few differences between patients undergoing modified radical mastectomy and those undergoing segmental mastectomy with radiation therapy. It is hard to believe that the fact of losing or keeping her breast makes no difference to the patient. Possibly, concerns about the integrity of the body are overshadowed by the existential threat of cancer diagnosis, at least in the beginning. It could also be that the assessment instruments are not sensitive and specific enough to this problem.

Psychosocial Factors as Prognostic Indicators

The controversy about psychosocial factors influencing disease course after initial treatment in breast cancer has been going on for years. The medical community and the public are divided into "believers" and "nonbelievers," and Discussions are usually highly emotional. A critical review of the literature demonstrates that the currently available studies do not yet give a final answer to this question, either positive or negative.

Treatment Side Effects

Nausea and vomiting are among the most common and most disturbing side effects of chemotherapy. In Redd et al.'s prospective study of 77 patients undergoing adjuvant cytotoxic treatment for breast cancer, 71% developed post-treatment nausea and vomiting and 57% anticipatory nausea and vomiting. These patients were characterized by greater expectations for experiencing side effects, anxiety about treatment, and actual experience of side effects after the first treatment. Anticipatory nausea and vomiting are a special variation of a ubiquitous biopsychological phenomenon: the conditioned response (Pavlov 1953). An initially neutral stimulus (the hospital environment) is repeatedly paired with a stimulus eliciting a subjective response (chemotherapy-induced nausea and vomiting) until the subjective response is conditioned, that is, elicited by the initially neutral stimulus alone.

Apart from implications for specific behavioral interventions to alleviate conditioned side effects, the conditioned response may also have a direct biological impact. Ader and Cohen (1975) have shown in animals that cell-mediated immune responses can be conditioned. Rats were repeatedly fed with a saccharine solution they especially like and simultaneously injected cytoxan intraperitoneally. Cytoxan elicited a taste aversion to saccharine and simultaneously a depression of cell-mediated immune responses by its cytotoxic effects. After several pairings of the two stimuli, the rats developed a reduction in cell-mediated immune response by being exposed to saccharine alone. Redd and his group in New York are currently approaching these questions by studying immune function in patients who are developing anticipatory nausea.

In conclusion, the four papers deal with quite different psychosocial aspects of adjuvant treatment in primary breast cancer, but they also have one thing in common. Since the integration of psychosocial aspects into research strategies in oncology is new, all researchers in this field are struggling with methodological problems. So far, the need not to confine ourselves to biomedical aspects of the adjuvant treatment in breast cancer, but also to consider psychological and social problems worthy for investigation is clear to many of us. However, developing a solid methodology that will enable us to investigate the problem of adjuvant chemotherapy integratively will need a lot of work and discussion in the future.

References

Ader R, Cohen N (1975) Behaviorally conditioned immunosuppression. Psychosom Med 37: 333–340
Brunner KW (1987) Evaluation criteria in comparative clinical trials in advanced breast cancer. In: Cavalli F (ed) Endocrine therapy of breast cancer II. Springer, Berlin Heidelberg New York, pp 47–51 (ESO monographs)
Gelber R, Goldhirsch A (1986) A new endpoint for the assessment of adjuvant therapy in postmenopausal women with operable breast cancer. J Clin Oncol 4: 1772–1779
Karnofsky DA, Burchenal JH (1949) The clinical evaluation of chemotherapeutic agents in cancer. In: MacLeod CM (ed) Evaluation of chemotherapeutic agents. Columbia University Press, New York, pp 191–205
Pavlov I (1953) Sämtliche Werke. Akademie, Berlin

Closing Summary and Outlook

J. H. Glick

Cancer Center, University of Pennsylvania, 3400 Spruce Street,
Philadelphia, PA 19104, USA

Introduction

Despite advances in early diagnosis and primary treatment of breast cancer with surgery, radiation therapy, or both modalities, more than one-third of newly diagnosed patients will develop recurrent or systemic disease and ultimately die of it. All of these patients are potential candidates for some form of systemic adjuvant therapy, which involves the use of cytotoxic drugs and/or endocrine therapy after definitive local treatment. The third International Conference on Adjuvant Therapy of Primary Breast Cancer in St. Gallen, Switzerland, brought together experts from all over the world to present their most recent data, which are collected in this volume, and to discuss the remaining challenges that confront both clinicians and basic scientists.

The data presented at the St. Gallen Conference allow us to pause and reflect on the changes that have taken place since September, 1985, when the National Institutes of Health Consensus Development Conference on the Adjuvant Therapy of Breast Cancer was held. The task of the NIH Consensus Panel in 1985 was much the same as the task presented in these closing remarks: examine the information available in the literature, and particularly the information presented at this conference, and make recommendations based on the data presented. This task results in two philosphical dilemmas: (a) it is possible to examine the same information and produce a set of divergent recommendations; and (b) well-supported data may exist that conflict with intuition about what the data will (should) demonstrate in the future.

The overall conclusions from the NIH Consensus Development Conference in 1985 are important and remain valid today:

1. Adjuvant chemotherapy and hormonal therapy are effective in the treatment of breast cancer patients with positive axillary lymph nodes.
2. While significant advances have been made in the past 5 years, optimal therapy has not been defined for any subset of patients.
3. For this reason, all patients and their physicians are strongly encouraged to participate in controlled clinical trials (NIH Consensus Conference 1985).

Recent Results in Cancer Research, Vol. 115
© Springer-Verlag Berlin·Heidelberg 1989

Table 1. NCI Consensus Development Conference: overall conclusions in 1985

Guidelines for patients treated outside the context of a clinical trial
  Premenopausal
    Node positive: Combination chemotherapy
    Node negative: Adjuvant therapy is not generally recommended. For high-risk patients,
      adjuvant chemotherapy should be considered.
  Postmenopausal
    Node positive, hormone receptor positive: Tamoxifen
    Node positive, hormone receptor negative: Combination chemotherapy should be
                                              considered but cannot be recommended as
                                              standard practice.
    Node negative: No indication for routine adjuvant therapy. For high-risk patients,
      adjuvant therapy may be considered.

Although these were the main conclusions from the NIH Consensus Panel, these statements were overshadowed by the Panel's published guidelines for patients treated outside the context of a clinical trial (Table 1). These guidelines were not intended to be a statement of standard care, nor were they intended to be inscribed in stone. The data presented at the St. Gallen Conference make it imperative to revisit the Consensus Development Conference and update these recommendations in 1988.

The goal of adjuvant therapy for breast cancer is to significantly prolong survival, while maintaining an acceptable quality of life. Three measures are important in evaluating whether this goal is met by specific treatments. Although overall survival remains the major end point, too great an emphasis on overall survival will obscure the benefit from many adjuvant trials. Disease-free survival, or the length of time free of any recurrence, has become a major end point in its own right, since prolonged periods of disease-free survival are advantageous, as quality of survival is generally better before than after recurrence. There continues to be accumulating evidence that longer periods of disease-free survival are translating into better overall survival rates. The data presented by Valagussa et al. (this volume, pp. 69–76) on survival after first relapse of breast cancer indicate that prior exposure to adjuvant cyclophosphamide + methotrexate + 5-fluorouracil (CMF) (compared with the no-treatment control group) does not adversely affect either salvage treatment response rates or overall survival. Finally, in choosing an adjuvant therapy program, any potential benefit must be balanced against both short-term and long-term side effects. Thus, the effect of the adjuvant regimen chosen on quality of life is an important end point for evaluating any adjuvant treatment program. The TWiST (Time Without Symptoms of Disease and Toxic Effects of Treatment) approach presented by Gelber and Goldhirsch for the Ludwig Group is an important attempt to quantify the benefit of adjuvant therapy, considering the balance in terms of reduction of symptoms of disease on the one hand and toxic effects of treatment on the other (Gelber and Goldhirsch, this volume, pp. 211–219). This methodology should be applied prospectively to more trials of adjuvant therapy.

The design and interpretation of adjuvant breast cancer trials has become more complicated in recent years. As we realize that breast cancer is an extremely heterogenous disease, prospective stratification factors become even more important.

In addition to the known prognostic variables of axillary lymph node status, hormone receptors (both estrogen and progesterone receptors), and histopathology (degree of differentiation, and the somewhat controversial and difficult to reproduce nuclear grade), the contributions presented in this volume debate the usefulness of subdividing patients by menopausal status or age. McGuire (this volume, pp. 170-174) also presents the large San Antonio experience with flow cytometry (ploidy and growth fraction) and oncogene amplification (*HER*-2/*Neu*), which are important new prognostic factors that must be considered in future trials.

Caveats in the design of adjuvant breast cancer trials include:

1. Were appropriate randomization procedures employed?
2. Is the question being addressed by the trial important or even answerable?
3. Were adequate patients accessioned to the trial?
4. Is there adequate follow-up to allow a definitive answer?

The time is long past when a trial of 100-200 patients randomized to two or three arms was sufficient to answer important questions that may have an impact on treatment patterns. Large-scale trials, prospectively stratified for important prognostic variables, which accession patients in a maximum of 2 or 3 years are necessary if we are to make progress within a reasonable time period.

Other caveats in the interpretation of adjuvant breast cancer data also exist. Henderson has identified both reader bias and publication bias as obstacles to a fair interpretation of worldwide data (Henderson 1987). Readers tend to remember positive results if they are of an activist mentality, while nihilists emphasize negative trials. This conference on which this volume is base was remarkably free from bias, as international breast cancer experts from around the world entered on a new phase of dialog – free from the polemic of the past. Although conflicting conclusions from trials addressing the same issues were actively discussed (e.g., the role of adjuvant chemotherapy in postmenopausal, node-positive, hormone-receptor-negative patients), more tolerance for divergent viewpoints was observed among the conference speakers and moderators.

Thus, in this volume, the role of randomized trials, compared with the overview analysis presented by Peto and colleagues, is discussed, with both felt to be important methodological approaches to the analysis of breast cancer trials. Although Tattersall raises the question "Why has adjuvant treatment failed?" (this volume, pp. 1-7), the majority of the contributions view this question in a different light. Specifically, progress has been made and survival has been improved with the use of adjuvant therapy, but not to the degree we all expected. We should not be satisfied with the advances made to date, since patients are still dying from breast cancer in even the most favorable subgroups. Thus, further clinical trials and basic laboratory investigation are mandatory.

Node-Positive Patients

Premenopausal

The data presented here continue to demonstrate that adjuvant chemotherapy produces a highly significant increase in disease-free survival and a significant reduction in mortality in premenopausal women with histologically positive axillary lymph nodes. Adjuvant chemotherapy remains the standard of care for these patients. The optimal drug combination has not been defined and is currently the subject of clinical investigation. Fisher et al. present the NSABP data suggesting that doxorubicin-containing combinations are superior for these premenopausal patients. Tormey reports the ECOG data, which show that premenopausal, estrogen-receptor-positive and -negative patients who develop amenorrhea from chemotherapy have significantly improved disease-free and overall survival (Tormey, this volume, pp. 106–112). However, Bonadonna et al. (this volume, pp. 113–117) are unable to detect an improvement in relapse-free survival in premenopausal women less than 40 years of age with CMF-induced amenorrhea as compared with those patients who do not develop amenorrhea.

Kaufmann presents the data of the Gynecological Adjuvant Breast Cancer Group for low-risk premenopausal patients one to three positive nodes and estrogen/progesterone receptor positive) (this volume, pp. 118–125). In this trial, CMF produced significantly improved disease-free and overall survival when randomized against tamoxifen alone for 2 years. In high-risk premenopausal patients (more than three positive axillary lymph nodes, or one to three positive nodes and receptor-negative tumors), there was no difference between patients randomized to doxorubicin-cyclophosphamide or to the same two drugs plus tamoxifen.

Mouridsen's overview of the premenopausal data observes that there appears to be no effect of tamoxifen when added to concurrent adjuvant chemotherapy (Mouridsen, this volume, pp. 132–135). The overview analysis of Peto tends to support this conclusion. However, no data are presented comparing the role of ovarian ablation and/or tamoxifen following adjuvant chemotherapy with a control group of chemotherapy alone. This important question remains to be solved by future randomized trials.

Postmenopausal: Hormone Receptor Positive

For the postmenopausal women with both positive axillary lymph nodes and positive hormone receptor levels, tamoxifen remains standard care. Both the data presented by Baum and Ebbs on behalf of the NATO trials (this volume, pp. 136–143), as well as the Scottish trials presented by Stewart (this volume, pp. 126–131), confirm both a disease-free survival benefit, as well as an overall survival benefit for 2 or more years of tamoxifen compared with a no-treatment control. Although the optimal duration of tamoxifen has not been defined, long-term (or indefinite) administration of tamoxifen appears to be indicated. The overview analysis presented by Peto continues to demonstrate an overall survival advantage for tamoxifen, which translates into a highly significant reduction in the odds of mortality.

The role of tamoxifen combined with chemotherapy compared with tamoxifen alone remains unresolved. Data from the current NSABP and the SWOG-ECOG trials using this study design are not presented. Fisher and Redmond report the updated NSABP data comparing PFT with PF in patients older than 50 years of age who are estrogen receptor positive or nuclear grade good. Tamoxifen improves both disease-free survival and overall survival in patients on the tamoxifen arm. Goldhirsch and Gelber (this volume, pp. 153–162) update the Ludwig III trial with estrogen-receptor-positive, node-positive, postmenopausal patients. At 7 years, the disease-free survival for the patients treated with cyclophosphamide + methotrexate + 5-fluorouracil + prednisone + tamoxifen (CMFpT) is significantly longer than for the observation group or patients treated with prednisone plus tamoxifen (p + T). However, there is no difference in overall survival at this point in time (Goldhirsch et al., this volume, pp. 153–162).

The issue of the timing of tamoxifen administration in patients receiving chemotherapy is discussed from the point of view that tamoxifen may well interact adversely with chemotherapy given simultaneously. Tamoxifen prolongs the G_0 phase, while cytotoxic agents are known to be active on cycling cells. Endocrine therapy slows the growth of cells and may protect against the action of cytotoxic chemotherapy. Fisher and Redmond observed that tamoxifen attenuates the cytotoxic effect of 5-fluorouracil and doxorubicin in vitro, while the combination of L-phenylalanine mustard (L-PAM) plus tamoxifen produces antagonist cytocidal effects. Thus, it would be important to initiate trials of tamoxifen alone compared with chemotherapy followed by tamoxifen, as this issue remains an open question.

Postmenopausal: Hormone Receptor Negative

With longer follow-up from three major cooperative group trials (NSABP, Ludwig III, and ECOG 4181), the benefits of adjuvant chemotherapy now appear to outweigh its short-term side effects (Goldhirsch and Gelber, this volume, pp. 153–162; Tormey, this volume, pp. 106–112). Improved disease-free survival and significantly improved overall survival have been demonstrated in the chemotherapy arms of these trials. Moreover, data from both the Ludwig and ECOG groups are demonstrating both a disease-free and overall survival advantage for the combination of CMF (or CMFp) plus tamoxifen in these node-positive, estrogen-receptor-negative patients. Although there has been controversy on this point, it now appears that adjuvant chemotherapy should be the control arm in future trials in this subset of patients. Again, the role of tamoxifen when given simultaneously with chemotherapy or chemotherapy followed by tamoxifen compared with chemotherapy alone remains to be determined by randomized controlled trials in the future. It is possible to conclude from data from both the NATO and Scottish trials of tamoxifen versus an observation group that tamoxifen prolongs disease-free and overall survival in estrogen-receptor-negative patients (Baum and Ebbs, pp. 136–143; Stewart, pp. 126–131). This lends additional support to the argument that tamoxifen does have some benefit even in this subgroup.

Node-Negative Patients

In 1985, the NIH Consensus Panel concluded that routine administration of adjuvant systemic therapy in women with histologically negative axillary lymph nodes could not be recommended at that time (NIH Consensus Conference 1985). The Panel did identify certain groups of high-risk node-negative patients who had a significantly greater chance of relapse (large tumor size, negative hormone receptors, younger age, higher degree of cellular proliferation). In these high-risk patients, the Panel concluded that adjuvant chemotherapy should be considered outside the context of a clinical trial. In this volume, McGuire provides a detailed overview of prognostic factors in node-negative breast cancer (Table 2). Estrogen receptor status and tumor size remain important prognostic parameters, as far as both disease-free and overall survival are concerned (McGuire, this volume, pp. 170–174). Newer data are presented by McGuire, indicating that approximately half of node-negative, estrogen-receptor-positive patients have aneuploid tumors based on flow cytometry determination. In addition, diploid patients with a high S-phase cutoff have significantly lower disease-free and overall survival than those with diploid tumors with a low S-phase cutoff. McGuire also presents data on oncogene amplification in patients with histologically positive axillary lymph nodes. In this subgroup, overexpression of *Her-2/Neu* predicted for a significantly lower disease-free and overall survival even within the same node subgroups (McGuire, this volume, pp. 170–174).

Bonadonna (this volume, pp. 175–179) updates the Milan randomized trial of 90 node-negative, estrogen-receptor-negative patients treated with either CMF adjuvant chemotherapy or observation. Patients with a high labelling index have significantly improved disease-free and overall survival with CMF. Jakesz presents the 7-year update from the Vienna trial, which also demonstrates improved survival in the chemotherapy-treated patients as compared with the control group (Jakesz et al., this volume, pp. 180–185). Both trials, however, have small numbers of patients entered into the study.

An important comment made by Fisher during the discussion at the St. Gallen conference related to preliminary data from the NSABP trial, which randomized both pre- and postmenopausal node-negative, estrogen-receptor-negative patients to either a no-treatment group or a group receiving sequential methotrexate-5-flurouracil plus leukovorin. Although these data were not formally presented, Fisher commented that in more than 600 of these patients, ther was a highly significant improvement in disease-free survival for the chemotherapy arm with both pre- and postmenopausal patients. No overall survival difference has been seen as yet because of the relatively short follow-up.

Thus, the benefits of adjuvant combination chemotherapy (improved disease-free survival) appear to outweigh the transient side effects from short-term treatment in node-negative, "high-risk" patients. Although the definition of "high risk" remains to be more fully elucidated using the prognostic factors summarized in Table 2, adjuvant chemotherapy is indicated for both pre- and postmenopausal high-risk, node-negative patients. Adjuvant chemotherapy should be considered as the control arm in future trials for this subgroup. Unanswered questions include whether there are subsets of "high-risk" patients who do not require chemothera-

Table 2. Prognostic factors in node-negative breast cancer

	Low risk	High risk
Estrogen receptors	Positive	Negative
Primary tumor size	<2.5 CM	>2.5 CM
Nuclear grade	Good	Poor
Histologic grade	Well differentiated	Poorly differentiated
Proliferative index	Diploid and low S-phase	Aneuploid; Diploid and high S-phase

py, the optimal duration and type of chemotherapy, and the role and timing of tamoxifen. Both the NATO and Scottish trials indicate a survival benefit from tamoxifen in the subset of patients who are node-negative. The Scottish trial includes a small number of premenopausal patients who are estrogen receptor negative and node negative, and this group has also benefited from adjuvant tamoxifen (Stewart, this volume, pp. 126–131).

Given the positive results from Ludwig and ECOG in node-positive, estrogen-receptor-negative, postmenopausal patients with the combination of chemotherapy and tamoxifen, the question naturally arises whether postmenopausal, estrogen-receptor-negative, node-negative patients might also benefit from the combination of chemotherapy plus tamoxifen or chemotherapy followed by tamoxifen. This question should be investigated in a future randomized trial.

"Low-risk" node-negative patients have a generally favorable prognosis, but Senn argued (at the conference) that a significant proportion of this subgroup still suffers recurrences and will eventually die. In this subgroup, the benefits of prolonged adjuvant tamoxifen (improved disease-free and overall survival) have been demonstrated for postmenopausal patients. Adjuvant tamoxifen can now be considered as standard care or the control arm for postmenopausal patients who are node-negative with a good prognosis (i. e., estrogen receptor positive, good nuclear grade, low proliferative index). Data from Baum and Ebbs and Stewart and White, which support this observation, have now been confirmed by a large randomized NSABP trial reported in the discussion period at the conference by Fisher. He noted that for postmenopausal patients who are estrogen receptor positive and node negative, there is a significantly improved disease-free survival advantage for the group receiving tamoxifen compared with a no-treatment control. Further, Fisher commented that this significantly improved disease-free survival is also observed in premenopausal, estrogen-receptor-positive, node-negative patients receiving tamoxifen.

Unanswered questions include whether there are any node-negative patients who should not be treated with adjuvant therapy, as well as for patients receiving tamoxifen, whether they should receive this hormonal agent on an indefinite basis. Finally, the role of chemotherapy in addition to tamoxifen, as opposed to tamoxifen alone for low-risk patients must be determined by future randomized trials.

Future Directions

Many questions have been left unanswered by the contributions in this important volume. Regarding adjuvant chemotherapy, the optimal therapeutic regimen remains to be determined. The role of doxorubicin is felt to be controversial, even though data from the NSABP are suggestive of an additive role for this drug. It would be ideal to define different chemotherapy regimens for specific subsets of node-positive patients, but this may prove to be a difficult question to answer in future clinical trials. Although there is sentiment for "more aggressive" chemotherapy regimens, the risk/benefit ratio for newer programs remains to be determined. No information is presented on noncross-resistant regimens (hybrids, sequential, or rotating regimens) and, thus, a true test of the Goldie-Goldman hypothesis, as far as adjuvant therapy of breast cancer is concerned, remains an open question (Goldie, this volume, pp. 8–16).

Although Hryniuk's retrospective review of the correlation between dose response, dose intensity, and prognosis is an important concept and intuitively appears correct, prospective data from randomized clinical trials confirming this theoretical observation are not presented (Hryniuk, this volume, pp. 17–24). The ongoing CALGB trial of different dose levels of (CAF) adjuvant therapy should help to answer this important question.

The role of perioperative chemotherapy also remains unresolved. Goldhirsch and Gelber (this volume, pp. 43–53) present the Ludwig V data, which demonstrate that one course of standard CMF adjuvant chemotherapy administered perioperatively is inferior to the same perioperative chemotherapy followed by standard adjuvant chemotherapy or standard adjuvant chemotherapy without perioperative treatment. Significant differences in favor of the standard adjuvant chemotherapy arms with respect to improved disease-free survival at 4 years have been observed. One cycle of perioperative chemotherapy administered in the manner given by the Ludwig group is clearly inadequate. Data are presented from the CRC (Clinical Trials Centre) using a 2×2 factorial design that appear to show no differences at 5 years between perioperative cyclophosphamide and a control group with respect to first-event (i.e., relapse) occurrence. However, when the CRC data are combined with the Scandinavian results using the overview methodology, there is a significantly reduced likelihood of a first event occurring in the cyclophosphamide-treated patients as compared with the no-treatment groups. The conclusion of Baum and Ebbs is that one course of perioperative cyclophosphamide significantly delays the risk of relapse, but as yet no significant effect on survival in the first 5 years has been observed. Thus, the issue of perioperative chemotherapy remains unresolved (Houghton et al.; Baum and Ebbs, both this volume, pp. 54–61, 136–145).

Similarly, there is no mature data from preoperative or neoadjuvant chemotherapy trials for clinical stage I or II patients. Ragaz presents the study design of the British Columbia trial, which utilizes fine-neddle aspiration to establish the diagnosis, followed by preoperative chemotherapy and then definitive local treatment (Ragaz et al., this volume, pp. 28–35). No data are available from this trial to date. For locally advanced breast cancer, including stage III and inflammatory disease, preoperative chemotherapy now appears to be effective and is a standard approach for cytoreduction prior to definitive local-regional therapy.

Newer chemotherapy approaches, especially for higher-risk, node-positive subsets (≥ 10 positive nodes for example), need to be explored. Cytoreductive chemotherapy followed by bone marrow harvest, preparative (supralethal) chemotherapy, and rescue with autologous bone marrow transplantation is being explored by several centers (Frei, this volume, pp. 25–27). The use of biologic response modifiers and combination chemotherapy is discussed, and one potential approach is the use of GM-CSF with chemotherapy in order to administer higher doses of drugs.

Conclusions: The Consensus Conference Revisited in 1988

Although adjuvant chemotherapy and hormonal manipulation are effective treatments for breast cancer patients with both positive and negative axillary lymph nodes, optimal therapy has not been defined for any subset of patients. Although all patients and their physicians are strongly encouraged to participate in controlled clinical trials, it is well recognized that only a small minority of patients in North America and in most of Europe actually enter clinical trials. Outside the context of a clinical trial and based on the research data presented at the 1988 St. Gallen Conference, we can revisit the NIH Consensus Conference guidelines and make personal recommendations in 1988 (Table 3).

1. For premenopausal, node-positive patients who are either hormone receptor positive or negative, adjuvant chemotherapy remains the standard of care and should be utilized in all patients.
2. For postmenopausal, node-positive, hormone-receptor-positive patients, tamoxifen should remain the control arm in future trials. There is evidence that chemotherapy plus tamoxifen is beneficial for the subgroup with four or more positive axillary lymph nodes. However, we must await the results of current and future trials comparing tamoxifen alone with tamoxifen plus chemotherapy or chemotherapy followed by tamoxifen before a definitive statement regarding the efficacy of chemotherapy for this subgroup of patients can be made.
3. For postmenopausal, node-positive, hormone-receptor-negative patients, the weight of evidence now favors adjuvant chemotherapy as the control arm for future trials. In this subset of patients, there is strong evidence that tamoxifen

Table 3. NIH Consensus Conference revisited in 1988

	Premenopausal	Postmenopausal
Node positive		
Receptor positive	Chemotherapy	Tamoxifen ± chemotherapy
Receptor negative	Chemotherapy	Chemotherapy ± tamoxifen
Node negative		
High risk	Chemotherapy	Chemotherapy ± tamoxifen
Low risk	Tamoxifen	Tamoxifen

may well be reinforcing chemotherapy as far as improved disease-free and overall survival is concerned, but further follow-up is required.

4. Although more data is required to define "high-risk" versus "low-risk" node-negative patients accurately, as well as to define an "intermediate" subgroup, the data presented here indicate that node-negative breast cancer is not a "benign" disease and that most node-negative patients should be treated with some form of adjuvant therapy, either chemotherapy and/or tamoxifen.

5. For the "high-risk" node-negative patient (estrogen receptor negative, larger tumor size, aneuploid, diploid with a high S-phase), adjuvant chemotherapy results in at least significantly improved disease-free survival. Thus, chemotherapy should be regarded as the control arm for these patients in future trials.

6. For the postmenopausal, node-negative, high-risk patient, the combination of chemotherapy plus tamoxifen must also be considered, but needs to be compared prospectively with chemotherapy alone for this subset.

7. The significantly improved disease-free survival for postmenopausal, node-negative, estrogen-receptor-positive patients treated with tamoxifen as compared with a no-treatment control has been confirmed in several trials. For this postmenopausal subset, tamoxifen is indicated outside of a clinical trial.

8. For the premenopausal, node-negative, low-risk patient, there is suggestive data that tamoxifen significantly improves disease-free survival and can be given outside of a clinical trial, although more information clearly needs to be presented.

9. It remains to be determined whether there is truly a "low-risk" subgroup that deserves no adjuvant therapy, given the low morbidity associated with tamoxifen.

It now appears in 1988 that almost all patients with clinical and pathologic stage I and II breast cancer, regardless of age, menopausal, nodal, or receptor status, will benefit from some form of adjuvant chemotherapy and/or hormonal therapy, in terms of both improved disease-free survival and overall survival. Thus, all patients with breast cancer should have a medical oncology consultation at the time of diagnosis to determine whether the patient is eligible for a clinical trial, which remains the first priority for both patients and physicians. However, given the common situation in which most patients are treated outside of a clinical trial, the burden of proof is now on the physician and patient as to why an individual patient should *not* receive some form of adjuvant therapy, which appears to be beneficial for all patients.

References

Henderson C (1987) Adjuvant systemic therapy for early breast cancer. Curr Probl Cancer 11 (3): 129–207

NIH Consensus Conference (1985) Adjuvant therapy for breast cancer. JAMA 254: 3461–3463

Subject Index